M000288443

STAFF

Senior Publisher
Matthew Cahill

Art Director
John Hubbard

Senior Editor
June Norris

Clinical Editors
Judith Schilling McCann, RN, BSN (clinical project editor), Beverly Tscheschlog, RN

Copy Editors
Cynthia C. Breuninger (manager), Lynette High, Doris Weinstock

Designers
Stephanie Peters (senior associate art director), Lorraine Lostracco

Photographer
John Gallagher

Typographers
Diane Paluba (manager), Elizabeth Bergman, Joyce Rossi Biletz, Phyllis Marron, Valerie Rosenberger

Manufacturing
Deborah Meiris (director), Pat Dorshaw (manager), T.A. Landis

Production Coordinator
Margaret A. Rastiello

Editorial Assistants
Beverly Lane, Mary Madden

Indexer
Barbara Hodgson

CCSKIL-010196

R A member of the Reed Elsevier plc group

Library of Congress Cataloging-in-Publication Data

Critical care skills: A nurse's photoguide.
    p.   cm.
  Includes index.
    1. Intensive care nursing—Atlases. 2. Emergency nursing—Atlases. I. Springhouse Corporation.
    [DNLM: 1. Emergency Nursing—methods—atlases.
    2. Critical Care—methods—nurses' instruction.
    3. Critical Care—methods—atlases.
    WY 17 C934 1996]
RT120.I5C784   1996
610.73'61—dc20
DNLM/DLC
ISBN 0-87434-847-1 (alk. paper)   95-46145
                                  CIP

CONTENTS

Respiratory Monitoring

Artificial Airways

Mechanical Ventilation

Neurologic Monitoring

Diagnostic Tests

Index

FOREWORD

With today's rapid advances in medical technology and older and more acutely ill patients, the boundaries of critical care are extending from the intensive care unit and emergency department to special care units, medical-surgical units, subacute units, and even the home.

No matter where you work, *Critical Care Skills*— with its step-by-step directions and over 1,200 photographs—will provide you with up-to-date information on the skills you need to care for critically ill patients.

The section called "Basic Cardiac Life Support" provides a comprehensive review of adult CPR procedures, including one- and two-person rescue, and instructions on how to clear a conscious or unconscious adult's airway. Especially valuable are the recent changes in CPR guidelines. "Advanced Cardiac Life Support" details the specific responsibilities of each code team member and includes a pictorial guide for performing defibrillation and synchronized cardioversion. "Respiratory Monitoring" covers $S\bar{v}O_2$ monitoring, pulse oximetry and capnography, and end-tidal carbon dioxide monitoring.

The photostories in "Pacemakers" show you how to use transcutaneous, transvenous, transthoracic, epicardial, and permanent pacing. "Cardiac Monitoring" discusses electrocardiography (ECG), the ECG grid, and the electrical basis of the ECG. Following this are photostories that explain how to perform hardwire, telemetry, and ST-segment monitoring.

The illustrated procedures in "Hemodynamic Monitoring" range from how to set up transducers and manage arterial and pulmonary artery lines to how to monitor central venous and left atrial pressures, perform thermodilution and thoracic electrical bioimpedance monitoring, and monitor cardiac output and $S\bar{v}O_2$ continuously.

"Artificial Airways" shows you how to establish oropharyngeal and nasopharyngeal airways. You'll also learn about endotracheal tube insertion and removal, endotracheal and tracheostomy tube care, and measuring tracheal cuff pressure.

"Mechanical Ventilation" describes the latest negative-pressure, volume-cycled, pressure-cycled, and high-frequency ventilators. Large, clear photographs show you how to prepare the ventilator, attach its components, and check and set its functions. Other key topics include how to maintain the ventilator and wean the patient.

"Neurologic Monitoring" teaches you the steps for setting up an intracranial pressure (ICP) monitoring system and assisting with catheter insertion, performing ICP monitoring, draining cerebrospinal fluid (CSF), and collecting a CSF specimen. This section also covers assisting with a lumbar puncture and monitoring cerebral blood flow.

Finally, "Diagnostic Tests" surveys test procedures, such as 12-lead, right chest-lead, posterior lead, signal-averaged, and atrial ECGs. This section also reviews arterial blood gas analysis, using a vascular intermittent access system to monitor blood chemistry results in a critically ill patient, and testing gastric contents.

Throughout the text, graphic logos call your attention to key information. *Clinical tips* gives you ways to avoid time-consuming missteps. *Complications* charts outline patient hazards during mechanical ventilation and other procedures. *Troubleshooting* charts list equipment problems, their causes, and corrective interventions. And *Insights and interpretations* deepens your understanding of specific techniques, such as how to interpret $S\bar{v}O_2$ tracings. Also, *Teaching aids* can be photocopied for your patient.

Critical Care Skills is particularly useful for new nursing graduates, patient care assistants, and technicians. They can benefit from the comprehensive descriptions of procedures and rationales. Experienced nurses will find this book helpful as a review for procedures they haven't done recently, when precepting new nurses, and when teaching during orientation and training.

Written by nurses with years of patient care experience, *Critical Care Skills* presents valuable information that will help you meet the needs of critically ill patients efficiently and effectively.

June Howland-Gradman, RN, MS, CCRN
Care Center Leader, Cardiac Services
University of Chicago Hospitals
Chicago, Illinois

Basic Cardiac Life Support

LEARNING ABOUT BASIC LIFE SUPPORT

Life-threatening emergencies represent a nurse's ultimate challenge. To rescue a patient who's choking or in cardiac or respiratory arrest, you'll need to bring all your skills into action—swiftly and expertly.

The American Heart Association (AHA) designates two types of emergency life-support procedures: basic life support (BLS) and advanced cardiac life support (ACLS). As emergency first aid, BLS aims to maintain life until the patient recovers or until ACLS can be implemented. You can perform BLS quickly, in almost any situation, without assistance or, if necessary, without equipment. ACLS includes BLS as well as procedures requiring special equipment or medications.

BLS includes performing cardiopulmonary resuscitation (CPR) and managing airway obstruction caused by a foreign body. As a nurse, you should be ready to perform BLS in any situation where you encounter a patient with an airway obstruction or in primary respiratory or cardiac arrest.

The sooner BLS begins, the better the patient's chances for survival. *Note:* For an adult who is outside of a hospital and unresponsive, the AHA recommends that a rescuer call emergency medical services. According to the AHA, this increases dramatically the person's chances for survival.

For patients in respiratory arrest or those with an airway obstruction, early intervention can prevent cardiac arrest. In primary respiratory arrest, the heart usually continues to pump blood for several minutes, giving you time to intervene and possibly prevent a cardiac arrest.

However, in primary cardiac arrest, blood doesn't circulate. Any oxygen stored in the lungs and other vital organs is quickly depleted. Although the patient's circulation stops, his heart may continue beating—though ineffectively.

C.P.R. BASICS

An emergency procedure, CPR seeks to restore and maintain the patient's respiration and circulation after his heart stops beating and his breathing ceases. It provides oxygen and blood flow to the heart, brain, and other vital organs until the patient recovers or until ACLS can begin.

Remember, the critical factor is time. If the patient's heartbeat and respirations stop for less than 4 minutes before intervention, he has a much better chance for complete recovery—provided that CPR efforts succeed. If his circulation stops for 4 to 6 minutes, he may suffer brain damage. If it stops for more than 6 minutes, he'll almost certainly suffer brain damage. Exceptions to these time frames include a drowning patient submerged in cold water or a patient with hypothermia. These patients may survive longer without oxygen because cold temperatures lower their metabolic rates.

INITIAL GUIDELINES

When deciding whether to start CPR, follow this guideline: Give CPR if you have any doubt about how long the patient has been without a pulse and respirations. Typically, you'll recognize a patient in cardiopulmonary arrest by these signs: He is unconscious, appears ashen or gray, has no palpable carotid or femoral pulse, and has no breath sounds or air movement through the nose or mouth.

To follow the correct sequence for CPR, remember the ABCs: open the airway, restore breathing, and restore circulation. For an adult, CPR can be performed by one or two rescuers.

You can perform CPR quickly in almost any situation without assistance. You'll need a firm surface for the patient to lie on so that you can deliver the most effective cardiac compressions.

If the patient is in a hospital bed, you may place the headboard under him to provide a firm surface. Or you may use a cardiac board, available in most units and included on most crash carts. If the patient is in a chair or elsewhere when the arrest occurs, position him on the floor or ground before beginning compressions.

If possible, use a one-way valve mask to perform rescue breathing. The mask helps to bar contact with potentially hazardous body secretions. Currently, the AHA recommends that health care professionals perform mouth-to-mask breathing through a one-way valve mask during a two-person rescue. Check the mask's location in your unit; it's usually included on the crash cart.

The following pages show how to perform CPR on an adult. Keep in mind that procedural changes occur periodically.

Judith S. McCann, RN, BSN, and *M. Christopher Saslo, RN, BSN,* contributed to this section. Ms. McCann is a clinical editor with Springhouse Corp., Springhouse, Pa. Mr. Saslo, a BCLS and ACLS instructor, is with Albert Einstein Medical Center, Philadelphia. The publisher also thanks *Laerdal Medical Corp.,* Armonk, N.Y., for its help.

ADULT C.P.R.: ONE-PERSON RESCUE

If you're the lone rescuer, follow this procedure to perform CPR on an adult. If gloves are available, use them when performing CPR. Gently shake the patient's shoulder (as shown) and shout, "Are you okay?" in both ears in case he has difficulty hearing. This simple action ensures that you don't start CPR on a conscious person. Quickly scan the patient for major injuries, particularly to the head or neck. Call for help. Ask the person who arrives to call a code. (If you're outside of the hospital and treating an unresponsive adult, call 911 or a similar local number for emergency help.)

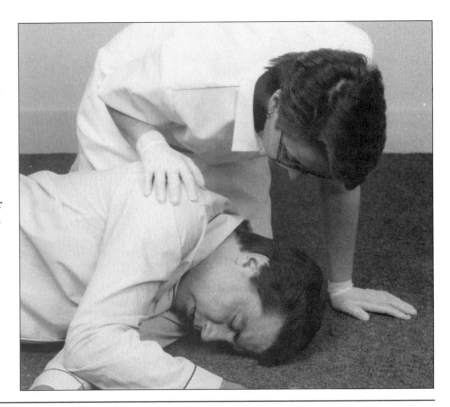

Position the patient supine on a hard, flat surface, such as the floor. If the patient is in bed, use a cardiac board or put the bed's headboard under him. If you suspect a head or neck injury, move the patient as little as possible to reduce the risk of paralysis. If you must move him, logroll him into the supine position, supporting his head and neck to keep his spinal column from twisting.

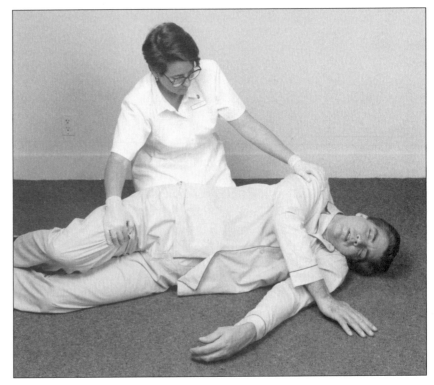

Opening the airway

To ensure an open airway, position yourself near the patient's shoulders, and perform the head-tilt, chin-lift maneuver (if you don't suspect a neck injury). Place one hand on the patient's forehead and the other hand on the bony portion of his chin near the jaw. Gently push his forehead back and pull upward on the chin, making sure the teeth are almost touching.

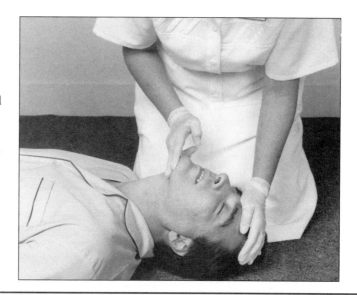

If you suspect a neck injury, open the airway using the jaw-thrust maneuver. Kneel behind the patient's head. Rest your thumbs on his lower jaw near the corners of his mouth. Your thumbs should point toward the patient's feet. Then place your fingertips around the lower jaw. With a steady, strong motion, lift the jaw upward and outward with your fingertips. This maneuver opens the airway without moving the neck.

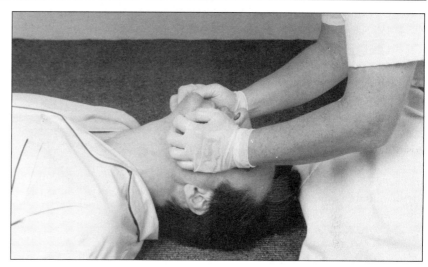

Restoring breathing

Keep the patient's airway open as you place your ear above his mouth and nose and look toward his feet. Listen for the sound of moving air, and watch for chest movement. You may also feel air on your cheek. If you detect signs of breathing, keep the patient's airway open and continue checking his breathing until help arrives.

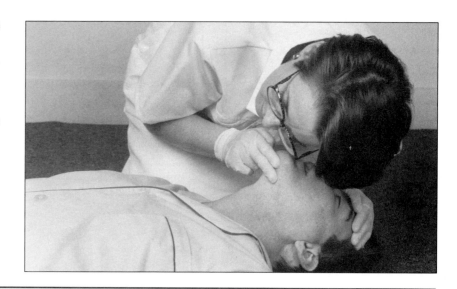

If breathing doesn't begin once the airway opens, start rescue breathing. Use the one-way valve mask as directed by your hospital's policy. If necessary, connect the one-way valve to the mask. Place the mask over the patient's nose and mouth.

Using your hand that's closest to the patient's chin, maintain the chin-lift position to keep the airway open. Place the palm of your other hand on the patient's forehead to stabilize the head. Use the index and middle fingers of this hand to seal the mask and to hold it in position.

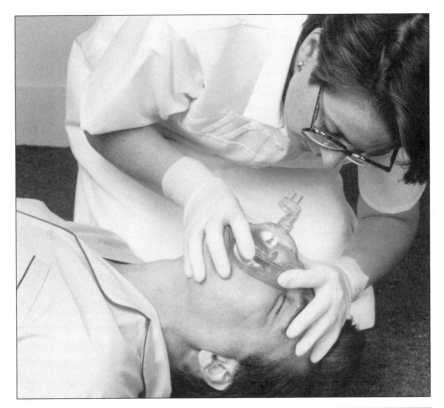

Take a deep breath and blow into the mask. Deliver two full ventilations, taking a deep breath after each. This allows time for the patient's chest to expand and relax and prevents gastric distention. Each ventilation should last 1½ to 2 seconds.

▶ *Clinical tip:* Although human immunodeficiency virus isn't known to be transmitted in saliva, you may be reluctant to give mouth-to-mouth rescue breaths. For this reason, the AHA recommends that all health care professionals use airway equipment, such as the one-way valve mask.

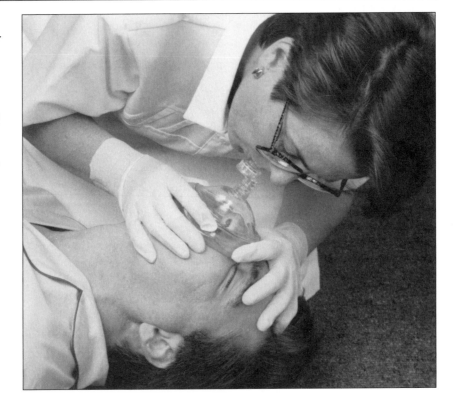

Without a mask, perform mouth-to-mouth rescue breathing. Once you've opened the patient's airway, pinch his nostrils shut with the thumb and index finger of the hand you had on his forehead.

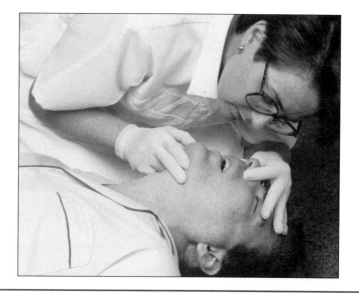

Take a deep breath, and cover the patient's mouth with yours. Aim for a tight seal. Deliver two full ventilations, taking a deep breath after each to allow time for the patient's chest to expand and relax and to prevent gastric distention. Each ventilation should last 1½ to 2 seconds. If this attempt fails, reposition the patient's head and try again. If that fails, suspect an airway obstruction. If a foreign body blocks the airway, follow the procedure for clearing a foreign body.

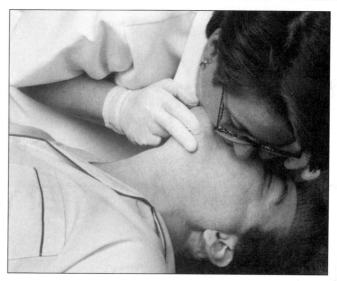

Restoring circulation

Keep one hand on the patient's forehead to keep the airway open. With your other hand, palpate the carotid artery closer to you by placing your index and middle fingers in the groove between the trachea and the sternocleidomastoid muscle. Palpate the artery for 10 seconds. If you detect a pulse, don't begin chest compressions. Instead, continue rescue breathing, giving 12 ventilations each minute (or one every 5 seconds). After every 12 ventilations, recheck the pulse.

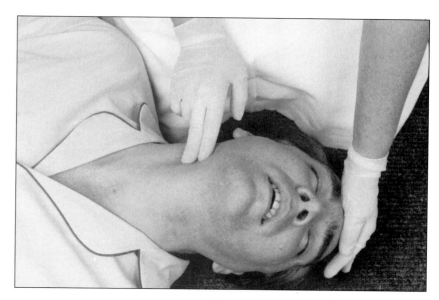

If you don't detect a pulse and help hasn't arrived yet, start chest compressions. Then, still kneeling, move to the patient's side. Spread your knees apart for a wide base of support. Next, using the hand closer to the patient's feet, locate the lower margin of his rib cage.

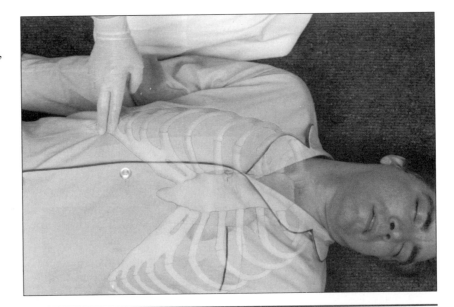

Move your fingertips along the margin to the notch where the ribs meet the sternum. Place your middle finger on that notch (the xiphoid process) and your index finger next to it. Your index finger should be on the bottom of the patient's sternum. Take care to find the correct hand position because improper placement can lead to complications.

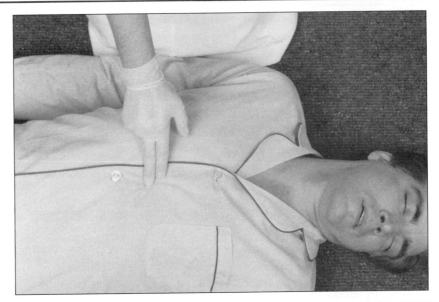

Put the heel of your other hand on the patient's sternum, next to your index finger. The long axis of the heel of your hand should align with the long axis of the sternum.

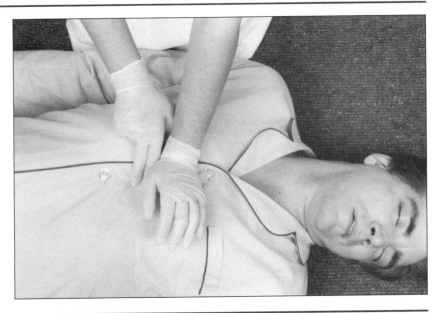

Take your fingers off the notch, and place that hand directly on top of your other hand. Make sure your fingers don't rest on the patient's chest. This keeps the force of the compressions on the sternum and reduces the risk of a rib fracture, lung puncture, or liver laceration. Keep in mind that liver laceration occurs more often with improper hand placement, especially if the hands are too low.

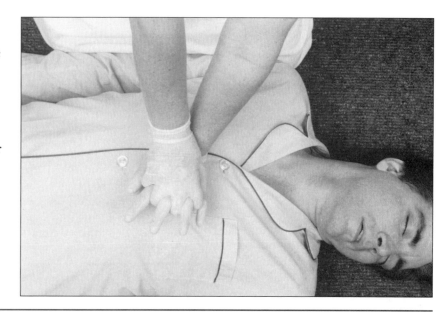

With your elbows locked, arms straight, and shoulders directly over your hands, you're positioned to start chest compressions. Using the weight of your upper body, compress the patient's sternum 1½″ to 2″ (3.8 to 5 cm), delivering the pressure through the heels of your hands. Don't let your fingers rest on the patient's chest.

After each compression, release the pressure and allow the chest to return to its normal position so the heart can fill with blood. To prevent injuries, don't change your hand position during compressions.

Give 15 chest compressions at a rate that simulates 80 to 100 heartbeats per minute. Count "one and two and three and" up to 15, compressing on the number and releasing the "and." After 15 compressions, give two ventilations. Reposition your hands properly and deliver 15 more compressions. Continue this pattern for four full cycles.

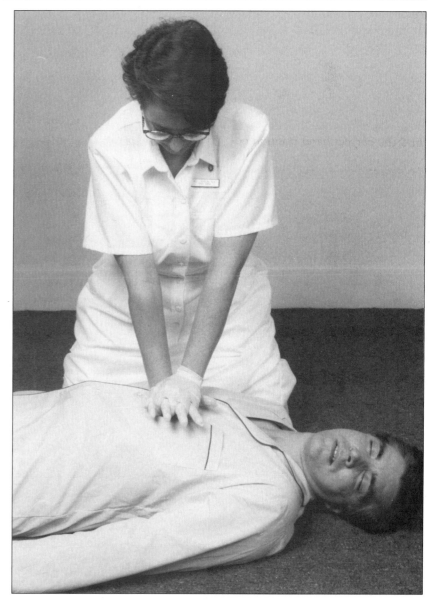

Palpate the carotid artery again. If you still don't detect a pulse, give two quick breaths and continue CPR in cycles of 15 compressions and two ventilations. Perform CPR for 1 more minute, check for a pulse, then call for help again. In most hospitals, help arrives promptly.

Without help, however, continue CPR. Check for renewed respirations and a pulse. If you feel a pulse but no breath, give 12 ventilations per minute, and monitor the pulse. Don't stop CPR until the patient's breathing and pulse resume, someone takes over for you, or exhaustion halts your effort.

If you detect both a pulse and respirations, position the patient on his side (turning his body as a unit), and monitor his condition.

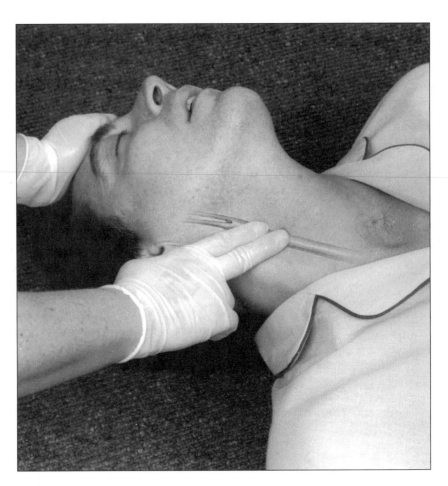

Reviewing recent CPR changes

In late 1992, the American Heart Association (AHA) revised its guidelines for performing cardiopulmonary resuscitation (CPR). Key changes include:
• All health care professionals should learn mouth-to-mask breathing (with a one-way valve mask).
• All health care professionals should wear gloves during CPR.
• Use a "phone first" protocol (for adults only). This advises a rescuer to call for emergency help immediately after confirming that the adult isn't breathing and has no pulse.
• All health care workers should demonstrate skill in using automated external defibrillators for basic cardiac life support. The use of these devices is expected to become commonplace in hospital units that don't have their own crash carts.

ADULT C.P.R.: TWO-PERSON RESCUE

Suppose you've discovered a patient in cardiac arrest and you've begun CPR. Now, help arrives and you'll be able to switch to two-person CPR momentarily. How should you proceed? If you're not in a medical facility or if you haven't contacted help, the second rescuer can do so now.

Continue one-person CPR until the second rescuer takes the proper position (at the patient's chest) opposite you. This tells you that he knows the standard AHA procedures for CPR.

The second rescuer can start assisting after you've finished a cycle of 15 compressions, 2 ventilations, and a pulse check. The second rescuer can check for a returning pulse while you perform chest compressions. If he feels a pulse, he may ask you to stop compressions for 5 seconds so that he can assess for an independent heartbeat.

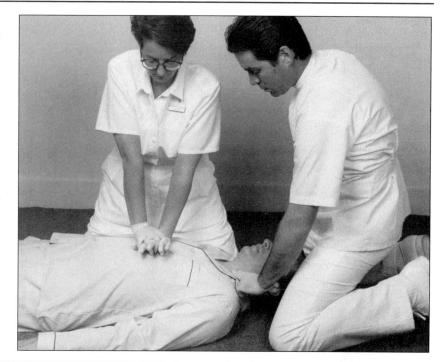

Move to the patient's head and check for a pulse while the second rescuer locates the correct hand position for delivering chest compressions.

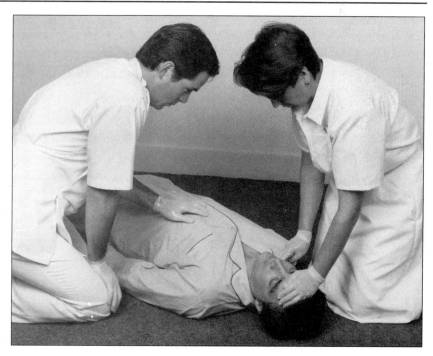

If you don't detect a pulse, say, "No pulse; continue CPR," and give one ventilation. Meanwhile, the second rescuer starts compressions at a rate of 80 to 100 per minute in a ratio of 5:1 (five compressions for each ventilation). The compressor (at this point, the second rescuer) should count "one and two and three and four and five" so that you know when to give the next ventilation. Then the second rescuer should stop compressions long enough for the patient's chest to rise and fall with a ventilation.

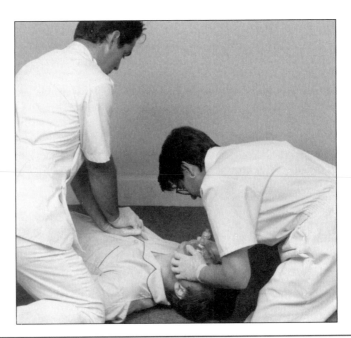

Periodically signal the compressor to stop for 5 seconds so you can check for breathing and a pulse.

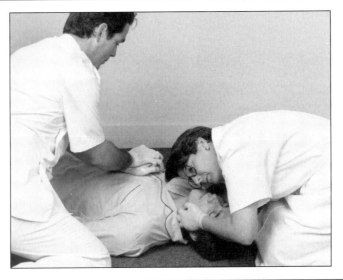

After a minimum of 10 cycles, the compressor may call for a change in positions by saying, "Switch and two and three and four and five." At that point, give a ventilation and move into place to deliver chest compressions.

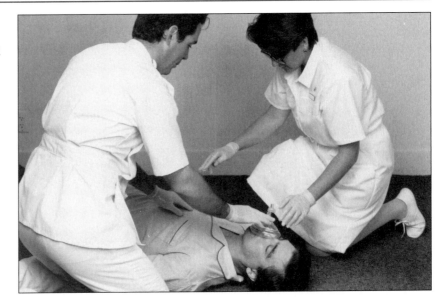

Now, the second rescuer moves to the patient's head to begin ventilations. First, he checks the patient's pulse for 5 seconds. If he doesn't find a pulse, he says, "No pulse" and gives a ventilation. Then you start compressions. Both of you should continue CPR until the patient's respirations and pulse return, ACLS can begin, or you both become exhausted.

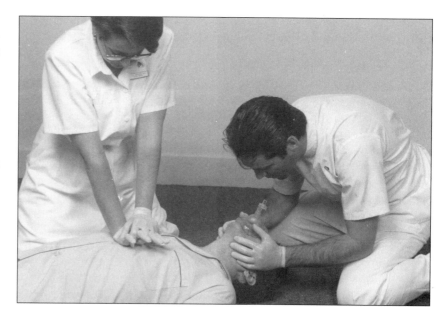

 COMPLICATIONS

Hazards of CPR

Although cardiopulmonary resuscitation (CPR) can save your patient's life, it can also cause internal injuries. To prevent complications, be sure to position your hands properly for chest compressions. And take care not to deliver excessive ventilation. If you suspect any of the following complications, notify the doctor—but don't stop CPR.

Fractured ribs

Once the patient's condition stabilizes, you can detect fractured ribs by palpating for bone displacement and crepitus (a crunching sound). The patient will need rest and analgesics for a fractured rib. If he has a serious fracture, his rib cage may need to be splinted.

Lacerated liver

Although rare, liver laceration poses a serious threat. It usually causes hemorrhage, resulting in shock and abdominal distention. You may have trouble distinguishing it from shock caused by respiratory or cardiac arrest. If you suspect liver laceration, tell the doctor. After the patient's condition stabilizes, the doctor may order diagnostic studies, such as peritoneal fluid analysis. Treatment includes fluid resuscitation and surgical repair.

Punctured lung

If a broken rib punctures the patient's lung, a tension pneumothorax may develop. With this complication, air enters—but can't escape—the pleural space. Positive pressure then builds in the thoracic cavity and collapses the lung.

Other signs of a tension pneumothorax include asymmetrical chest movement, no breath sounds on the side of the pneumothorax and, as the condition grows worse, a shift of the trachea away from the affected side. A chest X-ray can confirm the diagnosis.

Treatment involves inserting a chest tube or a large-bore needle into the pleural space (at about the second intercostal space) to relieve the pressure caused by trapped air.

Distended stomach

A common complication of CPR—also signaled by difficulty in giving resuscitative breaths—is gastric distention. Resulting from delivering too much air during ventilation, gastric distention can promote regurgitation, which increases the risk of aspiration.

If you notice the patient's stomach becoming distended during CPR, reposition his airway by retilting his head. Then make sure that his chest, not his stomach, rises and falls during ventilation. If distention confines the lungs and interferes with adequate ventilation, turn the patient on his side and apply pressure over the epigastrium to induce regurgitation. (The need for a continued air supply overrides the risk of aspiration.) In the unconscious patient, sweep out the airway or suction it, and continue CPR.

CLEARING AN OBSTRUCTED AIRWAY

You'll need to come quickly to the aid of a choking victim. That's because an airway obstruction causes anoxia, which, if uninterrupted, leads to brain damage and death in 4 to 6 minutes. A sudden airway obstruction may occur when a foreign body lodges in the throat or bronchus; when the patient aspirates blood, mucus, or vomitus; when the tongue blocks the pharynx; or when the patient experiences traumatic injury, bronchoconstriction, or bronchospasm.

In an adult, you may use one or more of the following maneuvers to relieve an airway obstruction: abdominal thrust, chest thrust, and finger sweeps. Each maneuver attempts to clear the airway and restore independent ventilation while preventing or reversing unconsciousness.

• The abdominal thrust (or Heimlich maneuver) creates sufficient diaphragmatic pressure below the obstruction to expel it.

• The chest thrust forces air out of the lungs, creating an artificial cough that expels the obstruction.

• The finger sweep (in an unconscious patient) manually removes the obstruction from the mouth.

If your initial efforts to clear the airway fail, keep trying. As oxygen deprivation increases, smooth and skeletal muscles relax, making your maneuvers more likely to succeed. However, avoid these maneuvers in a patient who has incomplete or partial airway obstruction and who has adequate ventilation and can still cough effectively. If he can speak or cough, encourage him to cough to expel the obstruction. On the other hand, if he can't speak, cough, or breathe, respond at once. This patient needs help to dislodge the obstruction.

Clearing the airway of a conscious adult

This maneuver requires only one person and no special equipment. If gloves are available, put them on. Begin by asking the patient, "Are you choking?" and then "Can I help?" If his airway is completely obstructed, he won't answer because airflow to his vocal cords will be blocked. But if he's making crowing sounds, his airway is only partially blocked. Encourage this patient to cough if he's indicated that you can help. Then if the airway becomes completely blocked, proceed.

▶ *Clinical tip:* Be sure the patient indicates that he wants your help. If he denies you permission and you help anyway, you risk a lawsuit for assault.

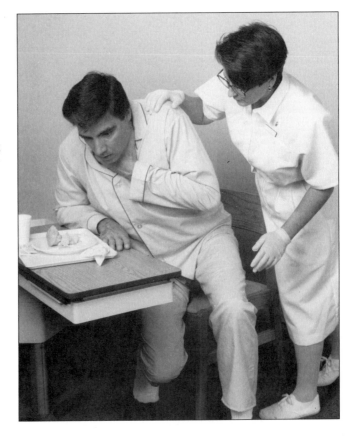

Tell the patient that you'll try to dislodge the foreign body. Stand behind him and put your arms around his waist. Make a fist with one hand. Place the top of the fist (thumb side) against the patient's abdomen, slightly above the umbilicus and well below the xiphoid process. Now grasp the bottom of the fist with the other hand.

▶ *Clinical tip:* When delivering abdominal thrusts, position your hands properly (midway between the xiphoid process and the umbilicus, at the beltline) to avoid injuring the patient. Never place them on the xiphoid process or the lower rib cage margins where the force of your thrusts may fracture the ribs or lacerate the abdominal or thoracic viscera.

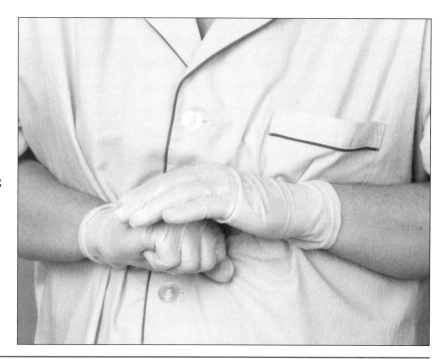

Squeeze the patient's abdomen 6 to 10 times with quick inward and upward thrusts. Each thrust should create an artificial cough with enough force to propel a foreign object from the airway.

▶ *Clinical tip:* When performing the thrusts, keep a firm grasp on the patient. Also be sure that you can provide support should he lose consciousness and need to be lowered to the floor. Scan the floor for a clear, safe area on which to place the patient if necessary.

If the patient loses consciousness, support him carefully. Gently lower him to the floor, using your leg as a sliding board. Remember to support his head and neck to prevent injury. Then take additional steps to clear his airway.

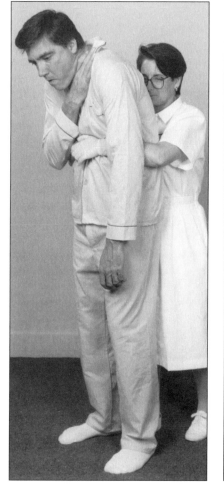

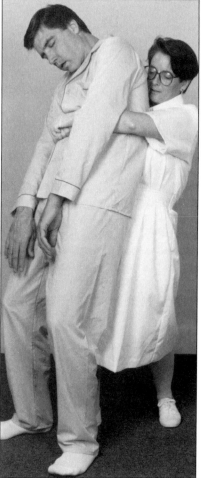

Clearing the airway of an unconscious adult

If you come upon an unconscious patient, ask any bystander to describe what happened. Then, begin CPR. Use the procedure for one-person rescue, and attempt to ventilate the patient. If you can't deliver ventilations, reposition his head and try again. If you still can't supply breaths, assume that his airway is obstructed.

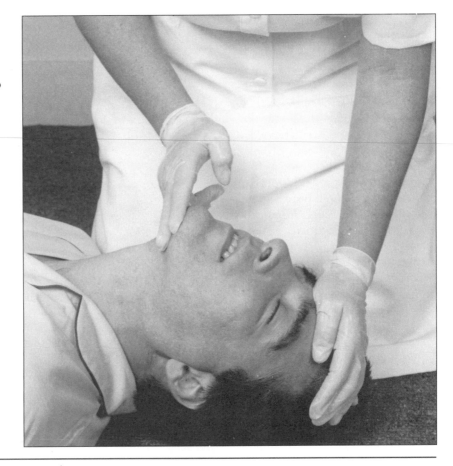

Kneel astride the patient's thighs. Place the heel of one hand on top of the other and put your hands on the patient's abdomen, between the umbilicus and the tip of the xiphoid process at his midline. Using quick thrusts, push inward and upward 6 to 10 times. Each thrust should be forceful enough to dislodge an obstructive foreign body. ▶ *Clinical tip:* If your patient vomits during abdominal thrusts, quickly wipe out his mouth with your fingers. Then resume the maneuver, as necessary.

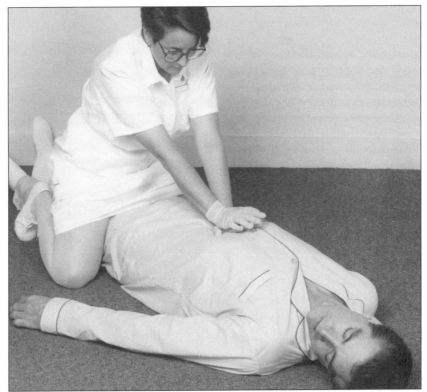

After giving abdominal thrusts, move to the patient's head. Now open his airway. To do so, grasp the tongue and the lower jaw between your thumb and fingers, then lift the jaw to draw the tongue away from the back of the throat and away from any foreign body.

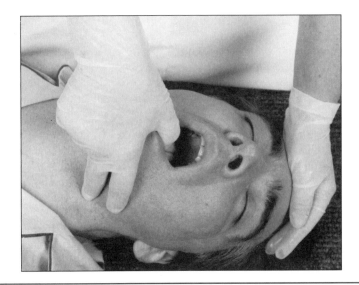

Insert your index finger deep into the patient's throat to the base of the tongue. With a hooking motion, scoop out the obstruction. Next try to ventilate the patient. If you can't, repeat abdominal thrusts until you can.

Keep in mind that some clinicians object to a blind finger sweep because your finger acts as a second obstruction. They believe that the tongue-jaw lift should be enough to dislodge the obstruction.

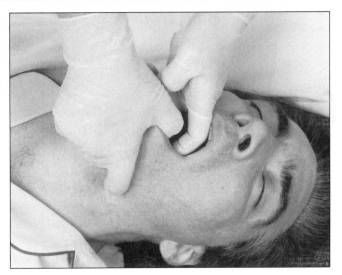

If you can ventilate the patient, assess for spontaneous respirations and check for a pulse. Proceed with one-rescuer CPR, if necessary. Ensure that the patient receives follow-up medical care.

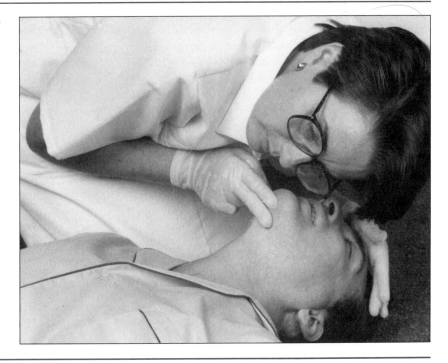

Clearing the airway of an obese or a pregnant patient

How can you clear the airway of a patient whose girth prevents you from encircling his midline with your arms? Or, how can you remove an obstruction from the airway of a pregnant patient when abdominal thrusts may harm the fetus?

In these situations, perform chest thrusts instead of abdominal thrusts. Put on gloves if available. Then place the top of your clenched fist (thumb side) against the middle of the patient's sternum. Put your other hand over the bottom of your clenched fist. Perform chest thrusts until the patient expels the object or the patient loses consciousness.

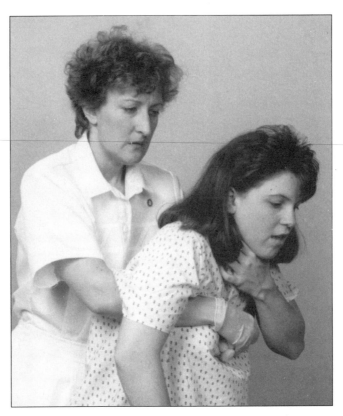

Position yourself at an unconscious patient's side. Place your hands on the chest as you would to perform chest compressions on a patient without a pulse. Give chest thrusts forceful enough to expel a foreign body.

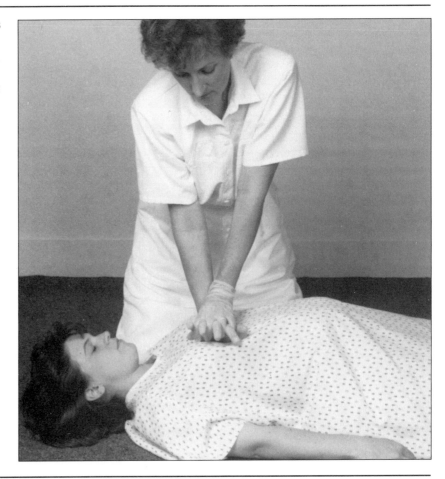

Advanced Cardiac Life Support

LEARNING ABOUT A.C.L.S. AND THE CODE TEAM

Advanced cardiac life support (ACLS) procedures treat the effects of cardiac or respiratory arrest by establishing and maintaining ventilation and circulation. ACLS also focuses on recognizing and treating the immediate causes of arrest. It provides step-by-step guidelines for treating different arrhythmias and for administering drugs, defibrillating, and establishing a patent airway.

To respond to cardiac and respiratory emergencies, most hospitals form code teams that are composed of staff members. The indications for calling a code are absent pulse, apnea, ventricular fibrillation, ventricular tachycardia, or asystole. Called to action by a hospital-determined code word over an address system, the team members come from such departments as anesthesia, respiratory therapy, electrocardiography, critical care, and I.V. therapy. Each of the team members plays a specific role in ensuring proper code management and life support for the patient.

The first two people on the emergency scene become team members simply by discovering the patient in distress and implementing lifesaving interventions, such as cardiopulmonary resuscitation (CPR). Other team members are assigned—usually according to hospital policy and each person's job and work schedule. Typically, the team member's assignment lasts for a specific time, ranging from one shift to several days.

These code team members act quickly in unison, anticipating the patient's needs. The equipment they need to revive the patient is a properly stocked, conveniently located emergency cart. The knowledge they need includes the American Heart Association's procedures for basic life support and ACLS. Once the patient's condition stabilizes, the underlying cause of cardiac or respiratory arrest can be assessed and treated.

IDENTIFYING CODE TEAM RESPONSIBILITIES

• When a nurse finds her patient unconscious in bed, she becomes *basic rescuer 1* because she's the first person on the scene. She assesses the patient's level of consciousness and his airway, breathing, and circulation. She also calls for assistance from another rescuer, calls the code team (if indicated by hospital policy), and begins one-person CPR.

• The nurse who responds to the call for help becomes *basic rescuer 2.* She usually brings the emergency cart and may be responsible for immediately calling the code team (if hospital policy delegates her this role). Then she begins performing CPR with basic rescuer 1.

• Within seconds, the rest of the team arrives. As basic rescuer 1 and basic rescuer 2 continue CPR, the newly arrived members set up the equipment and prepare the patient. The entire setup can be accomplished in 35 to 45 seconds, depending on the teammates' skills.

• The *nurse anesthetist,* the *anesthesiologist,* or the *respiratory therapist* moves quickly to the patient's head, relieves basic rescuer 1, and assumes responsibility for the patient's breathing. This team member maintains a patent airway, intubates the patient as necessary, administers oxygen, monitors respiratory status, and assesses breath sounds to ensure proper tube placement. In some cases, a nurse trained in ACLS will prepare for and assist with endotracheal intubation.

• The *team leader,* a doctor (although a nurse trained in ACLS procedures may act as team leader until a doctor arrives), has overall responsibility for managing the code team and its activities. This person directs resuscitation efforts and major lifesaving events.

When the team leader arrives on the scene, he applies the defibrillator paddles to the patient's exposed chest to obtain a quick look at the patient's cardiac rhythm. If he finds the patient in ventricular fibrillation, he will follow protocol and attempt to defibrillate the patient's heart.

• To further revive and support the patient, an *I.V. therapist* or a nurse trained in ACLS procedures starts two peripheral I.V. lines (in case one fails). For each line, she places a large-bore catheter in a large vein, such as the antecubital vein, if the patient doesn't already have an appropriate peripheral or central venous line in place.

• Meanwhile, the *medication nurse* or the pharmacist—depending on hospital policy—prepares the appropriate I.V. solution for infusion as soon as the I.V. catheter is in place. Typically, she'll infuse either 0.9% sodium chloride solution or lactated Ringer's solution to prevent circulatory collapse from hypovolemia.

Contributors to this section include *Linda C.D. Melly, RN, BSN, CCRN,* a clinical coordinator of critical care at Doylestown (Pa.) Hospital, and *Helen S. Adamson, RN,C, BSN,* a critical care educator at Grand View Hospital, Sellersville, Pa. The publisher thanks *Doylestown (Pa.) Hospital* for its help.

(*Note:* Although dextrose 5% in water [D₅W] is still acceptable for this procedure, recent ACLS guidelines encourage rescuers to avoid possible hyperglycemic effects by infusing 0.9% sodium chloride or lactated Ringer's solution instead.)

The medication nurse continues to administer and prepare needed medications throughout the rescue.

• The *equipment nurse* sets up such adjunctive emergency apparatus as suction and defibrillation equipment and takes vital signs. She also assists in preparing and administering medications when necessary.

• The *go-between nurse* helps as necessary. She may take vital signs, adjust equipment, or administer medications. Her other responsibilities may include transporting specimens to the laboratory for analysis and keeping the patient's family informed.

• The *recorder nurse* immediately takes the code record from the cart and begins to document resuscitation efforts. (See *Keeping the code record.*) She also writes postarrest progress notes.

Keeping the code record

If you're the recorder nurse on the code team, you'll keep a detailed record of the team's resuscitation efforts. The code record will include:
• patient's biographical data
• time of cardiac or respiratory arrest
• details of the arrest (for example, whether the arrest was witnessed or unwitnessed)
• kind of arrest—cardiac, respiratory, or both
• time that resuscitation began
• drug therapy data (time, dosage, route, and person administering drug)

• cardiac resuscitation measures (for example, details of rhythms generated)
• countershocks delivered, including energy level and outcome
• presence of spontaneous pulse and respirations
• special procedures performed
• patient status at end of arrest
• time that resuscitation ended
• names of all code team members.

PERFORMING DEFIBRILLATION

The American Heart Association (AHA) guidelines known as Advanced Cardiac Life Support (ACLS) are the standard for implementing emergency resuscitation procedures. Local AHA chapters teach ACLS techniques, as do AHA-authorized agencies. Caregivers learn to use equipment to support ventilation, control arrhythmias, and reestablish circulation, among other procedures.

One vital piece of equipment—the defibrillator—converts such life-threatening arrhythmias as ventricular fibrillation and pulseless ventricular tachycardia to stable, organized heartbeats. If you are responsible for operating the defibrillator, you'll need to know why and how it works.

Once activated, the defibrillator charges a large capacitor that fires a high-voltage electrical charge through two electrode paddles positioned on the patient's chest and across the heart muscle. The cur-

rent depolarizes the myocardium, allowing the sino-atrial node to resume control of the heart. Depending on the situation, the charge may be delivered asynchronously—as in defibrillation—or in synchrony with the QRS complex of the electrocardiogram (ECG)—as in synchronized cardioversion.

Because successful defibrillation requires a viable amount of myocardial tissue, early intervention is essential for patients with ventricular fibrillation or pulseless ventricular tachycardia. The longer the arrhythmia continues, the greater the damage to the heart.

Other factors that play an important role in successful defibrillation are the size, position, and pressure of the electrode paddles; the number of previous shocks; the intervals between the shocks; the voltage used; and electrical resistance. To perform defibrillation effectively, proceed as follows.

If you suspect that your patient is in ventricular fibrillation, take action at once. First, determine his responsiveness. Gently shake him, call his name, and assess his breathing and pulse. If he's unresponsive, call for help.

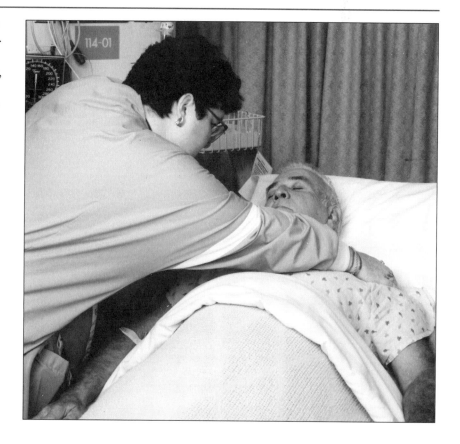

M. Christopher Saslo, RN, BSN, and *Helen S. Adamson, RN,C, BS,* contributed to this section. Mr. Saslo is a BCLS and ACLS instructor at Albert Einstein Medical Center, Philadelphia, and Ms. Adamson is a critical care educator at Grand View Hospital, Sellersville, Pa. The publisher thanks *Doylestown (Pa.) Hospital* for its help.

As soon as help arrives (usually within seconds in a hospital setting), place a backboard under the patient. In most cases, you can use the headboard or footboard of the bed. If help doesn't arrive immediately, place the backboard under the patient yourself. A hard surface is essential for effective chest compressions.

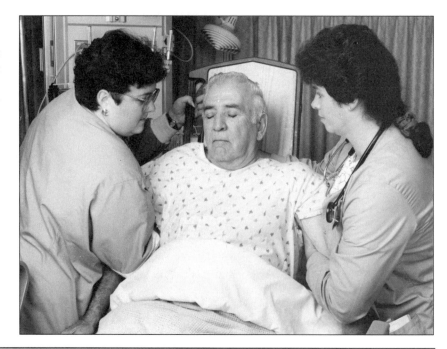

Put on gloves and begin performing cardiopulmonary resuscitation (CPR). Continue CPR while you wait for the emergency cart with the defibrillator to arrive.

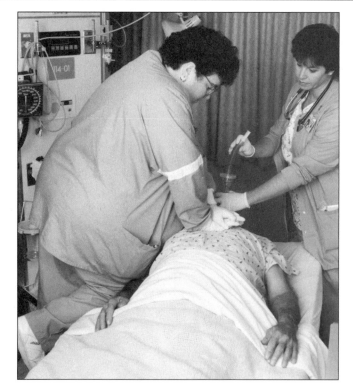

A nurse or another designated person will quickly bring the emergency cart into the room. The cart should include a defibrillator (such as the Physio-Control Lifepak 9P shown on the following pages), conductive gel pads, cardiac monitoring electrodes, and leadwires.

If the cart reaches the room before a backboard is placed under the patient, place the cardiac backboard attached to the cart under the patient.

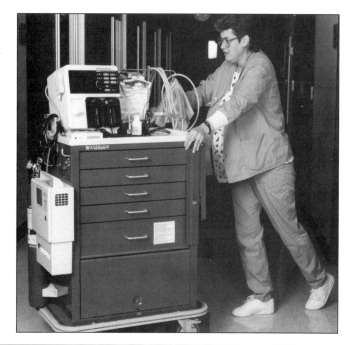

As soon as the emergency cart is positioned in the room, press the ON button on the defibrillator.

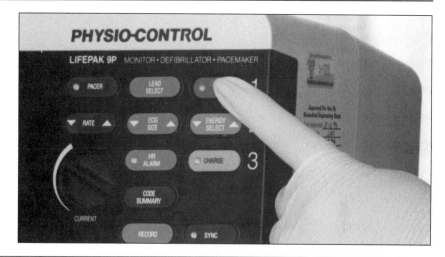

If the patient has an excessive amount of hair on his chest, quickly shave the chest areas where the electrodes will be placed. (A razor is kept on the emergency cart.)

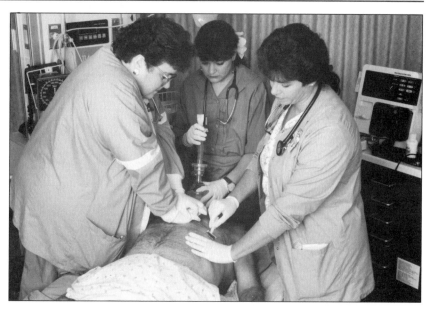

Place the electrodes from the defibrillator on the patient's chest, choosing an appropriate lead— usually lead II.

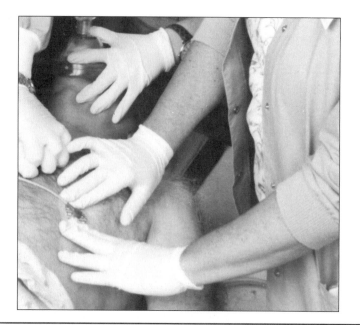

When the electrodes are in place, check the defibrillator monitor to ensure that the patient's heart is in ventricular fibrillation or pulseless ventricular tachycardia.

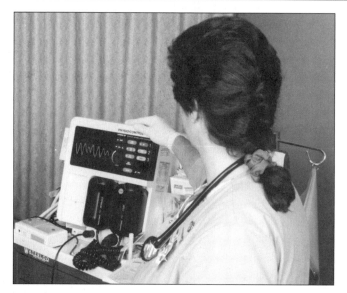

If the defibrillator you're using can also be used for synchronized cardioversion, check the mode before you use it. The SYNC light should be off.

▶ *Clinical tip:* The electrode paddles won't discharge current during ventricular fibrillation or pulseless ventricular tachycardia if the defibrillator is mistakenly set on the SYNC mode.

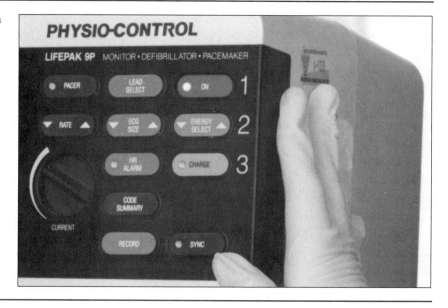

Place the conductive gel pads directly on the patient's chest. In a standard or anterolateral placement, place one pad slightly to the right of the midsternal area and the other pad at the fifth or sixth intercostal space on the left anterior axillary line (shown here). The gel pads reduce the risk of skin burns and avoid electrical current arcing.

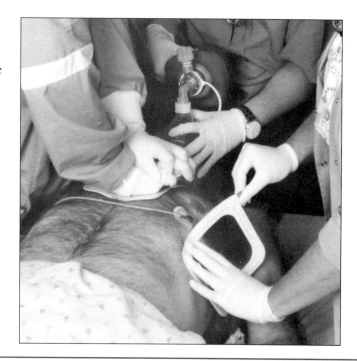

Using the ENERGY SELECT key, set the defibrillator to the appropriate energy level. For the initial defibrillation attempt, the AHA recommends 200 joules.

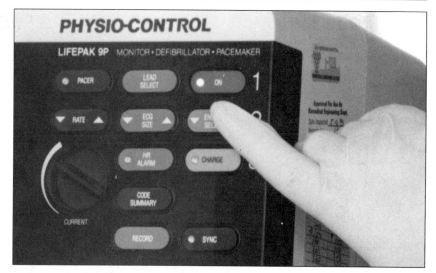

Next, charge the defibrillator (this may take a few seconds) by pressing the CHARGE button either on the defibrillator's panel or on the paddles. The light on the CHARGE button will flash while the paddles are charging. When the paddles are ready, the light will stop flashing and stay on.

▶ *Clinical tip:* On most defibrillators, the energy will drain after 1 or 2 minutes if it hasn't been discharged through the paddles.

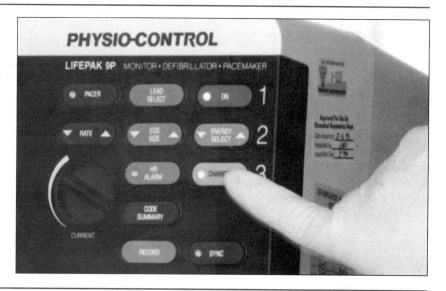

Place the electrode paddles on top of the gel pads. Don't place the paddles on the electrodes or the leadwires.

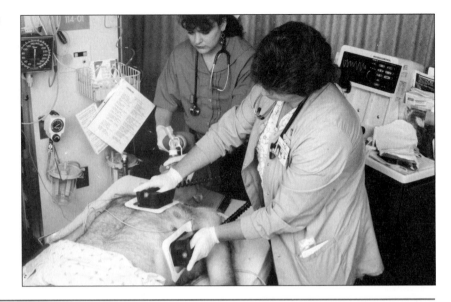

Reassess the patient's cardiac rhythm and level of consciousness to ensure that he still needs defibrillation. If he does, shout "Clear!" (as shown). Quickly look around to make sure that no one (including you) is touching the bed or anything connected to the patient. Also make sure that you're not standing in any fluid that may have dripped on the floor. Take these precautions to prevent accidental electric shock.

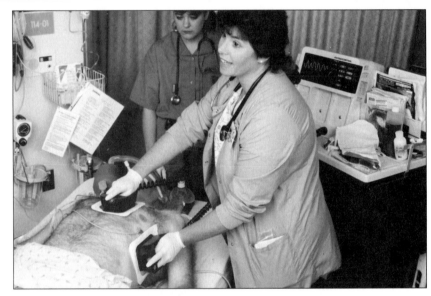

Apply firm pressure to the paddles to decrease transthoracic resistance. Then discharge the current by pushing the DISCHARGE button on both paddles simultaneously. As the shock is delivered, the patient's chest muscles will contract. Look at the monitor to determine whether the heart has returned to a normal rhythm.

▶ **_Clinical tip:_** If the paddles don't discharge, check the defibrillator quickly. Make sure that it isn't in the SYNC mode and that the power cord is still plugged in. If the defibrillator works by battery, make sure that the battery is sufficiently charged.

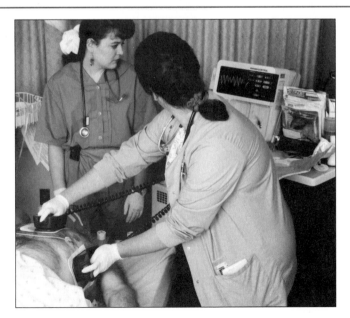

Assess the patient's pulse. If ventricular fibrillation or pulseless ventricular tachycardia persists, resume CPR, recharge the defibrillator, and administer a second shock at 200 or 300 joules. After the second defibrillation attempt, recheck the pulse and rhythm for change. If necessary, administer a third shock at 360 joules, following the same pattern of delivery.

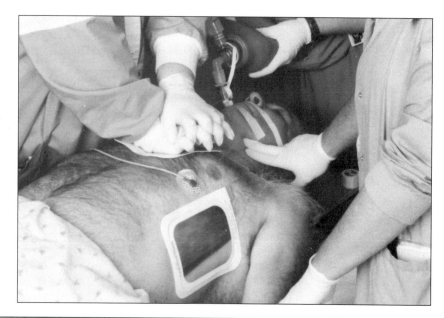

Tear off the ECG strip and put it in the patient's chart. Do this every time a rhythm change occurs. When the patient regains normal sinus rhythm, monitor him and provide supplemental oxygen and ventilation as needed. Continue to monitor his vital signs and cardiac rhythm, and give drugs as prescribed. Check his chest for burns, and treat them as necessary.

Explain to the patient and his family what happened, and provide emotional support. Make sure that the procedure is documented. Especially note the energy needed to convert the lethal rhythm to normal in case the arrhythmia recurs.

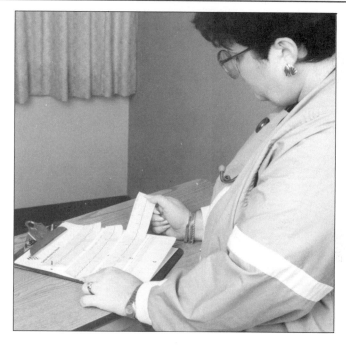

Recognizing ventricular fibrillation and ventricular tachycardia

Before beginning lifesaving treatment for such arrhythmias as ventricular fibrillation and ventricular tachycardia, learn to identify their characteristic features expertly.

Ventricular fibrillation

Defined as chaotic, asynchronous electrical activity within the ventricular tissue, ventricular fibrillation causes death if not corrected immediately. Disorders leading to ventricular fibrillation include myocardial ischemia, hypokalemia, cocaine toxicity, hypoxia, hypothermia, severe acidosis, and severe alkalosis.

Classic signs and symptoms result from lack of cardiac output. They include loss of consciousness, pulselessness, and respiratory arrest.

Electrocardiogram (ECG) characteristics include:
• atrial rhythm: can't be determined
• ventricular rhythm: no pattern or regularity
• atrial rate: can't be determined
• ventricular rate: can't be determined
• P wave: indiscernible
• PR interval: can't be measured
• QRS complex: duration indiscernible
• T wave: can't be determined
• QT interval: can't be measured.

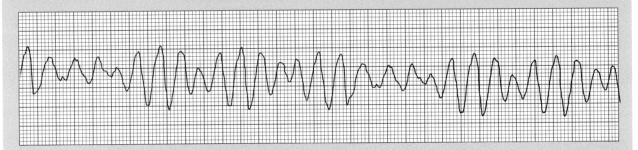

Ventricular tachycardia

This arrhythmia occurs when three or more premature ventricular contractions occur in a row and the ventricular rate exceeds 100 beats/minute. It may develop from enhanced automaticity or reentry within the Purkinje system. The rapid ventricular rate reduces ventricular filling time, atrial kick is lost, and cardiac output drops, putting the patient at risk for ventricular fibrillation.

Ventricular tachycardia typically results from acute myocardial infarction, coronary artery disease, congestive heart failure, cardiomyopathy, an electrolyte imbalance (such as hypokalemia), or drug toxicity (for example, from digitalis glycosides, procainamide, quinidine, or disopyramide).

Signs and symptoms of decreased cardiac output include hypotension, pulselessness, confusion, vertigo, and syncope. Some patients tolerate ventricular tachycardia briefly; others become unresponsive immediately. ECG characteristics include:
• atrial rhythm: can't be determined
• ventricular rhythm: usually regular but may be slightly irregular
• atrial rate: can't be determined
• ventricular rate: rapid (100 to 200 beats/minute)
• P wave: usually absent but may be obscured by QRS complex; retrograde P waves may be present
• PR interval: not measurable
• QRS complex: duration greater than 0.12 second; bizarre appearance, usually with increased amplitude
• T wave: in opposite direction of QRS complex
• QT interval: not measurable.

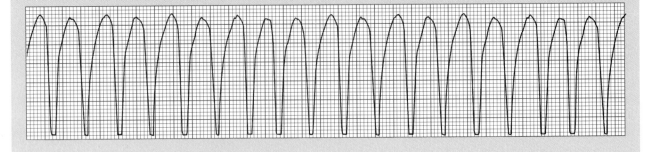

PERFORMING SYNCHRONIZED CARDIOVERSION

Like defibrillation, synchronized cardioversion involves delivering an electric current to the heart to correct an arrhythmia. However, synchronized cardioversion uses much lower energy levels, and the burst of electricity—or shock—is timed precisely to coincide with the peak of the R wave on the ECG.

When successful, the procedure corrects such arrhythmias as atrial flutter, rapid-rate atrial fibrillation, asymptomatic ventricular tachycardia, and paroxysmal supraventricular tachycardia. All of these arrhythmias may be associated with low cardiac output and hypotension.

According to the AHA's Advanced Cardiac Life Support protocols, synchronized cardioversion generally should follow this standard sequence of energy levels: 100, 200, 300, and 360 joules. The exceptions are the energy levels used to convert atrial flutter and paroxysmal supraventricular tachycardia. These arrhythmias usually respond to current starting at 50 joules.

Synchronized cardioversion may be performed as an elective or an emergency procedure. Usually, you'll assist the doctor, although a specially qualified nurse may perform emergency cardioversion. After the procedure, be prepared to intubate the patient in case the arrhythmia recurs or the patient's condition deteriorates further.

In an emergency, rush the following equipment to the patient's bedside: the emergency cart with a defibrillator, conductive gel pads, cardiac monitor electrodes, and leadwires. You'll also need the prescribed sedative.

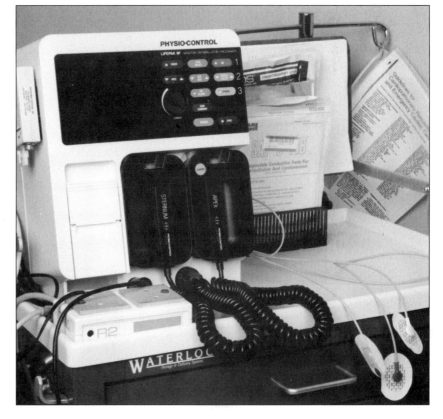

In a nonemergency situation, explain the procedure to the patient and make sure that he has signed an informed consent form.

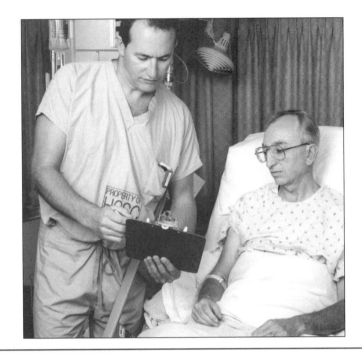

Put on gloves and apply the monitoring electrodes and leadwires of the defibrillator unit to the patient so that the unit can sense the R waves. Turn the monitor on by pressing the ON button. Remove any telemetry and bedside monitors to avoid damaging them during cardioversion.

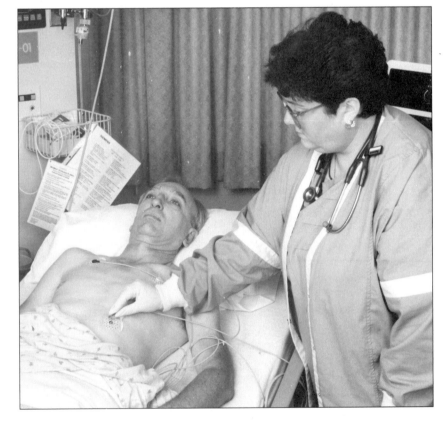

Double-check the waveform on the monitor, and reposition the electrodes if the waveform isn't satisfactory. You should see tall, distinct R waves and much smaller T waves without artifact.

▶ *Clinical tip:* Remember to keep the electrodes away from the areas where you'll place the defibrillator paddles.

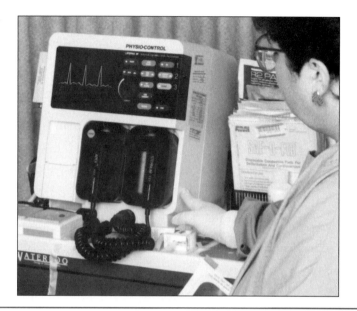

Make sure that the patient's I.V. line is patent, or establish I.V. access as ordered. Administer the prescribed sedative.

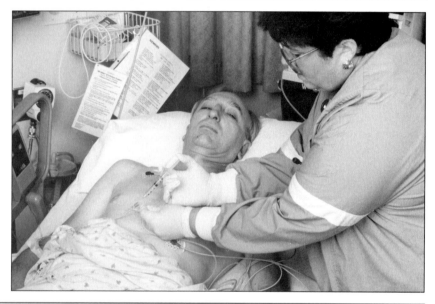

Next, press the SYNC button on the defibrillator unit. This synchronizes the unit with the patient's QRS complexes so that the shock isn't timed concurrently with the vulnerable T wave. Delivering a shock at the wrong time can trigger ventricular fibrillation. The SYNC button flashes each time the machine senses a QRS complex.

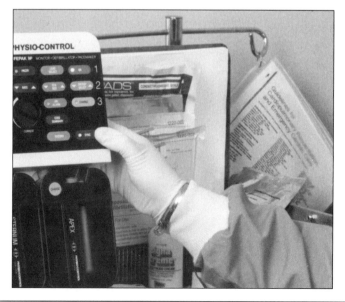

Use the ENERGY SELECT button to set the ordered amount of energy.

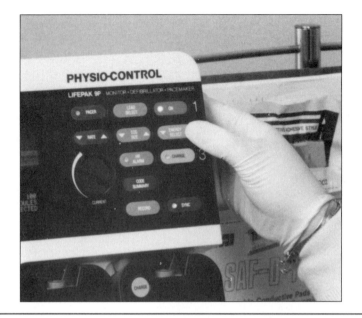

Lower the bed until the patient is lying flat. To reduce the patient's risk of skin burns, apply conductive gel pads to his chest. Place one pad over the sternum—slightly to the right and just below the right clavicle—and the other at the fifth or sixth intercostal space on the left anterior axillary line.

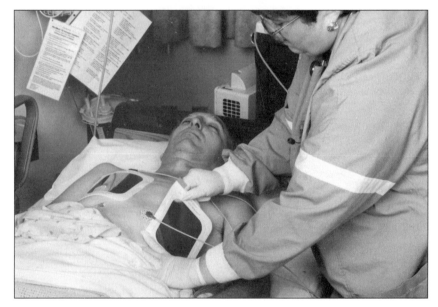

Charge the paddles by pressing the CHARGE button either on the defibrillator panel or on the paddles. A blinking light on this button signals that the paddles are charging. When they're fully charged, the light will stop blinking and remain on.

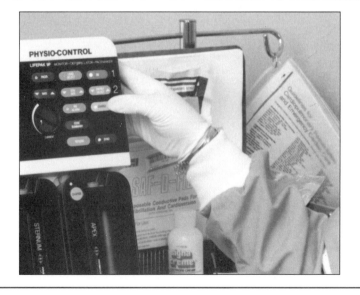

Place the paddles on the conductive gel pads. Reassess the patient's cardiac rhythm to make sure that he still needs synchronized cardioversion. If he does, shout "Clear!" (as shown) and quickly look around to make sure that no one (including you) is touching the bed or anything connected to the patient.

Also make sure that you're not standing in any fluid that may have dripped on the floor. Take these precautions to protect yourself and other caregivers from accidental electric shock.

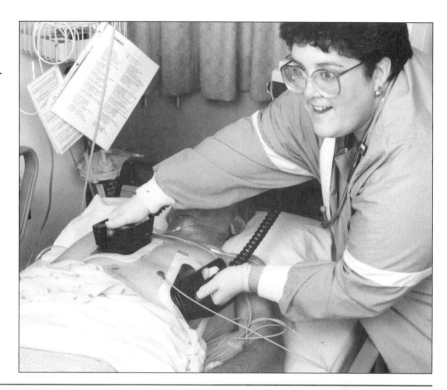

Apply firm pressure to both paddles; then discharge the current by pushing both paddle DISCHARGE buttons simultaneously. The electric shock won't be delivered immediately, as it is in defibrillation; instead, you'll notice a slight delay while the defibrillator synchronizes with the R wave.

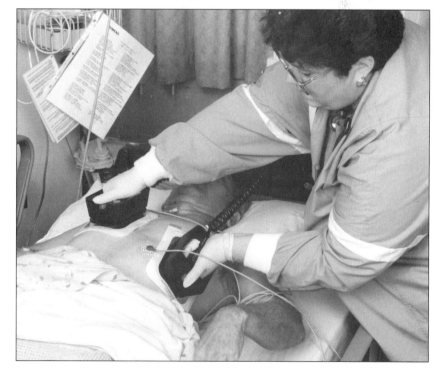

Check the waveform on the monitor. If sinus rhythm hasn't been restored, prepare the paddles again, increase the energy as ordered by pressing the ENERGY SELECT button (as shown), and repeat the procedure.

▶ **Clinical tip:** If synchronized cardioversion results in ventricular fibrillation or pulseless ventricular tachycardia, turn off the SYNC button and perform defibrillation.

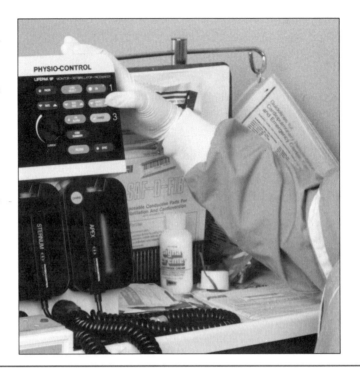

When sinus rhythm has been restored, give the patient supplemental oxygen as prescribed. Remove the gel pads and check his chest for burns. Provide treatment as necessary and continue to monitor his vital signs (as shown). Offer emotional support and document the procedure.

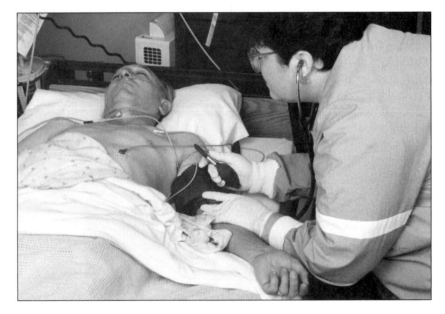

Recognizing atrial flutter, atrial fibrillation, and PSVT

Synchronized cardioversion may be used to treat these common arrhythmias—atrial flutter, atrial fibrillation, and paroxysmal supraventricular tachycardia (PSVT). Review the information and sample waveforms below to reinforce your recognition of these arrhythmias.

Atrial flutter

Characterized by a rapid atrial rate, atrial flutter originates in one atrial focus. This arrhythmia results from circus reentry and, possibly, from increased automaticity. As with any tachycardia, the decreased ventricular filling time may reduce cardiac output.

If the patient's apical or peripheral pulse rate and rhythm remain normal, he may exhibit no signs or symptoms of atrial flutter. On the other hand, if he has a high pulse rate, he'll probably have signs and symptoms of decreased cardiac output, such as dizziness, light-headedness, or low blood pressure. Characteristic features of the patient's electrocardiogram (ECG) include the following:
• atrial rhythm: regular
• ventricular rhythm: depends on atrioventricular (AV) conduction pattern—typically regular, but cycles may alternate
• atrial rate: 250 to 400 beats/minute
• ventricular rate: depends on degree of AV block; usually from 60 to 100 beats/minute but may be 125 to 150 beats/minute, especially during acute episodes. Consider atrial flutter controlled if the ventricular rate falls below 100 beats/minute and uncontrolled if the rate exceeds 100 beats/minute.
• P wave: saw-toothed appearance, referred to as F (flutter or fibrillatory) waves
• PR interval: not measurable
• QRS complex: duration usually within normal limits but may be widened if F waves are buried in QRS complex
• T wave: not identifiable
• QT interval: not measurable because T wave isn't identifiable.

Atrial fibrillation

Atrial fibrillation results from impulses in many circus reentry pathways in the atria. These impulses usually fire at a rate of 400 to 600/minute, causing the atria to quiver rather than contract regularly. Chronic obstructive pulmonary disease, congestive heart failure, coronary artery disease, and stimulants (such as caffeine and nicotine) can cause atrial irritability.

The patient has an irregular pulse rhythm with a normal or abnormal rate. If atrial fibrillation is acute and the ventricular rate is rapid, the patient has signs and symptoms of decreased cardiac output. He also runs the risk of developing pulmonary, cerebral, or peripheral emboli. Typical ECG characteristics include:
• atrial rhythm: grossly irregular
• ventricular rhythm: grossly irregular
• atrial rate: almost indiscernible; usually more than 400 beats/minute
• ventricular rate: usually ranges from 100 to 150 beats/minute but can be less than 100 beats/minute. Consider atrial fibrillation controlled when the ventricular rate drops below 100 beats/minute and uncontrolled when the rate exceeds 100 beats/minute.
• P wave: absent; erratic baseline F waves appear in their place
• PR interval: indiscernible
• QRS complex: usually normal duration and configuration
• T wave: indiscernible
• QT interval: not measurable.

(continued)

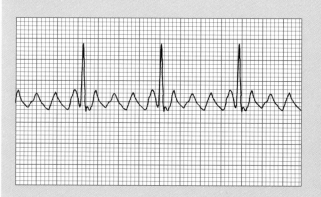

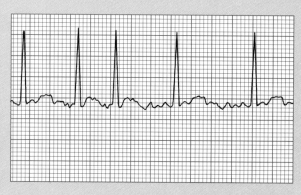

Recognizing atrial flutter, atrial fibrillation, and PSVT (continued)

Paroxysmal supraventricular tachycardia
Typically starting and stopping suddenly, PSVT may be caused by a sinoatrial (SA) node or an AV node reentry mechanism.

PSVT from an SA node reentry mechanism may be initiated by a sinus beat or a premature atrial contraction with sudden onset and cessation of sinus tachycardia. Typical signs and symptoms include jugular vein pulsations, dyspnea, angina, perspiration, fatigue, anxiety, and dizziness. Characteristic ECG features include the following:
• atrial rhythm: regular
• ventricular rhythm: regular
• atrial rate: 100 to 150 beats/minute
• ventricular rate: 100 to 150 beats/minute
• P wave: may be similar to sinus P waves
• PR interval: within normal limits
• QRS complex: normal duration and configuration
• T wave: normal size and configuration
• QT interval: within normal limits and constant.

PSVT from an AV node reentry mechanism may be initiated by an ectopic beat arising in the AV junction.

The patient's ECG may feature:
• atrial rhythm: regular
• ventricular rhythm: regular
• atrial rate: 170 to 250 beats/minute
• ventricular rate: 170 to 250 beats/minute
• P wave: inverted, resulting from retrograde activation of the atria from the junction; may be hidden in QRS complex
• PR interval: can't be determined
• QRS complex: normal size and configuration
• T wave: normal size and configuration
• QT interval: within normal limits and constant.

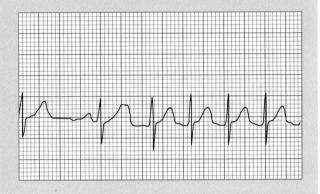

Pacemakers

LEARNING ABOUT PACEMAKERS

When cardiac output and blood pressure plummet, a temporary or permanent pacemaker can restore a normal heart rate by stimulating cardiac muscle contractions. Typically used in an emergency, a temporary pacemaker may be removed after 2 or 3 days. If the heart still needs pacing, a permanent pacemaker can be inserted surgically under the skin.

Both temporary and permanent pacemakers deliver an electrical stimulus to the heart muscle when some phenomenon impairs the intrinsic electrical stimulus or alters normal conduction. (See *Comparing pacemaker types,* page 43.)

HOW PACEMAKERS WORK

All pacemakers share certain basic components. All have a *pulse generator,* which houses a battery and electrical circuitry that directs the pacemaker's function. All have a *pacing lead* (or an electrode wire) that carries an electrical stimulus to the heart muscle from the pulse generator. This lead consists of a conductive wire with exposed metal surfaces called *electrodes.* Located at the distal end of the pacing lead, these electrodes are positioned next to the heart muscle. Through the electrodes, the electrical current enters and exits the heart.

Polarity

A unipolar lead system has one distal negative electrode, whereas a bipolar lead system has two electrodes at the distal end of the pacing lead. The electrode at the distal catheter tip has a negative charge and is called the *cathode.* Several millimeters proximal to the tip is the positive electrode called the *anode.* (See *A look at unipolar and bipolar pacing systems,* page 43.)

ECG characteristics

The pacing stimulus, or *pacer spike,* appears as a vertical spike on the electrocardiogram (ECG) of a patient with a pacemaker. Unipolar pacing catheters produce a larger spike than bipolar ones. A unipolar lead system may be used after cardiac surgery and for permanent pacemakers. Most temporary pacemakers have bipolar electrodes. With bipolar pacing, the second electrode functions as a backup if the first electrode fails.

PACEMAKER MODES AND CODES

Pacemakers function in a demand or fixed mode. The *demand* (or *synchronous*) *mode* delivers an electrical stimulus to the heart at a predetermined rate when the pacing lead senses no intrinsic heart rhythm. The *fixed* (or *asynchronous*) *mode* also provides an electrical stimulus to the heart at a predetermined rate but doesn't have the capacity for sensing intrinsic heart rhythm. The demand mode is usually chosen because the patient is safer with a pacemaker that senses the patient's own electrical activity and fires only when needed.

A five-letter coding system, known as the NBG system, provides a simple description of pacemaker modes and capabilities. The first three letters pertain to the pacemaker's basic functions, including the heart chamber being paced, the chamber being sensed, and the pacemaker's response to the sensed event. The remaining two letters relate to special programmable and antitachyarrhythmia functions. (See *Understanding pacemaker codes,* page 44.)

Among common pacemaker modes are AAI, VVI, DVI, and DDD. AAI—or atrial demand—is used most commonly after cardiac surgery when sinus bradycardia occurs and a faster heart rate is desired. For AAI to be effective, conduction from the atrioventricular (AV) node must be normal.

VVI—or ventricular demand—is the most commonly used pacemaker mode. It's used for various rhythm disturbances, including sick sinus syndrome, junctional rhythms, AV blocks, ventricular rhythms, and atrial fibrillation or flutter with a slow ventricular response. Its main disadvantage is that ventricular pacing doesn't maintain AV synchrony. The atrial contribution to cardiac output, or atrial kick, may be as much as 30% of the total amount of blood lost from atrial contraction, and this loss may not be tolerated by many cardiac patients.

DVI, or AV sequential pacing, is used most often after cardiac surgery during which atrial and ventricular wires are easily inserted. This mode maintains AV synchrony during pacing in most instances. Disadvantages arise because the pacemaker doesn't sense atrial activity and isn't readily available for temporary transvenous pacing.

Contributors to this section include *Sandra J. Bixler, RN, MSN, CCRN; Cynthia Possanza, RN, MSN, CCRN;* and *Linda S. Baas, RN, PhD, CCRN.* Ms. Bixler is a clinical nurse specialist with Berks Cardiologists in Reading, Pa. Ms. Possanza is a nursing consultant for Springhouse Corporation. Ms. Baas is an assistant professor at the University of Cincinnati College of Nursing and Health. The publisher thanks *Medtronic, Inc.,* Minneapolis, for its help.

DDD, or AV universal pacing, is typically the mode of choice for permanent pacemakers and for pacing during cardiac surgery because its action replicates natural cardiac conduction more closely than other pacemaker modes. It maintains AV synchrony and can pace at different rates in response to varying atrial activity. High and low rate limits are set, providing the flexibility to meet individual needs during sleep, exercise, fever, and other stressful activities and conditions.

INDICATIONS

Typically, a temporary pacemaker is inserted when a patient shows signs of an inadequate heart rate, such as decreased blood pressure, diaphoresis, dizziness, light-headedness, and syncope.

The most common causes of rhythm disturbances requiring temporary pacing include acute myocardial infarction, valvular disorders, and the use of certain cardiac drugs. Other causes include coronary artery disease, respiratory failure, pulmonary embolism, and multisystem organ failure. Rhythm disturbances also may occur after surgery or trauma.

Additional rhythm disturbances calling for pacing include sinus arrest or pause; sinus bradycardia; second-degree (Mobitz II) and third-degree heart block; junctional, idioventricular rhythm; ventricular standstill; and asystole. Temporary pacing may also be used for atrial flutter and ventricular tachycardia to override the atrial or ventricular rate, break the cycle of tachycardia, and restore normal rhythm.

A temporary pacemaker may also be used as a backup in high-risk cardiac patients undergoing anesthesia, elective cardioversion, cardiac drug administration, and certain diagnostic procedures, such as cardiac catheterization and electrophysiologic testing. In these cases, noninvasive pacing is beneficial.

Pacemaker glossary

Review the following glossary of common terms related to cardiac pacing and pacemakers.

Artifact. The vertical spike recorded on the electrocardiogram (ECG) depicting the energy discharged from the pulse generator

Asynchronous pacing. The activity initiated by a pacemaker stimulating the heart at a fixed rate regardless of the heart's electrical or mechanical activity; also known as fixed pacing

AV interval. The time period from atrial stimulation to ventricular stimulation; appears as the PR interval on the ECG

Bipolar lead. A pacing lead (or electrode wire) having two electrodes near the distal end of the pacing catheter

Capture. The electrical activation of the atria (P wave) or the QRS complex following an electrical pacing stimulus

Dual-chamber pacemaker. A pacemaker that provides electrical stimulation of the atria and ventricles

Electrode. A thin, electrically conductive wire that's enclosed within the leadwire of the pacing system; or the skin patch used with transcutaneous pacemakers through which the electrical current passes

Fusion beat. An intrinsic (heart-generated) electrical stimulus occurring simultaneously with a paced (pacemaker-generated) electrical stimulus

Inhibited rhythm. A programmed electrical inhibitor that prevents the release of a stimulus when the pacemaker senses intrinsic electrical activity

Intrinsic rhythm. A naturally occurring electrical stimulus from within the heart

Milliampere. A unit of measure of electrical current delivered to the heart through the electrode wire

Mode. The capability of a pacemaker to supply artificial electrical stimuli to the heart; identified by three- to five-letter codes

Pulse generator. A device that includes the power source and circuitry for transmitting pacing signals and for sensing the heart's intrinsic activity

Pulse width. The time (measured in milliseconds) from the onset of electrical stimulation to capture

Sensing. The ability to recognize the electrical signal that stimulates (or inhibits) the discharge of electrical energy by the pulse generator

Synchronous pacing. The activity initiated by a pacemaker delivering an electrical stimulus as needed when the heart's intrinsic rhythm fails or isn't sensed; also known as demand pacing

Unipolar lead. A pacing lead having one electrode at the distal end of the pacing catheter

Comparing pacemaker types

Temporary pacemakers are used primarily in emergencies or experimentally to observe their effect before inserting a permanent pacemaker. Permanent pacemakers are usually implanted when the heart's natural pacing mechanism is irreversibly impaired.

Temporary pacemakers
• *Transcutaneous pacemakers* consist of two electrode patches connected to a combined monitor and pulse generator. These noninvasive devices are easily applied to the skin in hospital or other settings.
• *Transvenous pacemakers* are probably the most common and reliable of the temporary pacemakers. Usually performed at the bedside or in a fluoroscopy suite, insertion involves advancing a balloon-tipped catheter into the right ventricle through the subclavian or jugular vein.
• *Transthoracic pacemakers* may restore heart rhythm after cardiac arrest when other methods have failed. This kind of pacing involves inserting an electrode wire directly into the heart.
• *Epicardial pacemakers* are implanted during cardiac surgery and are used most commonly in the early postoperative period. The surgeon brings the electrode wires out through the chest below a mediastinal incision and attaches them to a pulse generator. The wires are gently withdrawn around the 5th postoperative day or when pacing is no longer required.

Permanent pacemakers
After giving the patient a local anesthetic, the doctor usually implants a permanent pacemaker transvenously. He inserts an endocardial electrode wire into the right ventricle and connects the other end of the wire to a pulse generator placed subcutaneously below the right clavicle. Batteries last from 6 to 10 years and are easily replaced. Hand-held programmers are available to adjust pacemaker functions.

A look at unipolar and bipolar pacing systems

This illustration shows a unipolar pacing system and a bipolar pacing system (inset, right). In both systems, the pulse generator is positioned outside of the heart in the anterior chest.

Unipolar system
In unipolar systems, electrical current moves from the pulse generator through the leadwire to the cathode (the negative pole), stimulates the heart, and returns to the pulse generator's metal surface (the anode, or positive pole) to complete the circuit.

Bipolar system
In bipolar systems, current flows from the pulse generator through the leadwire to the cathode at the tip, stimulates the heart, and then flows to the anode (also located at the leadwire's tip) to complete the circuit.

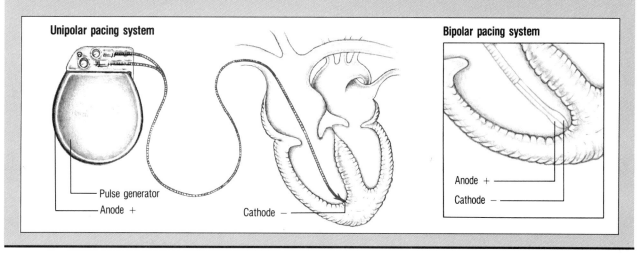

Unipolar pacing system
Pulse generator
Anode +
Cathode −

Bipolar pacing system
Anode +
Cathode −

Understanding pacemaker codes

The five-letter pacemaker coding system describes a pacemaker's capabilities. The first letter identifies the heart chamber being paced; the second letter, the heart chamber that the pacemaker senses; and the third letter, the pacemaker's response to any sensed activity or inactivity. The remaining two letters relate to special programmable functions and antitachyarrhythmia functions.

Examples of typical modes are AAI, VVI, DVI, and DDD. In AAI, the atrium is the chamber both paced and sensed, and the pacemaker's response to sensed activity is inhibited. In VVI, the ventricle is both paced and sensed, and the pacemaker's response to sensed activity is also inhibited. In DVI, both chambers are paced but only the ventricle is sensed. In DDD, both the atria and ventricles are paced and sensed, and the pacemaker's response to sensed activity may be inhibited or triggered, depending on cardiac activity. A pacemaker in the DDD mode is fully automatic.

LETTER 1: CHAMBER PACED	LETTER 2: CHAMBER SENSED	LETTER 3: RESPONSE TO SENSING	LETTER 4: PROGRAMMABLE FUNCTIONS AND RATE MODULATION	LETTER 5: ANTITACHYARRHYTHMIA FUNCTIONS
V — ventricle	V — ventricle	T — triggers pacing	P — programmable rate, output, or both	P — pacing (antitachyarrhythmia)
A — atrium	A — atrium	I — inhibits pacing	M — multiprogrammability of rate, output, sensitivity, and so forth	S — shock
D — dual (A and V)	D — dual (A and V)	D — dual (T and I)	C — communicating functions (telemetry)	D — dual (P and S)
O — none	O — none	O — none	R — rate modulation	O — none
			O — none	

USING A TRANSCUTANEOUS PACEMAKER

Also known as an external, external transthoracic, noninvasive, or transdermal pacemaker, a transcutaneous pacemaker works by using two electrode patches and an external pulse generator–monitor unit. The electrode patches are applied to the patient's chest and back. Then, electrical current passed through the electrodes stimulates the heart, causing it to depolarize and contract.

Unlike early transcutaneous pacemakers, current devices avert skeletal muscle stimulation and skin burns by using large electrode patches and ECG filtering. This makes transcutaneous pacing a primary emergency treatment for bradycardia and asystole. The American Heart Association's guidelines for advanced cardiac life support include transcutaneous pacing protocols.

Quickly established in emergency or hospital settings, transcutaneous pacing is cost-effective and carries none of the risks and complications of invasive techniques.

Setting up transcutaneous pacing

Take the necessary equipment to the patient's room: an external pulse generator–monitor unit, such as the Physio-Control Lifepak 9P shown here; electrode patches; a skin preparation kit or shaving supplies; and a towel to dry the skin at the electrode application area. Have emergency resuscitation equipment nearby.

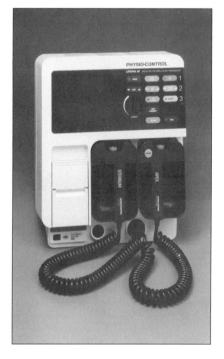
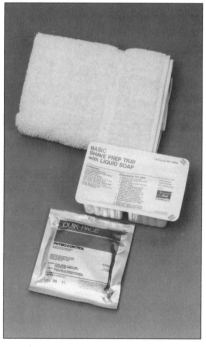

Before transcutaneous pacing, explain the procedure to the patient and his family. For example, describe the pacing sensation as a pectoral muscle twitch or a hiccuplike feeling. Then turn on the power to the pulse generator–monitor unit.

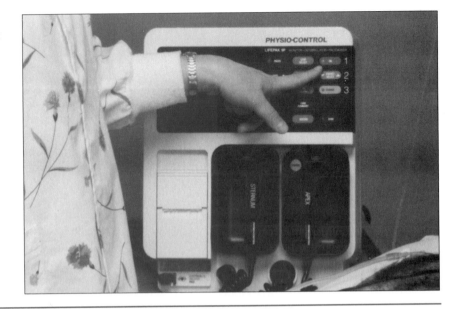

Open the skin preparation kit and fill the basin with warm water. Clean and dry the center of the left anterior chest and the corresponding area on the back—beside the left spine and just below the left scapula—where you'll place the electrodes. If necessary, clip or shave excess hair to decrease skin resistance to the flowing electrical current and to minimize discomfort when you remove the electrode patches.

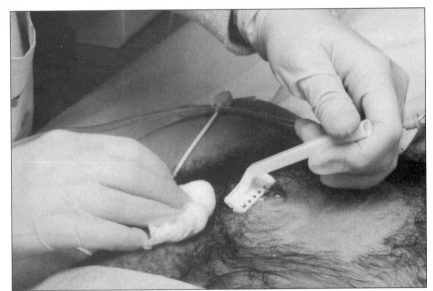

Attach the pacing cables from the pulse generator to the electrode patches.

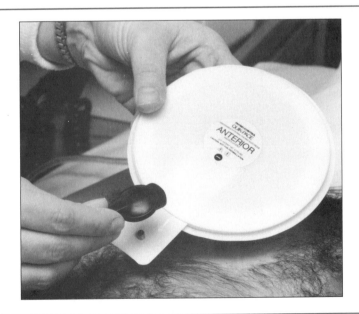

Then apply the electrode patch marked "ANTERIOR" or "NEGATIVE" on the center of the left anterior chest at the fourth intercostal space, just to the left of the sternum (the V_2 position).

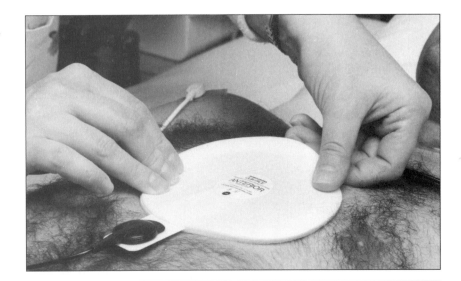

Place the center of the second electrode patch marked "POSTE-RIOR" or "POSITIVE" on the patient's back beneath the scapula and to the left of the spine (on the heart side).

If you're using a bridging cable (commonly called an ECG slave) to connect the bedside monitor to the transcutaneous monitor, remove the bedside monitor electrodes from the patient.

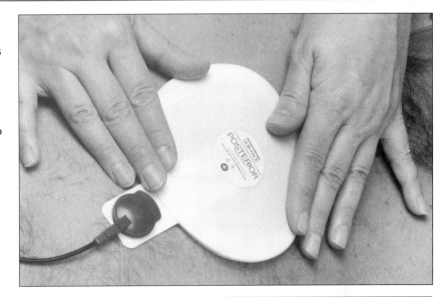

Alternatively, place the electrode patches in the anterolateral position. If you select this position, put the negative electrode on the left side of the chest at the midaxillary area, over the fourth intercostal space, and put the positive electrode on the upper right side of the anterior chest just below the clavicle.

▶ *Clinical tip:* This alternative position is usually less desirable; if you need to initiate defibrillation, you must remove the electrode patches and replace them with the defibrillator paddles.

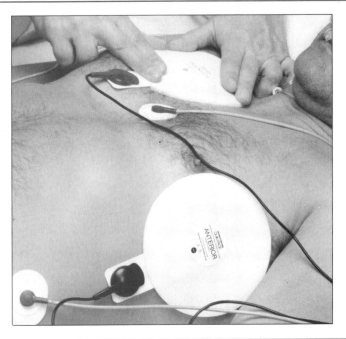

After you've positioned the electrode patches, set the pacemaker mode to DEMAND or FIXED by pressing the PACER key. The option you choose will depend on the clinical situation and available equipment. Set the initial pacing rate at 70 (beats per minute) and the generator output at 0 (MA, or milliamperes).

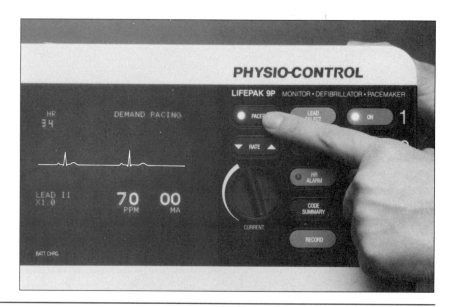

Watch for capture on the ECG monitor. At the same time, slowly advance the MA setting until 100% capture occurs. Usually, 55 to 90 milliamperes will produce capture. After complete capture occurs, the doctor will order settings to maintain pacing. The settings may reflect adjustments tailored to the patient's condition.

Finally, evaluate and document the patient's response to pacing and tolerance of it. Verify adequate perfusion by taking his blood pressure, and mount an ECG strip on his chart.

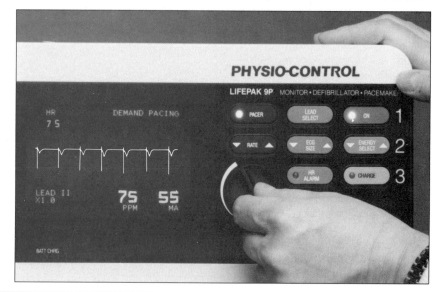

Maintaining transcutaneous pacing

Check the cardiac monitor frequently, noting the patient's underlying cardiac rhythm. Press the RECORD key to obtain a 1-minute rhythm strip, and determine the percentage of beats that require pacing.

If the pacemaker activity varies widely, obtain a second rhythm strip and recalculate. Also check the pacemaker's electrodes and settings. Be sure to document the MA setting and the pacing rate every hour or as designated by your hospital's policy.

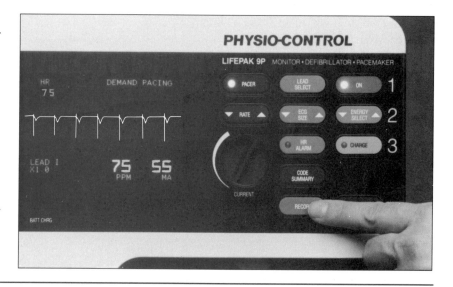

Applying new electrode patches

Change electrode patches every 24 hours or according to hospital protocol. To do this, first remove the electrode cable from the electrode patch on the patient's chest, and quickly attach it to a new electrode patch.

▶ *Clinical tip:* If the patient requires the pacemaker all the time and has no intrinsic cardiac rhythm, remove the patches only when they no longer adhere to his skin.

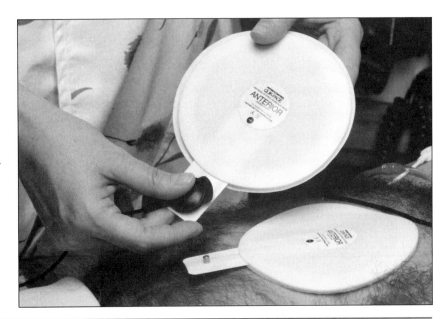

Apply the new electrode patch to the chest slightly away from the original position to prevent skin breakdown. Repeat the procedure to replace the posterior electrode patch.

Check the monitor to make sure that the pacemaker is functioning properly. Also note the readings on the pulse generator–monitor to ensure that the settings are correct.

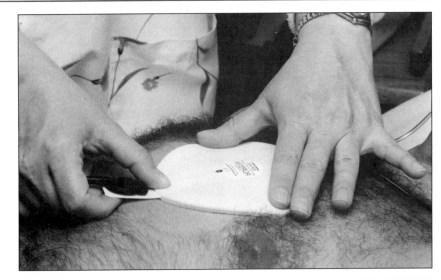

Performing defibrillation

If defibrillation becomes necessary, place the paddles in the standard locations. Use the defibrillation settings as usual if the patient has pacing electrodes on his chest and back.

Turn off the pacemaker before defibrillation; some pacing equipment must be disconnected to avoid damaging the generator.

▶ *Clinical tip:* Don't defibrillate with the paddles on the pacing electrodes. If the patient has pacing electrodes in the anterolateral positions, remove them before defibrillating.

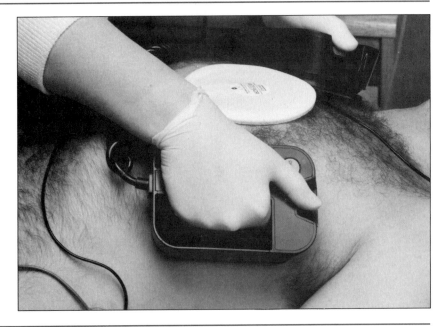

Discontinuing transcutaneous pacing

To stop pacing, first verify the doctor's order and then turn the MA setting and the pacing rate to OFF.

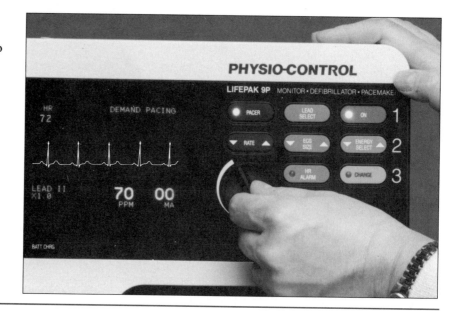

Remove and discard the electrode patches, and return the remaining equipment to storage. Finally, evaluate and document the procedure and the patient's response.

Be ready to assist with transvenous pacemaker insertion or to prepare the patient for permanent pacemaker insertion.

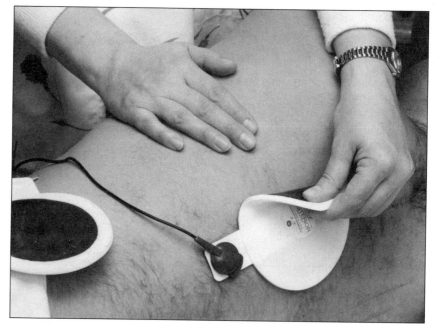

USING A TRANSVENOUS PACEMAKER

Transvenous pacing is the most reliable method of maintaining an adequate heart rate when a temporary rhythm disturbance occurs. In this procedure, the doctor uses an introducer to insert a pacing catheter (most have a balloon tip to ease insertion) into a vein leading to the right ventricle. Once the catheter enters the vessel, blood flow carries it past the tricuspid valve and into the right ventricle. The jugular and subclavian veins are the most commonly used insertion sites; however, the brachial or femoral veins also may be used.

An alternative device, the thermodilution pacing catheter combines cardiac pacing and pulmonary artery pressure monitoring in one catheter.

To initiate pacing, the doctor may insert the catheter at the bedside, guided by fluoroscopy or an ECG. In special circumstances, or when using a catheter without a balloon tip, the doctor *must* use fluoroscopy. For bedside insertion, the doctor typically uses the ECG-guided technique described on the following pages.

Take the necessary equipment to the patient's room. You'll need a semifloating pacing catheter or a semifloating thermodilution pacing catheter with an additional port through which a pacing catheter can be inserted.

You'll also need an introducer kit, a pulse generator, a bridging cable, double-ended alligator clips, linen-saver pads, a skin preparation kit, 4" × 4" gauze pads, sterile gloves, a gown, and a face shield. Additional equipment includes a 12-lead ECG machine or a 5-lead bedside monitor.

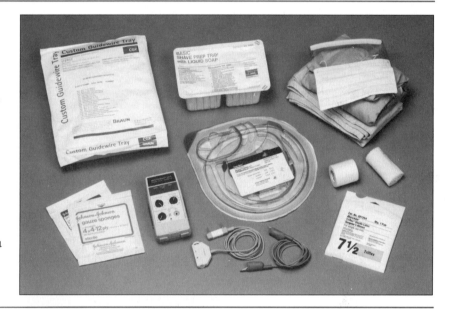

Explain the procedure, keeping in mind that the doctor will have the patient (or a responsible party) sign a consent form. Then prepare the monitor to display two leads: lead II and a V lead.

Place the patient in a supine position with the insertion site exposed. Place the linen-saver pad under the catheter insertion site. If necessary, shave or clip the hair around the insertion site. Open the introducer kit onto an overbed table, or place the necessary equipment on a sterile towel. Then put on the gown, face shield, and gloves.

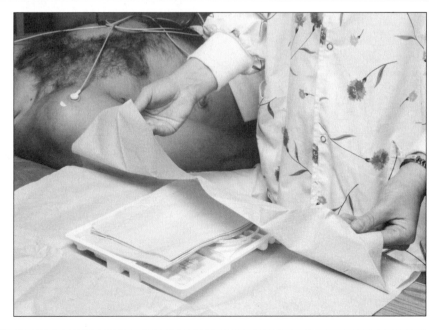

Turn the patient's head away from the insertion site. Using sterile technique and a circular motion, the doctor will wipe the skin at the insertion site with a povidone-iodine swab. Then he'll cover the site with a sterile fenestrated drape and administer a local anesthetic.

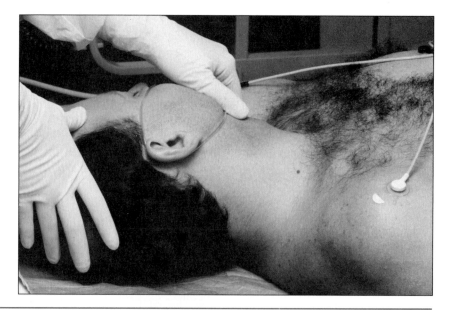

After the doctor numbs the site, he'll insert the introducer into the selected vein. As he does this, open the pacing catheter package. Once the introducer's position is verified by blood return, hold the package so that the doctor can withdraw the catheter.

▶ **Clinical tip:** Be prepared to place the patient in Trendelenburg's position, if requested, before the doctor inserts the introducer. This position promotes venous engorgement, which eases insertion.

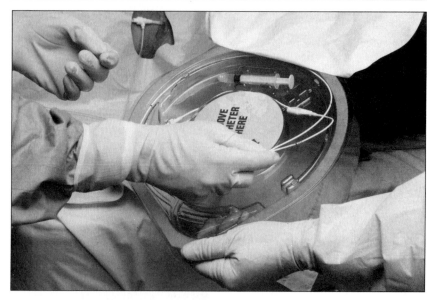

If requested, attach alligator clips to the distal port of the pacing catheter and to the V lead of the ECG equipment, whether it's a 12-lead ECG machine or a 5-lead bedside monitor.

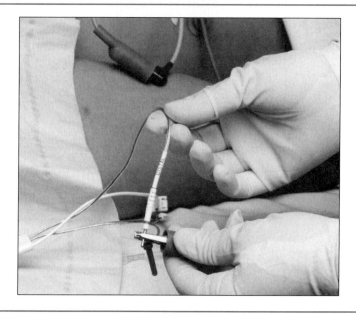

Observe the II and V lead tracings on the bedside monitor for changes in cardiac rhythm.

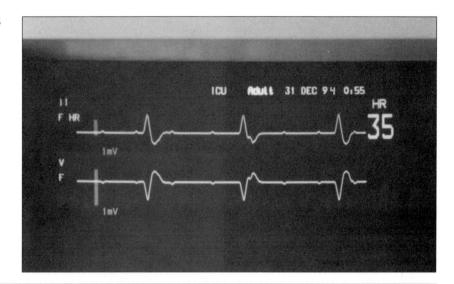

Watch the ECG tracing as the doctor inserts the pacing catheter and injects air into the port to inflate the catheter's balloon tip. Be alert for arrhythmias as the catheter floats from the right atrium to the right ventricle. The tip of the catheter may irritate the heart muscle and cause premature ventricular contractions (PVCs), as shown, or ventricular tachycardia (VT), in which case the doctor may administer lidocaine. If sustained VT occurs, the doctor may withdraw the catheter into the right atrium until VT subsides.

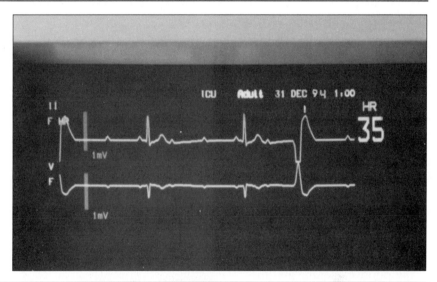

Check the V lead tracing on the monitor to verify proper catheter placement. As the catheter passes through the right atrium, expect to see large P waves and small QRS complexes. When it reaches the right ventricle, expect to see large QRS complexes with ST-segment elevation. This indicates that the catheter is in contact with the heart muscle.

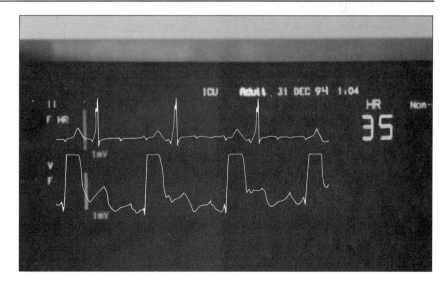

When the catheter reaches the heart muscle, the doctor will deflate the balloon tip and remove the alligator clips. Next, you or the doctor will attach the pulse generator to the pacing catheter. To do this, press the thumb release at the top of the pulse generator while simultaneously inserting first one pacing catheter and then the other (as shown). Remember that the positive (proximal port) and negative (distal port) connections must be correctly aligned.

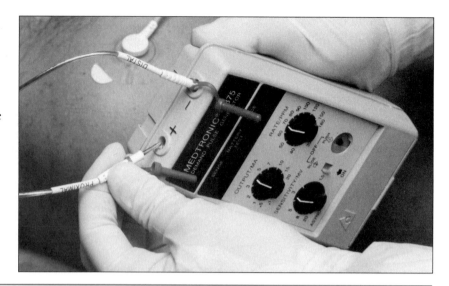

In some cases, you may connect a bridging cable between the pacing catheter and the pulse generator. (This cable provides slack between the catheter and the generator and, thereby, reduces the risk of accidental catheter displacement.)

To do this, insert each pacing catheter into the patient end of the bridging cable. Then press the thumb release at the top of the pulse generator while simultaneously pressing the pulse generator end of the bridging cable into the pulse generator (as shown). Make sure to put the positive pin in the positive opening and the negative pin in the negative opening.

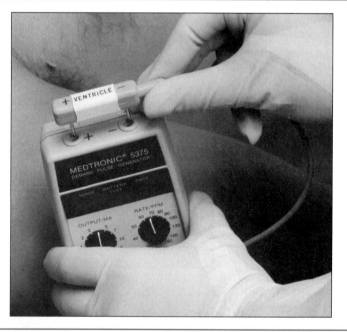

Adjust the pacemaker rate, output (MA), and sensitivity as the doctor prescribes.

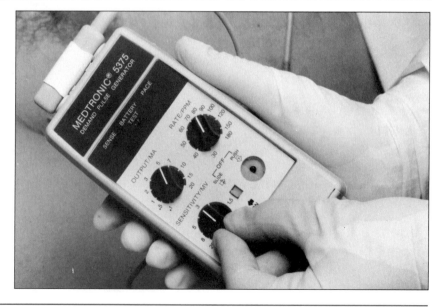

Monitor the ECG for capture. Also monitor the patient's pulse rate and blood pressure. Determine the stimulation threshold by turning the MA from 0 to the setting at which 100% capture occurs. Set the MA to at least two times the threshold to ensure that pacing remains reliable. Normal thresholds for a transvenous pacemaker range between 0.1 and 1.5 MA.

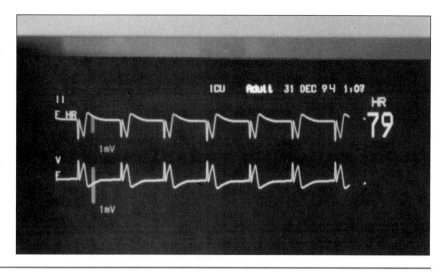

With the final settings determined and pacing established, the doctor will suture the introducer to the skin. When he finishes, cover the site with a 4″ × 4″ sterile occlusive dressing secured with tape or a transparent dressing. Label the dressing with the date and time.

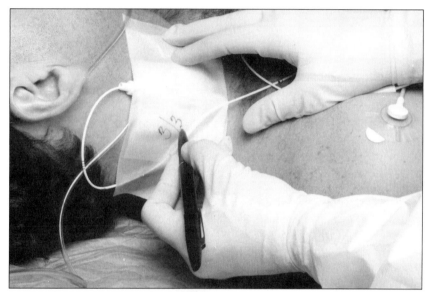

Anchor the pacing catheter with a piece of tape just below the dressing to prevent accidental catheter removal.

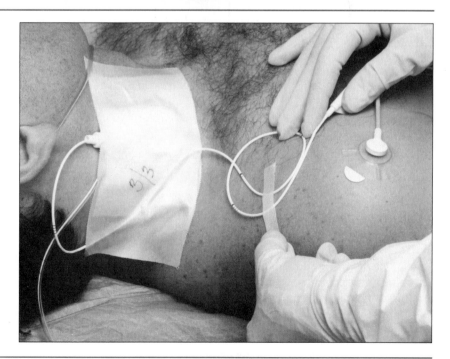

Secure the pulse generator to the patient's chest, waist, upper arm, or leg with tape, muslin, or a Velcro strap. To use muslin, insert one end through the pulse generator's bracket (as shown) and tie the piece to the bracket. Then pass the muslin around the patient's limb or waist, through the pulse generator's other bracket, and tie the muslin securely.

If the doctor used a femoral or brachial vein, ask the patient not to use that limb if possible because doing so would increase the risk of dislodging the catheter and impairing circulation to the limb.

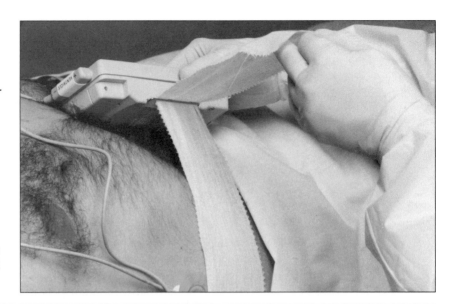

Alternatively, you can place the pacemaker in a strapped pouch specially designed to secure pacemakers. These products are available at some hospitals.

Arrange for an immediate bedside chest X-ray to verify catheter placement. Then document the procedure and the patient's tolerance of it.

▶ *Clinical tip:* If a cover cap is available, place it over the pacemaker controls to avoid accidental setting changes or exposure to moisture.

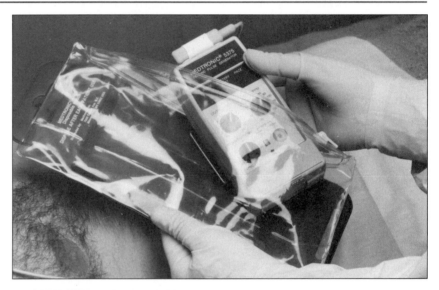

Once the patient's rhythm disturbance resolves, the doctor may remove the pacing catheter. Wearing gloves, he'll withdraw the pacing catheter from the introducer. Then he'll disconnect the catheter from the bridging cable and the pulse generator and discard it according to hospital protocol.

Put on gloves and use a prescribed solution to clean the pulse generator and bridging cable after each use. When you're finished, remove and discard your gloves. Document the patient's tolerance of the procedure, and continue assessing his condition according to hospital protocol.

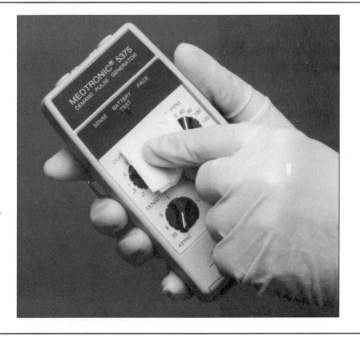

Providing care during transvenous pacing

When caring for a patient with a transvenous pacemaker, your priorities include assessment, safety measures, and documentation. Here are some guidelines.

Assessment
• Carefully assess the patient for signs and symptoms of complications, such as infection, pneumothorax, thromboembolism, right ventricular perforation, and cardiac arrhythmias. Although uncommon, these complications may arise from problems related to pacemaker insertion or maintenance.
• Assess for signs of pacemaker malfunction, such as failure to capture, failure to sense, and loss of pacer artifact.
• Assess the insertion site, pacemaker settings, and cardiac rhythm as often as required by your hospital's policy.

Safety measures
• Change the dressing at the pacing catheter insertion site according to hospital protocol. Change transparent dressings every 72 hours or more often if the dressing isn't intact.
• Observe precautions during pacing, such as making sure that all electrical equipment is properly grounded. Transthoracic and transvenous pacemakers take a direct path to the heart; even a small

amount of extraneous electrical current can reach the heart and cause serious arrhythmias.
• Advise the patient not to use nonessential electrical equipment, such as razors, while he has a temporary pacemaker.
• Keep the pacemaker wires, connections, and box dry because moisture promotes conductivity.
• Make sure that anyone who touches the pacemaker connections wears gloves, thereby decreasing the chance of any current being transmitted by hand contact. Some hospitals recommend insulating the connections with rubber gloves. Check your hospital's policy for specific recommendations for maintaining an electrically safe environment.
• Check any pacemaker generators and batteries not in regular use, preferably every shift when the emergency cart is checked.

Documentation
• After pacemaker insertion, document the patient's tolerance of the procedure and the pacemaker.
• Document the percentage of pacing required and the patient's underlying rhythm once every shift or more frequently if necessary. This information reveals the patient's degree of dependence on the pacemaker and helps determine whether a permanent pacemaker will be needed.

Managing pacemaker malfunction

MALFUNCTION	TYPICAL RHYTHM STRIP	INTERVENTIONS
Failure to capture ECG pacer spikes occur at the appropriate rate set on the pacemaker but aren't followed by a P wave in atrial pacing or by a QRS complex in ventricular pacing. When the patient's intrinsic rhythm is slow or absent, patient deterioration will follow.	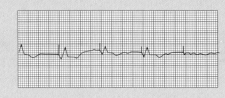	• Provide emergency treatment, as indicated by the patient's condition. • Reposition the patient. • Increase the output (MA) setting. • Administer atropine or other cardiac drugs, as prescribed, or apply a noninvasive pacemaker.
Failure to sense ECG pacer spikes appear where they don't belong; this occurs in demand pacing only. Ventricular pacing spikes that occur on the T wave of an intrinsic beat can trigger ventricular tachycardia and ventricular fibrillation.	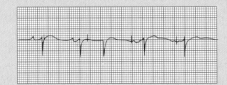	• Make sure the sensitivity dial is set correctly. • Notify the doctor. • Lower the pacing rate if intrinsic activity is regular and consistent.
Loss of artifact When pacer spikes are absent from the ECG tracing, suspect loss of artifact. Potential causes include loose connections from the pacing catheter to the pulse generator, battery failure, very low output (MA), or electromagnetic interference.	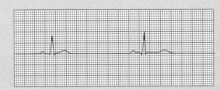	• Check all connections and the MA setting. • If necessary, change the battery or pulse generator.

USING A TRANSTHORACIC PACEMAKER

Transthoracic pacing is used only for a patient in cardiac arrest after all other attempts to restore heart rhythm have failed. This type of pacing may cause severe complications if the needle inadver-tently strikes structures such as coronary arteries. Once cardiopulmonary resuscitation (CPR) efforts succeed, prepare the patient for insertion of a trans-venous pacemaker.

During cardiac arrest, gather the equipment from the emergency cart, as ordered, and take it to the patient's room. You'll need a trans-myocardial pacing kit, a pulse gen-erator, povidone-iodine swabs, sterile 4″ × 4″ gauze pads or sponges, tape, gowns, clean gloves, and sterile gloves (for the doctor).

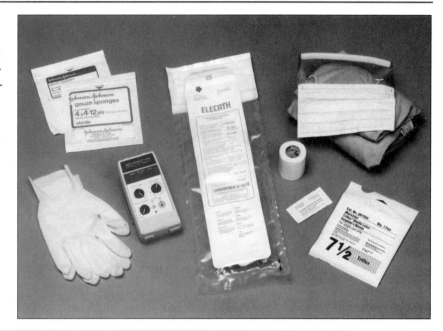

Put on a gown and clean gloves. Open the package of povidone-iodine swabs and use the swabs to prepare the skin area to the left of the xiphoid process (unless the doctor prefers to do this himself).

Open the outer wrapper of the pacing kit, and hand the kit to the doctor so that he can remove the inner sterile package.

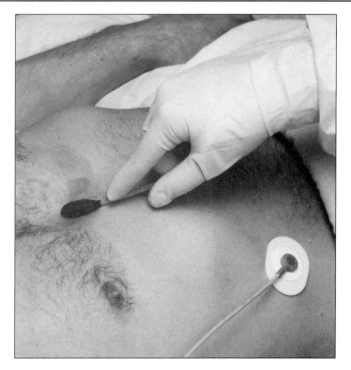

Once the doctor inserts a transthoracic needle into the myocardium, he'll pass an electrode wire through the needle into the heart muscle. After this, you can connect the electrode wire coming from the patient to the adapter (as shown).

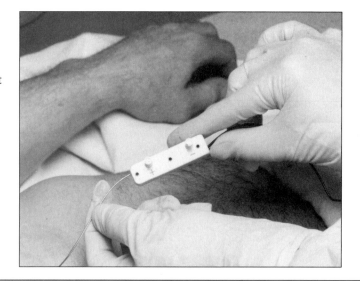

Connect the electrode wire to the pulse generator. Make sure that the proximal (positive) and distal (negative) ends are connected properly.

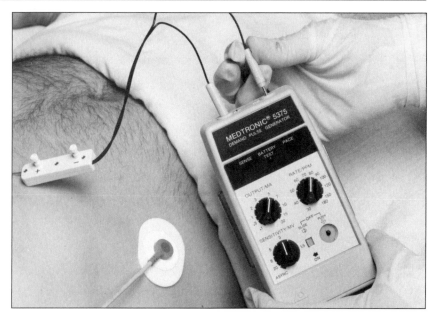

Set the pacing mechanism as follows: output (or MA for milliamperes) at the maximum; rate between 70 and 100; and sensitivity, asynchronous.

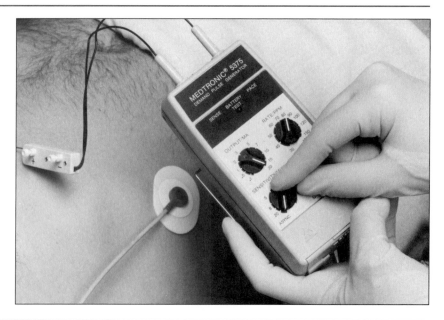

Look for signs of ventricular pacing and capture on the ECG and the monitor. Palpate for a carotid or femoral pulse, as appropriate. Check the patient's blood pressure and level of consciousness. If you can't palpate a pulse, continue CPR and advanced cardiac life support measures.

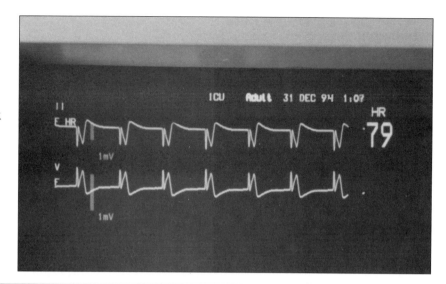

If you can palpate a pulse, and the monitor indicates successful pacing, cover the insertion site with a sterile 4″ × 4″ gauze pad and tape to create an occlusive dressing or use a transparent dressing. Be sure to use aseptic technique. Then remove and dispose of your gloves and gown and document the procedure.

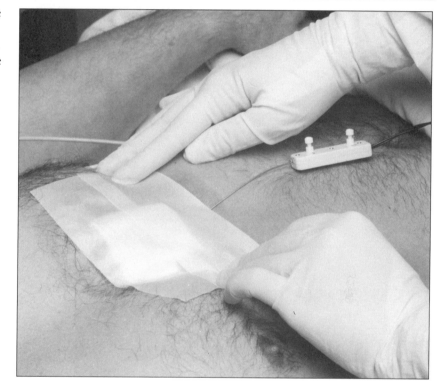

USING AN EPICARDIAL PACEMAKER

To prevent life-threatening arrhythmias, which occur commonly in the first 2 or 3 days after cardiac surgery, the surgeon may place a temporary epicardial pacemaker on the heart during surgery. That way, the pacemaker can be activated rapidly, safely, and effectively if needed.

Epicardial pacemakers have several diagnostic and therapeutic functions. They help diagnose cardiac arrhythmias with an atrial electrogram, initiate cardiac pacing to manage bradycardia and conduction disturbances, correct atrial tachyarrhythmias through rapid atrial pacing, and can increase the heart rate and cardiac output in normal sinus rhythm.

Epicardial electrode wires may be unipolar or bipolar, depending on the patient's needs and the surgeon's preference. In most cases, the surgeon places two to four wires on the right atrium and the right ventricle. A unipolar lead system usually involves placing one wire (or negative electrode) on the heart chamber and one wire (or positive electrode) on the skin.

A bipolar lead system, which is more reliable, typically involves placing two atrial and two ventricular wires directly on the heart, although other configurations may be used.

The electrode wires are inserted into the epicardium and held in place by various methods. Some wires have flanged tips; others may be curled or bent to hold them in place. Occasionally, wires may be loosely sutured in place; the opposite ends of the wires are then tunneled through the skin and exit below the sternotomy incision. Atrial wires are directed to the right of the patient's incision and ventricular wires to the left. Sutures fasten the wires to the skin, preventing accidental removal. Color-coding helps to distinguish atrial from ventricular wires.

Epicardial pacemakers typically remain in place for 3 to 5 days but, in some cases, may be used for up to 10 days. If pacing is required after this time, the patient will receive a transvenous or permanent pacemaker.

Epicardial wires can pace the atria, the ventricles, or both. Commonly used pacing modes are AAI, VVI, DVI, and DDD. The pulse generator with DDD pacing is one of the most commonly used in temporary pacing.

Most patients entering the postanesthesia room from the operating room have a pulse generator attached to the epicardial electrode wires. The pulse generator is detached at the discretion of the nurse or doctor. In the initial postoperative or step-down periods, be prepared to reestablish cardiac pacing when indicated.

Initiating temporary epicardial pacing

Take the necessary equipment to the patient's bedside: a pulse generator, bridging cables, clean gloves, 3″ × 3″ or 4″ × 4″ gauze pads, and tape.

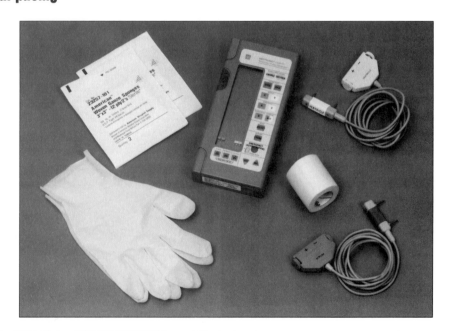

Put on clean gloves and remove the dressings from the atrial and ventricular wires.

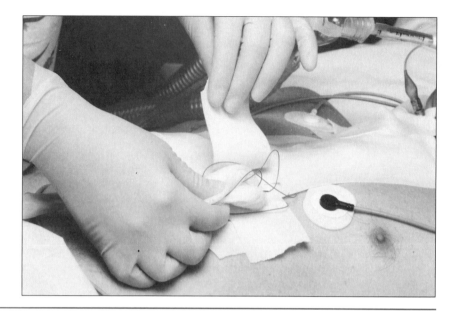

Put one atrial wire in the negative port of the bridging cable and the second atrial wire in the positive port of the bridging cable. Make sure the connections are tight.

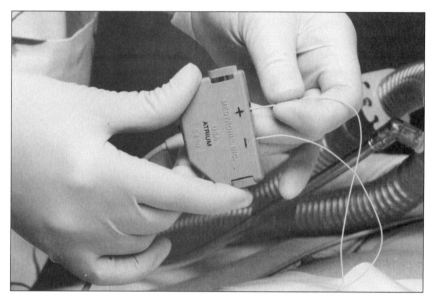

Place the atrial pins located at the opposite end of the cable in the pulse generator port labeled ATRIUM. To do this, press the thumb of one hand on the pin release at the top corner of the pulse generator while placing the atrial pins in the generator with the other hand.

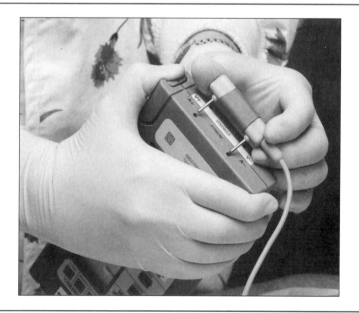

Put the ventricular electrode wires in the bridging cable and the ventricular pins at the opposite end of the cable in the pulse generator port labeled VENTRICLE. To do this, press the pin release at the top corner of the pulse generator with the thumb of one hand while you place the ventricular pins in the generator with your other hand.

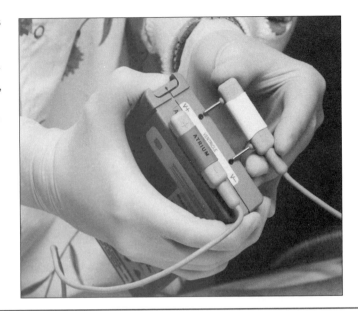

Wrap the electrode wires and the bridging cable connection in a 3″ × 3″ or 4″ × 4″ gauze pad. Then tape the pad to the patient's chest.

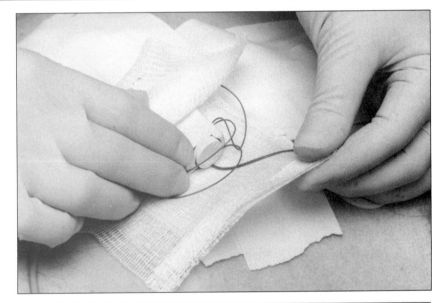

Turn on the pulse generator by pressing the PRESS & HOLD key on the side of the generator. Simultaneously press the key at the bottom of the pulse generator to choose the type of pacing that's indicated by the clinical situation: either A-VPACE (as shown) or VPACE. Next, press the mode key to select the pacemaker mode. Once activated, the mode code will appear on the pulse generator display screen.

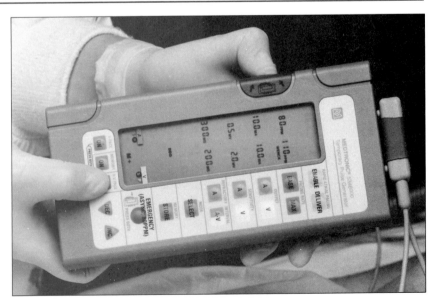

For DDD pacing, check the following parameters, known as default parameters: pacing rate; atrial and ventricular outputs, sensitivities, and pulse widths (if available on your generator); atrial refractory (A Ref) period; and A-V interval. These parameters will automatically appear on the pulse generator display screen when you select the DDD mode (as shown). If you're using another mode, the appropriate parameters for that mode will appear on the display screen.

▶ *Clinical tip:* Epicardial pacing requires much higher output (MA) settings than does transvenous pacing. An MA range of 10 to 20 is not unusual.

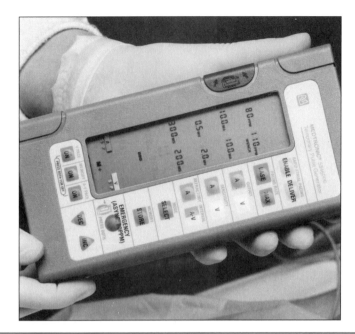

Adjust settings as prescribed or according to hospital protocol. To do this, press the PRESS & HOLD key while simultaneously making parameter adjustments by pressing the PARAMETER key. Then, continue to press the PRESS & HOLD key while using the MAX or BASE key to obtain the desired setting.

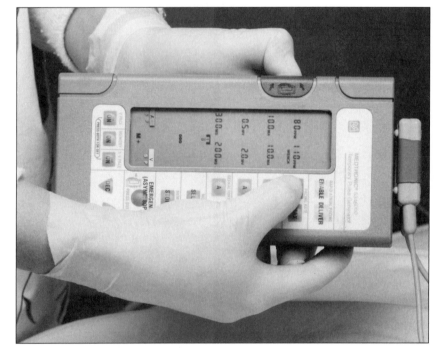

While the patient remains on bed rest, place the pulse generator on his bed (as shown). When he gets out of bed, secure it to his chest or gown.

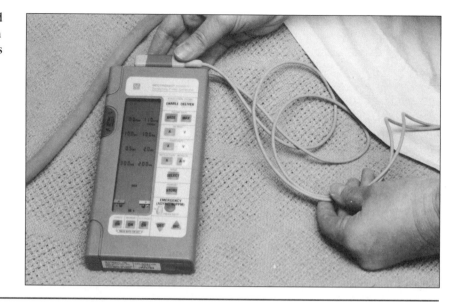

Evaluate the effectiveness of pacing as often as ordered. Check the patient's pulse, blood pressure, and other hemodynamic parameters, such as central venous pressure, pulmonary artery pressure, and cardiac output. Document the reason for initiating pacing, the pacemaker settings and mode, and the patient's response. Record an ECG strip. Also be sure to check the patient's underlying cardiac rhythm and stimulation thresholds at least daily.

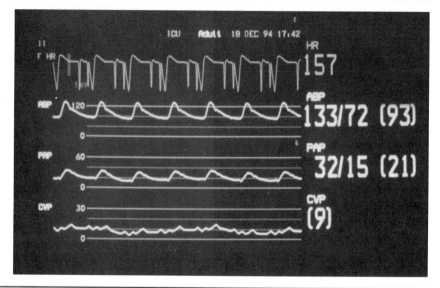

Maintaining an epicardial pacemaker

When caring for a patient with an epicardial pacemaker, you must maintain an electrically safe environment, provide meticulous wound care at the pacemaker insertion site, and ensure that the pacemaker runs smoothly. To do so, wear gloves when handling wires and make sure that all wires stay dry. Besides gloves, you'll need povidone-iodine ointment, 3″ × 3″ or 4″ × 4″ gauze pads, and tape.

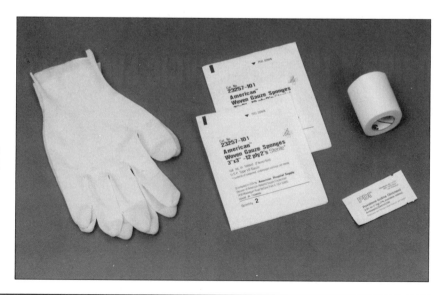

Changing dressings

Change the dressing at the pacemaker site daily until the pacing wires are removed, regardless of whether or not you use them. Put on clean gloves and remove the old dressing and tape. Apply povidone-iodine ointment to the site, and cover it with a 3″ × 3″ or 4″ × 4″ gauze pad and tape. Then wrap the atrial wires in a gauze pad, as shown. (The gauze helps to keep the pacing wires isolated from all other wires and catheters.)

Tape the covered wires in place on top of the chest dressing and label the site "A" for "atrial wires." Do the same to the ventricular wire site, and label it "V."

▶ *Clinical tip:* To keep all wires accessible in an emergency, avoid using a bulky dressing and excess tape to cover the wires.

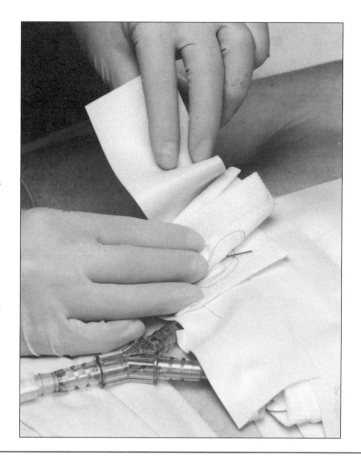

Ensuring smooth operation

A handy feature of electronic pacemakers is the display symbol for a low battery. Once this symbol appears, the battery will continue operating for 16 to 24 hours before failing. This provides plenty of time to obtain a 9-volt alkaline replacement battery.

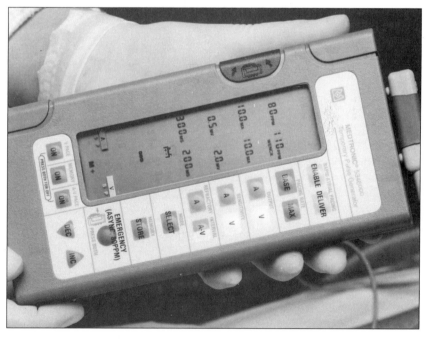

If possible, change batteries routinely before pacemaker use. If you need to change the battery during pacemaker operation, locate the battery storage chamber on the side of the generator, and press the bottom button to open the chamber.

Take out the old battery and put in the new one by lining up the negative (−) and positive (+) ports. Close the chamber. To ensure uninterrupted pacing, complete the change in 1 to 2 minutes.

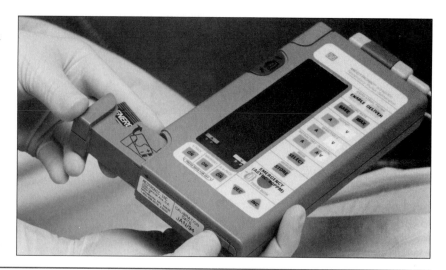

Discontinuing epicardial pacing

Once the patient no longer needs epicardial pacing, put on gloves and disconnect the bridging cable from the pulse generator.

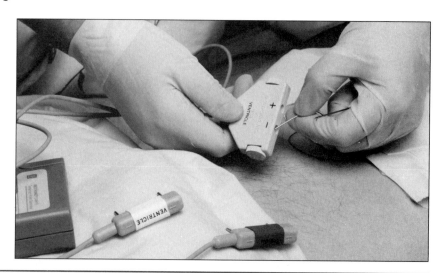

Reassure the patient and assist as needed when the doctor removes the pacing wires—usually between the 3rd and 5th postoperative day. With the patient supine, the pacemaker dressing removed, and the sutures clipped, the doctor will withdraw the wires gently and steadily. The site can be left open to the air if it's dry.

Keep the patient in bed for 2 hours after the wires are removed. Check his vital signs every 30 minutes for the first 2 hours and hourly thereafter. Monitor him for signs and symptoms of cardiac tamponade, such as hypotension, decreased pulse pressure, pulsus paradoxus, neck vein distention, and diaphoresis.

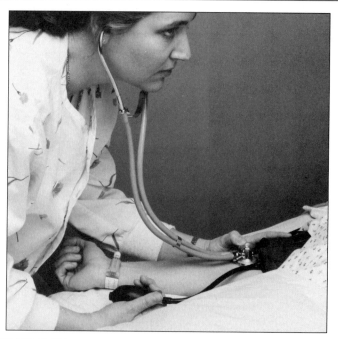

MONITORING A PERMANENT PACEMAKER

When a patient has an irreversible arrhythmia, the doctor may insert a permanent pacemaker. Arrhythmias that respond to this kind of extrinsic pacing include chronic bradycardia and primary conduction disturbances, such as Mobitz II heart block, complete heart block, bifascicular block, sinus bradycardia, junctional rhythm, and sick sinus syndrome.

The pacemaker is inserted after medication or a temporary pacemaker stabilizes the patient's condition.

PACEMAKER COMPONENTS

Primary pacemaker parts include a pulse generator and a leadwire. The pulse generator houses a battery and electrical circuitry that determines how the pacemaker functions. The circuitry directs the pacemaker to sense and pace one or both heart chambers. The most common pacing modes are VVI for single-chamber pacing and DDD for dual-chamber pacing (see *Understanding pacemaker codes,* page 44 in this section). The number of chambers paced depends on the patient's condition and on the type of arrhythmia. (See "Learning About Pacemakers," pages 41 to 44 in this section.)

Typically made of lithium, the battery's lifespan ranges from 7 to 12 years—depending on the complexity of the circuitry and the pacemaker's use. Abrupt failure seldom occurs because the battery's gradual power loss and consequent slowing can be detected by medical follow-up (during an office visit or by telecommunication devices).

A unipolar or bipolar leadwire, which transmits the electrical stimulus to the heart, typically has fixation devices near the electrode tip that reduce the risk of dislodgment. These devices, which may be tines, screws, barbs, wedges, or coils, ensure continuous contact with the heart chamber.

TECHNOLOGICAL ADVANCES

Today's technology has produced advanced electrical circuits that allow rate-responsive pacemakers to pace the heart according to different levels of sensed activity. Available in VVIR and DDDR modes, these pacemakers have a special material in the pulse generator that responds to activity or motion.

Another kind of pacemaker currently in clinical evaluation paces the heart according to sensed changes, including alterations in respiratory rate, temperature, oxygen saturation level, right ventricular stroke volume or pressure, or venous pH value.

Current multiprogrammable pacemakers provide a noninvasive method for changing pacemaker settings. The doctor simply places a hand-held programmer on the skin over the pulse generator and adjusts the dials or presses a key to obtain the desired settings. Programmable settings usually include sensitivity, pacing rate, atrioventricular (AV) interval, pulse width, refractory periods, and modes.

NURSING CONSIDERATIONS

To provide the complex nursing care that pacemaker patients require, you must be familiar with pacemaker function, insertion, and aftercare. (See *Permanent pacemaker insertion,* page 70.)

Before surgery, you'll prepare the patient for pacemaker insertion and provide supportive care. (See *Preparing the patient for pacemaker insertion,* page 71.) After surgery, you'll monitor the patient's condition for about 24 hours, watching for changes in vital signs and for arrhythmias and assessing the effectiveness of pacing. In patients whose intrinsic heart rate exceeds the pacemaker's rate, you'll use a pacemaker magnet, as directed by the doctor. Supplied by the manufacturer, this magnet, which usually fits over the pulse generator, can convert the pacing mode to a fixed (or asynchronous) mode.

Note: The pacemaker's firing rate, which is set by the manufacturer and unalterable, is known as the magnet rate. In many cases, the magnet rate differs from the rate programmed for operation.

During the patient's convalescence, intervene appropriately if you detect signs of pacemaker malfunction (such as failure to capture, failure to sense, and loss of pacemaker artifact) or signs and symptoms of complications. (See *Managing pacemaker malfunction,* page 58 in this section.)

Finally, before the patient is discharged, provide him with instructions to promote safety and reduce his anxiety about home care. Use the patient-teaching aids *Caring for your pacemaker,* page 75, and *Checking your pacemaker by phone,* page 76.

Linda S. Baas, RN, PhD, CCRN, and *Cynthia Possanza, RN, MSN, CCRN,* contributed to this section. Ms. Baas is an assistant professor at the University of Cincinnati College of Nursing and Health. Ms. Possanza is a nursing consultant for Springhouse Corporation. The publisher thanks *Hewlett-Packard Co.,* McMinnville, Ore., and *Medtronic, Inc.,* Minneapolis, for their help.

Permanent pacemaker insertion

Considered a minor surgical procedure, permanent pacemaker insertion is performed by a surgeon or cardiologist in the operating room or in the cardiac catheterization or electrophysiology laboratory. Typically, the patient receives a sedative and a local anesthetic before the procedure.

A look at the pacemaker

Depending on the patient's condition and other factors, the pacemaker will be unipolar or bipolar and will have one or two leadwires for positioning in an atrium, a ventricle, or both. The leadwires are insulated and have exposed metal-tip electrodes on the heart end and connectors on the pulse generator end.

The electrical current generated by the pacemaker flows through the connector to the exposed metal-tip electrodes, which conduct electricity through the heart. After stimulating the heart muscle, the current flows to the anode to complete the electrical circuit.

Implanting the pacemaker

The surgeon or cardiologist usually inserts the pacemaker leadwires transvenously, completing the procedure in about 30 minutes. To begin, he makes a small incision in the left or right upper chest below the clavicle. Then, guided by fluoroscopy, he advances the electrode tip of the leadwire through the cephalic or jugular vein into the appropriate heart chamber. If he cannot locate either of these veins, he may insert the leadwire through the subclavian vein.

Next, he tests the device to make sure that it works properly. Then he connects the opposite end of the leadwire to the pulse generator and places the pulse generator (which is a little larger than a man's wristwatch) in the subcutaneous pocket created by the incision. He closes the incision and applies a dressing.

When he can't implant the pacemaker transvenously, the surgeon or cardiologist may perform a thoracotomy or make a subxiphoid incision and place the electrodes on the heart's epicardial surface. If the patient needs the pacemaker during cardiac surgery, the surgeon or cardiologist may place the electrodes on the heart's surface at that time.

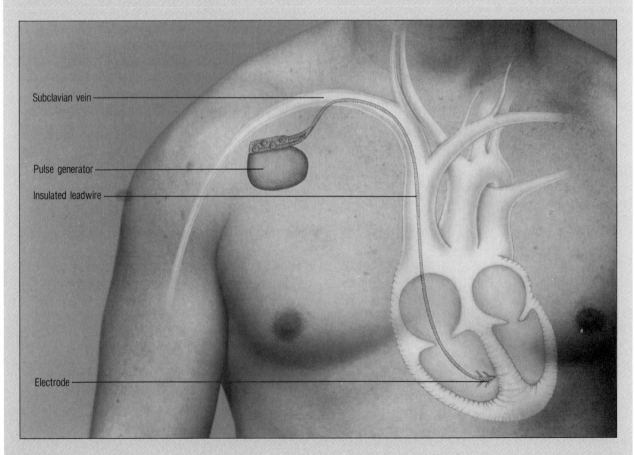

Subclavian vein

Pulse generator

Insulated leadwire

Electrode

Preparing the patient for pacemaker insertion

Before the patient undergoes pacemaker insertion, make sure that he and his family understand the procedure. Tell him what to expect before and after the surgery and what to expect when he goes home. Reinforce the doctor's explanation, if needed, and answer any questions. As appropriate, review cardiac activity and conduction as it relates to pacemaker function.

Check your preparations by asking yourself the following questions:

☐ Has the patient signed the proper informed consent form authorizing the procedure?

☐ Can he recount instructions and other information given in patient-teaching sessions? For example, can he describe the pacemaker and explain why he needs it? Can he describe the procedure? Can he relate his understanding of postprocedural self-care?

Does he have visual aids or other up-to-date patient-teaching materials to refer to if necessary?

☐ Has the patient refrained from eating or drinking anything after midnight?

☐ Is the surgical site properly cleaned and prepared?

☐ Is the patient's I.V. line in place and patent?

☐ Have all medications, including an I.V. antibiotic and a sedative, been administered as prescribed?

☐ Did the patient void as directed?

☐ Is he wearing the correct identification bracelet?

☐ Are his baseline vital signs on record? Have subsequent vital signs data been updated and charted?

☐ Does the patient's chart include all current diagnostic test results, such as blood and electrolyte analyses and chest X-ray findings?

☐ Is the cardiac monitor set up and ready to travel with the patient to the operating room?

Checking pacemaker function with a magnet

When the patient's intrinsic heart rate exceeds the pacemaker rate, the doctor may direct you to use a special magnet to evaluate pacemaker function. Doing so involves recording electrocardiograms (ECGs) with and without the magnet.

Take the necessary equipment, including a 12-lead ECG machine and the appropriate magnet, to the patient's bedside.

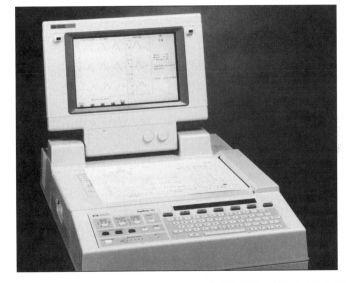

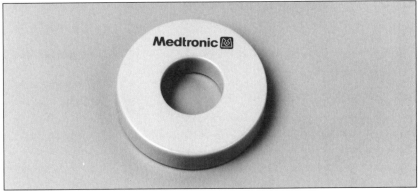

Explain the procedure to the patient. Then attach the limb leads and the precordial leads from the ECG machine as you would to obtain a standard 12-lead ECG.

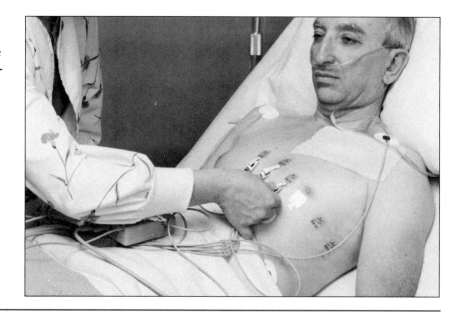

Turn on the ECG machine, and enter the information required by the machine you're using, such as the patient's name and identification number.

Once you complete the preparations, press the START key (as shown) to obtain a 12-lead ECG tracing.

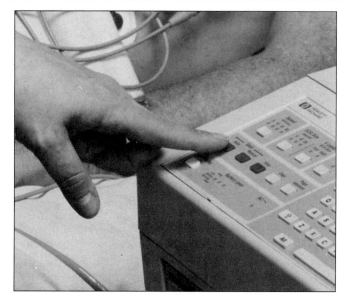

Then place the magnet on the patient's skin directly over the pulse generator.

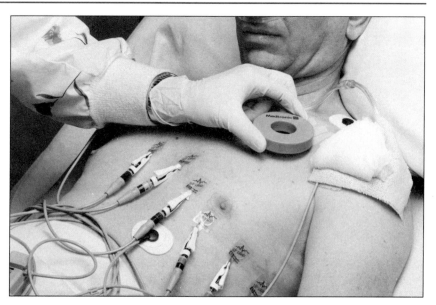

Press START again to obtain a second 12-lead ECG tracing.

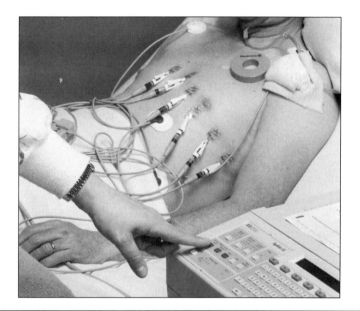

Remove the magnet and the ECG leads from the patient. Review and interpret the ECG tracing. A normal tracing will show pacemaker spikes occurring at the magnet rate (as shown). If the tracing doesn't show this, the pacemaker isn't functioning properly.

Inform the doctor of any abnormal findings—for example, the absence of pacemaker spikes or loss of capture. Though you'll usually detect capture when nothing else competes with the intrinsic heart rate, you may not always be able to detect loss of capture.

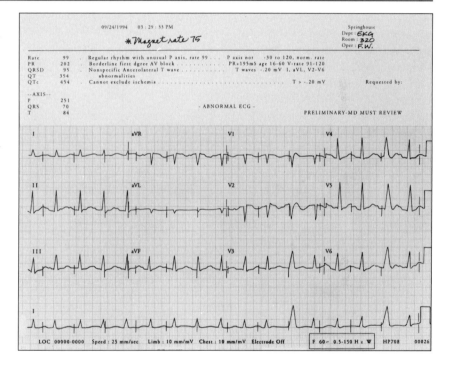

Managing problems of permanent pacemakers

Insertion of a permanent pacemaker places the patient at risk for certain complications, such as infection and lead displacement. Here's how to deal with the most common complications.

Perforated ventricle and cardiac tamponade
When the patient returns from the operating room, watch for signs and symptoms of these complications, including persistent hiccups, distant heart sounds, pulsus paradoxus, hypotension with narrow pulse pressure, increased venous pressure, cyanosis, distended neck veins, decreased urine output, restlessness, or complaints of chest fullness. If these problems develop, notify the doctor at once.

Infection
Some patients may experience sepsis or local infection of the pacemaker pocket after pacemaker insertion. Signs and symptoms include redness, swelling, warmth, pain, and discharge at the insertion site.

To intervene, change the dressing, administer prescribed antibiotics, or prepare the patient for surgery, as ordered, to replace the pulse generator.

Lead displacement
A displaced lead is most likely to occur soon after pacemaker insertion. If chaotic pacing and sensing occur, notify the doctor, who may order a chest X-ray to confirm the lead's location. To correct this problem, he may reposition or replace the lead, possibly with a fixation-type lead.

Lead fracture and disconnection
Suspect these unusual problems when most other causes of sensing and pacing problems have been ruled out.

If these problems occur, notify the doctor, who may order a chest X-ray to confirm that the lead has been fractured and disconnected. To correct the problem, he may replace the lead or manipulate the pulse generator.

Twiddler's syndrome
This problem occurs if a pulse generator is too mobile within the subcutaneous pocket and the patient twists and turns it. The manipulation may cause a lead to twist, fracture, or disconnect from the pulse generator.

Intervene by either notifying the doctor or, if the patient is at home, directing him to notify the doctor about the loosely positioned pulse generator. The doctor may order a chest X-ray to confirm the problem. Then, if indicated, he may reposition the device.

PATIENT TEACHING

Caring for your pacemaker

Dear Patient:

Your doctor has inserted a pacemaker in your chest to generate the electrical impulses needed to help your heart beat evenly. Here are some tips to help you care for yourself and your pacemaker.

Daily care
• Clean your pacemaker site gently with soap and water when you take a shower or a bath. Leave the incision exposed to the air.
• Inspect your skin around the incision. A slight bulge is normal, but call your doctor if you feel discomfort or notice swelling, redness, discharge, or other problems.
• Check your pulse for 1 minute as your nurse or doctor showed you — on the side of your neck, inside your elbow, or on the thumb side of your wrist. Your pulse rate should be the same as your pacemaker rate or faster. Contact your doctor if you think your heart is beating too fast or too slow.
• Take your medications, including those for pain, as prescribed. Even with a pacemaker, you still need the medication your doctor ordered.

Safety and activity
• Keep your pacemaker instruction booklet handy, and carry your pacemaker identification card at all times. This card has your pacemaker model number and other information needed by health care personnel who treat you.
• You can resume most of your usual activities when you feel comfortable doing so, but don't drive until the doctor gives you permission. Also avoid heavy lifting and stretching exercises for at least 4 weeks or as directed by your doctor.
• Try to use both arms equally to prevent muscle stiffness. And check with your doctor before you golf, swim, play tennis, or perform other strenuous activities.

Electromagnetic interference
• Fortunately, today's pacemakers are designed and insulated to eliminate most electrical interference. You can safely operate common household electrical devices, including kitchen appliances, microwave ovens, razors, and sewing machines. And you can ride in or operate a motor vehicle without it affecting your pacemaker.
• Take care, however, to avoid direct contact with large running motors, high-powered CB radios and other similar equipment, welding machinery, and radar devices.
• If your pacemaker activates the metal detector in an airport, show your pacemaker identification card to the security official.
• Because the metal in your pacemaker makes you ineligible for certain diagnostic studies, such as magnetic resonance imaging (MRI), be sure to inform your doctors, dentist, and other health care personnel that you have a pacemaker.

Special precautions
• If you feel light-headed or dizzy when you're near any electrical equipment, moving away from the device should restore normal pacemaker function. Check with your doctor if you have questions about particular electrical devices.
• Notify your doctor if you experience any signs of pacemaker failure, such as palpitations, a fast heart rate, a slow heart rate (5 to 10 beats less than the pacemaker's setting), dizziness, fainting, shortness of breath, swollen ankles or feet, anxiety, forgetfulness, or confusion.

Checkups
• Be sure to schedule and keep regular checkup appointments with your doctor.
• If your doctor checks your pacemaker status by telephone, keep your transmission schedule and instructions in a handy place.

Checking your pacemaker by phone

Dear Patient:

Your doctor wants to check your pace-maker regularly by telephone. Doing this helps him to monitor pacemaker function and battery strength while you stay at home. Here's how to use your pacemaker's transmitter.

Insert the battery
Before using your transmitter for the first time, remove the battery cover and insert the battery supplied by the manufacturer. You'll need to replace the battery every 2 or 3 months.

Set up the transmitter
When you're ready, take the transmitter out of its case. Also take the electrode cable from the case, and plug the cable into the jack on the transmitter.

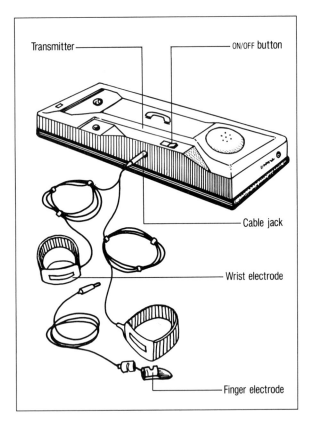

Place the electrodes on your fingers or on your wrists.

Turn on the transmitter and listen for the tones indicating that the power is on.

Phone in your electrocardiogram
Dial the telephone number of your doctor's office or pacemaker clinic, and listen for instructions.

When directed, place the telephone handset in the pacemaker transmitter. Stay still (for up to 60 seconds) to minimize interference with the signals from your heart.

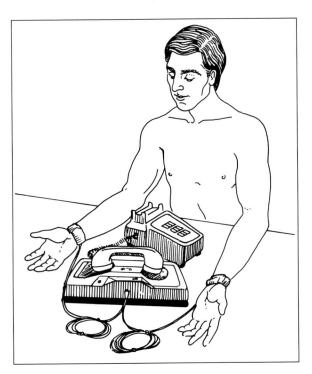

Wait for further instructions. For example, the doctor may ask you to use a special magnet that's in the transmitter's case. To do so, simply hold the magnet over the pacemaker and transmit your electrocardiogram as before.

When you finish transmitting, take off the electrodes and turn off the transmitter. Place the equipment in the storage case until the next time you use it.

USING RAPID ATRIAL PACING

Rapid atrial pacing (also called overdrive atrial pacing) may be performed on a cardiac surgery patient to convert an atrial tachyarrhythmia to normal sinus rhythm. It may also be used to convert an atrial tachyarrhythmia to atrial fibrillation, which is managed more successfully with medication or cardioversion.

Rapid atrial pacing is most successful in converting atrial flutter to normal sinus rhythm when flutter waves are uniform and the heart rate is under 340 beats/minute. It's also effective in converting paroxysmal atrial tachycardia and arrhythmias associated with Wolff-Parkinson-White syndrome to normal sinus rhythm. Attempts to convert atrial fibrillation to normal sinus rhythm with rapid atrial pacing have been unsuccessful.

HOW RAPID ATRIAL PACING WORKS

To implement rapid atrial pacing, the atrial wires inserted during open-heart surgery are connected to an external atrial pulse generator. This raises the abnormal atrial rate and causes the abnormal rhythm to revert to normal. The pacing stimulus may be applied once or several times to interrupt the abnormal circuit.

Rapid atrial pacing's chief advantage is that it can be applied immediately after the abnormal atrial rhythm is detected. What's more, it doesn't cause the patient discomfort, and it eliminates the need for the sedatives and anesthetics typically used during cardioversion. The procedure also reduces traumatic injury, eliminates chest burns and, for a patient on digoxin, eliminates the risk of ventricular arrhythmias that may follow cardioversion.

Among rapid atrial pacing's potential disadvantages are these: The pacemaker may fail to capture the atrium and, consequently, fail to interrupt the tachyarrhythmia. This problem may occur if the epicardial wire is not properly positioned. The patient's ventricular rate may also accelerate, which may be detrimental. Finally, rapid atrial pacing can't convert all tachyarrhythmias to normal sinus rhythm.

Take the necessary equipment to the patient's bedside. You'll need an atrial pulse generator (which can deliver up to 800 impulses/minute), gloves, 3″ × 3″ or 4″ × 4″ gauze pads, tape, and a marking pen.

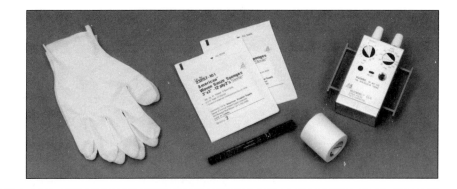

Explain the procedure to the patient. Wash your hands, put on gloves, and remove the dressing from the atrial wires (which the doctor is responsible for correctly identifying). Usually, the atrial wires are located on the right side of the chest just next to the sternum. Put the wires into the negative (−) and positive (+) ports of the pulse generator.

Be sure to avoid using the ventricular wires by mistake. Rapid ventricular pacing will cause ventricular fibrillation.

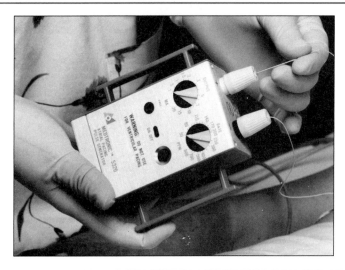

Check the pacemaker's output (MA) setting, which the doctor usually establishes.

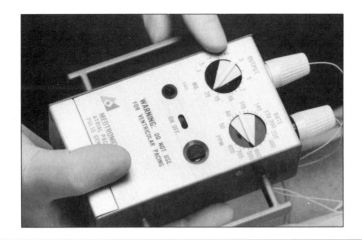

Continuously record an electrocardiogram (ECG) as the doctor alters the MA and the rate.

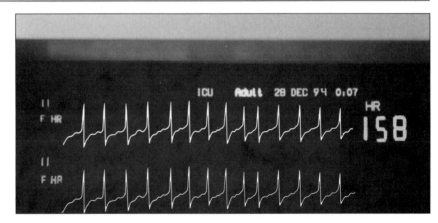

Monitor the ECG until the doctor completes the procedure, which usually takes a few seconds but sometimes takes 1 minute. Note the return to sinus rhythm on the monitor. Check the patient's heart rate and blood pressure. The ventricular rate should not accelerate during the procedure because the atrioventricular node usually won't conduct impulses to the ventricles beyond a range of 150 to 200 per minute.

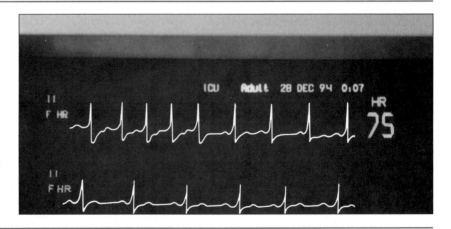

Disconnect the pacing wires from the atrial pulse generator, and wrap them in a finger cot and then in a sterile 3″ × 3″ or 4″ × 4″ gauze pad. Tape the pad to the patient's chest, and label the dressing "A" to identify the atrial wires.

Be prepared for the doctor to implement the procedure again if the arrhythmia recurs. Finally, document the patient's response to the procedure and identify the cardiac rhythm established.

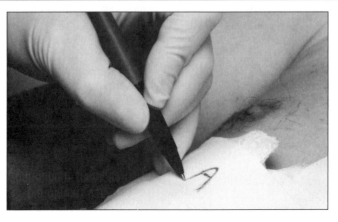

Cardiac Monitoring

LEARNING ABOUT CARDIAC MONITORING

When patients die from acute myocardial infarction, arrhythmias are the most common culprit. These cardiac disturbances usually result from thrombi or from an abrupt increase in myocardial oxygen demand. To identify arrhythmias promptly and allow early treatment, you can use cardiac monitoring. Such monitoring allows continuous evaluation of the heart's electrical activity.

Patients with arrhythmias aren't the only ones who may need cardiac monitoring. The procedure is commonly performed after major surgery and chest trauma. It's also performed for patients with severe electrolyte disturbances, major organ failure, and hemodynamic instability.

Besides providing clues that help you determine the patient's underlying problem, continuous cardiac monitoring helps you select the most appropriate intervention. What's more, it helps you evaluate the effects of therapy.

ELECTROCARDIOGRAPHY

The basis for cardiac monitoring is electrocardiography (ECG) — a representation on the body's surface of the heart's electrical activity (see *Understanding the ECG grid*, page 2). Although the ECG portrays this electrical activity, its appearance also depends on the sequence of electrical activation by the heart's chambers, the adequacy of the blood supply to the heart muscle, and the ability of the conducting system to initiate and transmit the electrical impulse.

The electrical activity produces a distinctive graphic pattern based on the sequence of depolarization and repolarization through the atria and the ventricles. Depolarization refers to the process by which the resting potential of a polarized cell becomes less negative. Repolarization, in turn, refers to the process by which a depolarized cell returns to its resting state. (See *Reviewing the electrical basis of the ECG*, page 3.)

To perform cardiac monitoring, you'll apply electrodes to the patient's chest. The electrodes sense the heart's electrical activity and relay the information to a cardiac monitor (an oscilloscope), where the impulses appear as a continuous ECG waveform.

MONITOR FEATURES

Besides providing a visual display of the patient's heart rate and rhythm, most monitors produce a printed record, known as a rhythm strip. By analyzing the rhythm strip, you can evaluate conduction patterns, estimate heart size, assess heart muscle function and size, and recognize abnormalities in electrolyte balances.

Another common monitor feature is an alarm that signals when the heart rate rises above or falls below set limits. Some monitors also recognize and count abnormal beats and activate an alarm when abnormalities occur. Cardiac monitors may have one or more channels, allowing them to survey cardiac activity in one or more patients.

MONITOR TERMINOLOGY

Operating a cardiac monitor isn't difficult once you learn the technique and become familiar with the following terms:
• *artifact* — incidental, extraneous electrical activity apparent on the ECG tracing and typically caused by electrical interference
• *electrodes* — adhesive pads that detect the heart's electrical activity
• *gain* — adjustment of the monitor's ability to sense the amplitude (size) of the QRS complex
• *ground* — ECG lead that prevents electrical interference ("noise") from entering the monitoring circuit
• *lead* — both the actual color-coded wire that connects the electrode to the monitor cable and the placement of the wire and electrode, which provides different views of the heart's electrical activity. Each lead consists of a positive pole and a negative pole that sense the amplitude and direction of electrical current within the heart. Standard ECG leads reflect 12 views of cardiac activity and are known as leads I, II, III, aV_R, aV_L, aV_F, V_1, V_2, V_3, V_4, V_5, and V_6.

Marilyn Sawyer Sommers, RN, PhD, CCRN, who contributed to this section, is an assistant professor in the College of Nursing and Health at the University of Cincinnati. The publisher also thanks *Hill-Rom,* Batesville, Ind., and *Hewlett-Packard Co.,* Waltham, Mass., for their help.

Understanding the ECG grid

To decipher your patient's electrocardiogram (ECG), begin with the paper it's printed on. Composed of parallel horizontal and vertical lines that form a grid, ECG paper allows you to measure time and amplitude. You need to know these two values to identify certain cardiac irregularities and the patient's heart rate.

To understand the grid, place a strip of ECG graph paper in front of you. Look at the configuration of the squares. Notice how the darker horizontal and vertical lines define large square boxes containing 25 small squares.

Measuring time

The ECG machine traces electrical activity onto the ECG paper at a standard speed of 25 mm/second. Each small square on the horizontal plane represents 0.04 second. Similarly, five small squares represent 0.2 second, and five large squares measure 1 second. You'll use these squares to compute the PR interval and the duration of the QRS complex.

Measuring amplitude

The ECG paper's vertical plane quantifies the amplitude of cardiac electrical activity. Each vertical line falls 1 mm from the next vertical line, with each small square measuring 1 mm × 1 mm. These squares join to form the height and width of a large box. On the vertical plane, these blocks measure the magnitude (or voltage) of a QRS complex, for example. Typically, a 1-millivolt (mV) electrical charge produces a 10-mm deflection on the ECG grid.

Applying the information

Printed along the upper edge of the ECG paper are regularly spaced, short vertical lines denoting additional intervals. With the ECG machine set at standard paper speed, the distance between two consecutive short vertical lines is 75 mm, or 3 seconds, and between every third short vertical line 150 mm, or 6 seconds. By counting the cardiac cycles in one 6-second interval and then multiplying that sum by 10, you'll learn the patient's heart rate.

ECG graph paper

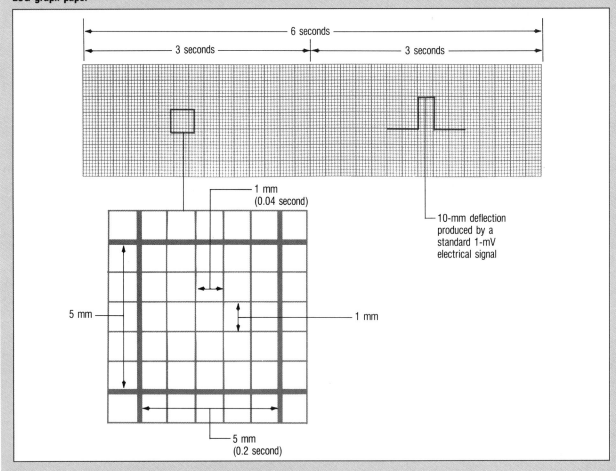

INSIGHTS AND INTERPRETATIONS

Reviewing the electrical basis of the ECG

The graphic waves on your patient's electrocardiogram (ECG) show the direction and magnitude of electrical current, which is generated by atrial and ventricular depolarization and repolarization. Each part of the ECG shows a different phase of cardiac activity.

As shown here, the P wave represents atrial depolarization. The Ta wave—obscured by the QRS complex—represents atrial repolarization, which occurs at the same time as ventricular depolarization (reflected in the QRS complex). The T wave represents ventricular repolarization.

Other factors affecting the ECG waveform include the adequacy of cardiac perfusion and the heart's ability to initiate and conduct the electrical impulse.

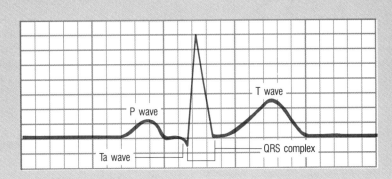

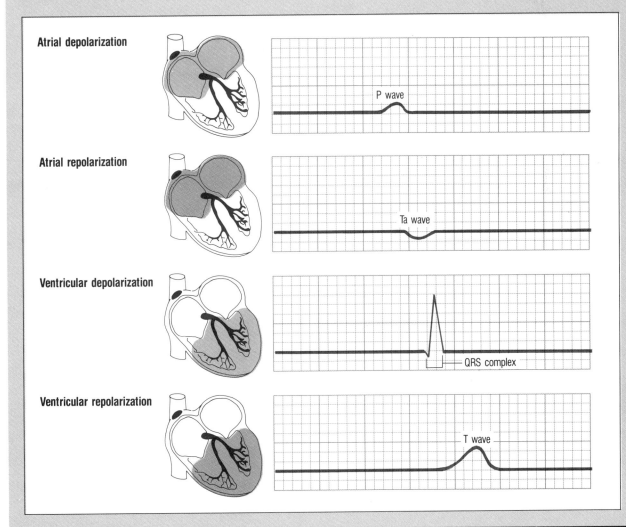

PERFORMING HARDWIRE MONITORING

With hardwire monitoring, your patient and the cardiac monitor are connected by electrodes, leadwires, and a cable. Most hardwire monitors are mounted permanently on a shelf or a wall near the patient's bed. However, some may be mounted on an I.V. pole (for portability), and some may include defibrillators.

The monitor continuously displays the patient's cardiac rhythm and transmits the electrocardiogram (ECG) tracing to a console at a main control station on the nursing unit. Used most commonly in critical care units and emergency departments, hardwire monitoring allows continuous observation of one or more patients from more than one area in the unit.

FEATURES

To track cardiac activity, most hardwire monitors include a three-electrode system, consisting of a positive lead, a negative lead, and a ground lead.

By repositioning these leads, you can detect electrical activity in different areas of the patient's heart. Less prevalent but even more precise are other hardwire systems that use four or five leads. These systems allow you to assess cardiac activity in various areas of the heart without repositioning the electrodes. (See *Comparing lead placement systems*.)

Besides monitoring cardiac rhythm, most monitors available today can track other critical functions, such as pulmonary artery pressure, arterial blood pressure and central venous pressure, cardiac output, body temperature, respiratory rate, and oxygen saturation. Some monitors extend these capabilities to include the analysis of ST segments and the measurement of carbon dioxide pressure in the patient's airway.

Of the available hardwire monitoring systems, some are easier to use than others. For example, adjustments and selections on Siemens and SpaceLabs systems can be made by touching the monitor screen rather than by manipulating knobs and buttons.

Comparing lead placement systems

For most cardiac monitoring, you'll use a three-electrode system. But to increase monitoring capability, you may use a four- or five-electrode system.

Three-electrode system
This system has one positive electrode, one negative electrode, and a ground. Typically, you'll place these electrodes in lead II position, although sometimes you'll use modified chest lead (MCL) placements—specifically MCL_1 or MCL_6. The following describes the differences in leads:
• Lead II records the electrical potential difference between the right arm (negative lead) and the left leg (positive lead). This lead produces clear QRS complexes (which reflect ventricular activity) and positive P waves (showing atrial activity).
• MCL_1 records the sequence of ventricular depolarization more clearly than the other leads, making this

lead a better choice for differentiating between right or left bundle-branch block and ectopy.
• MCL_6, another modified chest lead, clearly visualizes tall QRS complexes, making this the lead of choice for identifying right bundle-branch block, ST-segment abnormalities, and T-wave changes.

Four- and five-electrode systems
In a four-electrode system, a right leg electrode becomes a permanent ground for all leads. In a five-electrode system, an additional exploratory chest lead allows you to monitor any of six modified chest leads as well as the standard limb leads.

Preparing the equipment and the patient

To evaluate your patient's ECG with hardwire monitoring, you'll need a cardiac monitor. You'll also need a monitor cable, leadwires, electrodes, a dry washcloth or gauze pad, alcohol sponges, and the patient's medical record.

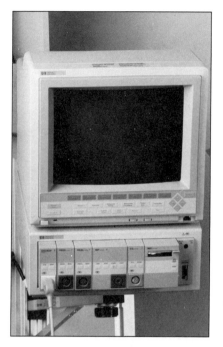
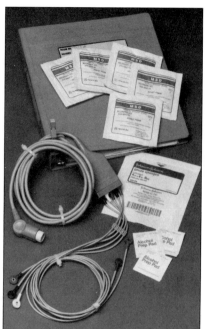

Plug in the monitor and switch on the power. If the cable isn't already connected to the monitor, attach it now.

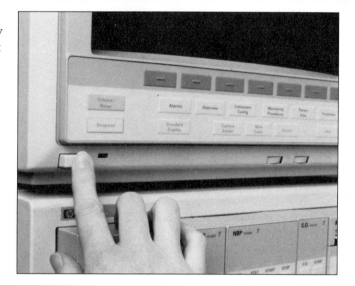

Connect the leadwires to the correct positions on the cable (as shown). If you must connect individual leadwires to the cable and the wires and cable are color-coded, make sure that the color on the leadwire matches the color on the cable. If they're not color-coded, check carefully to make sure that you attach the right arm (RA) wire to the RA outlet on the cable, the left arm (LA) wire to the LA outlet, and so on.

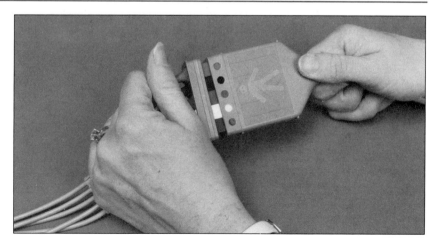

Open the package of electrodes, and attach an electrode to the end of each leadwire.

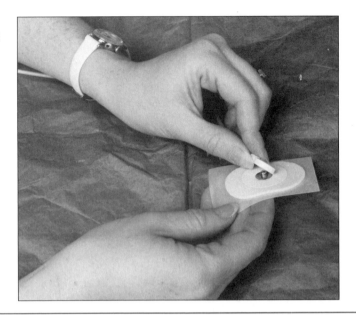

Wash your hands. Explain the procedure to the patient and provide privacy. Expose the patient's chest, and select the electrode sites for the chosen lead arrangement. Then, using a special rough patch on the electrode, a dry washcloth, or a gauze pad, briskly rub each site (as shown) until it reddens. Be sure not to damage or break the skin. Rubbing the skin promotes better electrical contact because this removes dead skin cells. If the patient has an extremely hairy chest, shave about 4″ (10 cm) of hair from each site. Dry these areas.

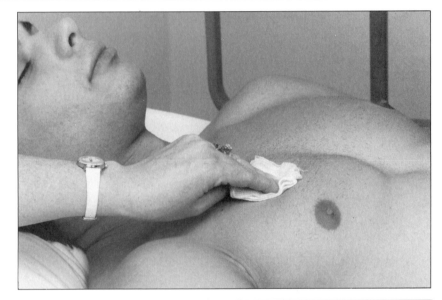

If the patient has oily skin, clean each site with an alcohol sponge. Let the areas dry completely to ensure proper adhesion and to prevent alcohol from becoming trapped underneath the electrode, which could irritate the skin and cause breakdown.

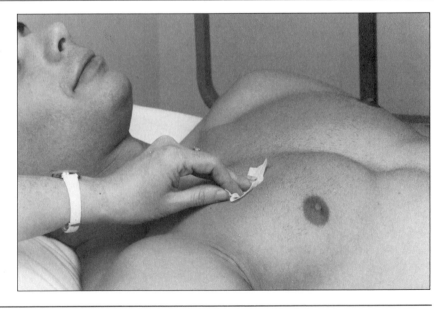

Remove the backing from the pre-gelled electrode. Check the gel. It should be moist. If it's dry, discard the electrode and obtain another one.

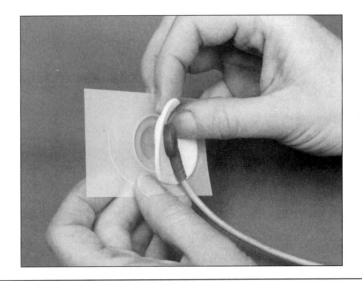

Apply one electrode to each site. To do so, press one side of the electrode against the patient's skin, pull gently, and then press the opposite side of the electrode against the skin. Then use two fingers (as shown) to press on the electrode in a circular pattern. This fixes the gel and stabilizes the electrode. Repeat this process for each electrode.

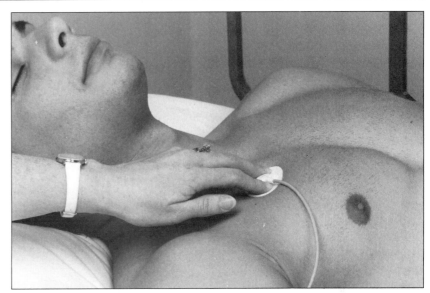

Placing the electrodes

To monitor leads I, II, and III with a three-electrode system, place the color-coded electrodes in the following areas: white electrode just below the right clavicle, black electrode just below the left clavicle, and red electrode on the lower left anterior rib cage. Then turn the lead selector on the monitor to the desired setting (lead I, II, or III). *Note:* The photos use these abbrevations: RA, right arm; LA, left arm; RL, right leg; LL, left leg; and C, chest.

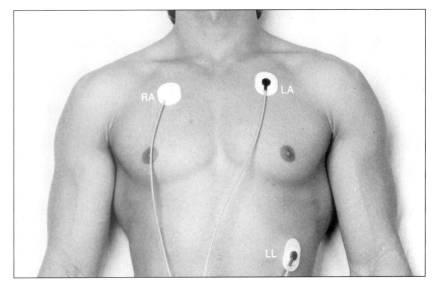

To monitor modified chest lead I (MCL$_1$) with a three-electrode system, turn the lead selector on the monitor to MCL$_1$. If the monitor doesn't have an MCL$_1$ selection, turn the selector to lead III. Then place the white electrode just below the right clavicle, the black electrode just below the left clavicle, and the red electrode over the fourth intercostal space at the right sternal border.

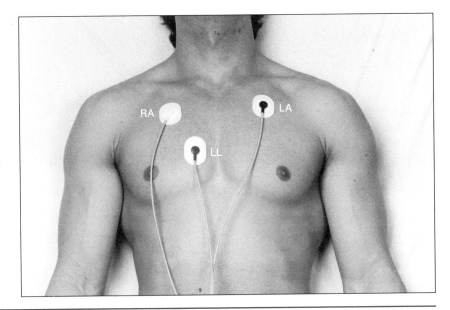

To monitor MCL$_6$ with a three-electrode system, turn the lead selector to MCL$_6$. If the monitor doesn't have an MCL$_6$ selection, turn the selector to lead III. Then place the white electrode just below the right clavicle, the black electrode just below the left clavicle, and the red electrode over the fifth intercostal space at the left midaxillary line.

▷ *Clinical tip:* When placing electrodes, select sites over soft tissue or close to bone. Avoid placing electrodes over muscle, bony prominences, or skin folds because these placements may produce waveform artifacts.

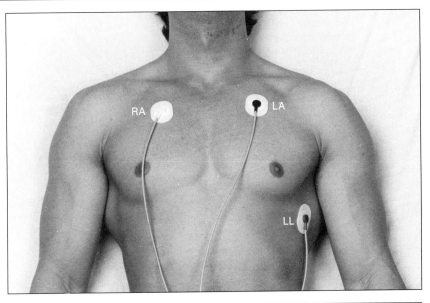

You can monitor any of the 12 standard leads, MCL$_1$, or MCL$_6$ with a five-electrode system. To monitor common leads I, II, III, and MCL$_1$, turn the lead selector on the monitor to the appropriate lead. Then place the white electrode just below the right clavicle, the black electrode just below the left clavicle, the green electrode on the right lower anterior rib cage, the red electrode on the left lower anterior rib cage, and the brown electrode over the fourth intercostal space at the right sternal border (the V$_1$ position).

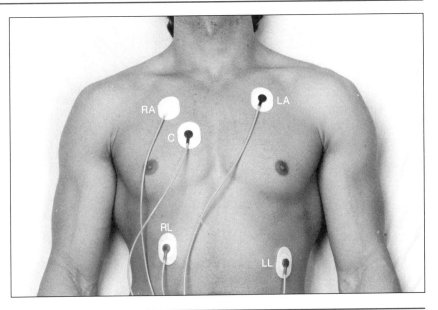

To monitor MCL₆ with a five-electrode system, turn the lead selector to MCL₆. If the monitor doesn't have an MCL₆ selection, turn the selector to lead III. Then place the white electrode just below the right clavicle, the black electrode just below the left clavicle, the green electrode on the right lower anterior rib cage, the red electrode on the left lower anterior rib cage, and the brown electrode over the fifth intercostal space at the left midaxillary line.

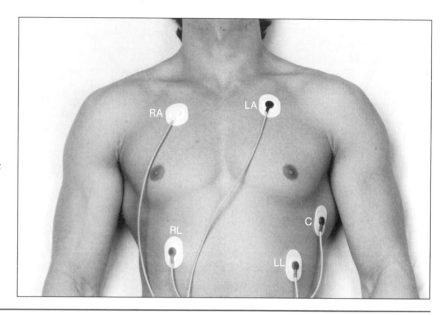

Adjusting the monitor and obtaining a rhythm strip

After you've applied all of the electrodes, observe the monitor screen. You should see the patient's ECG waveform. Assess the quality of the waveform. If the size of the tracing is too large or too small, change the size by adjusting the gain control. If the waveform appears too high or too low on the monitor screen, use the position dial to adjust the position.

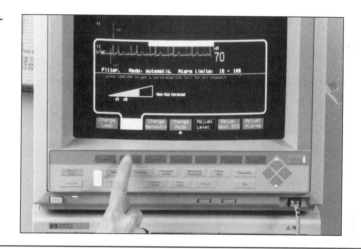

Verify that the monitor detects each heartbeat by taking the patient's apical pulse and comparing it with the digital heart rate display.

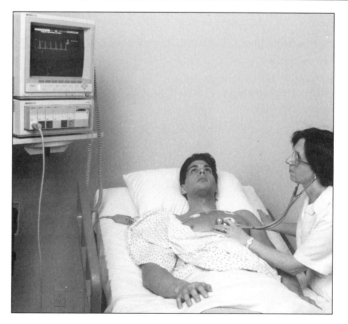

Set the upper and lower limits of the heart rate alarm on the cardiac monitor according to your hospital's policy.

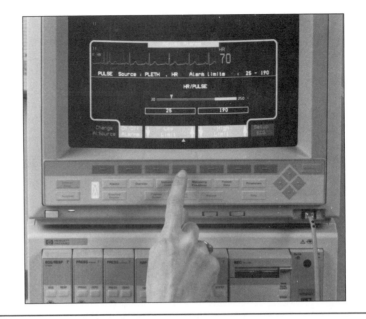

To obtain a printout of the patient's cardiac rhythm, press the RECORD control on the monitor.

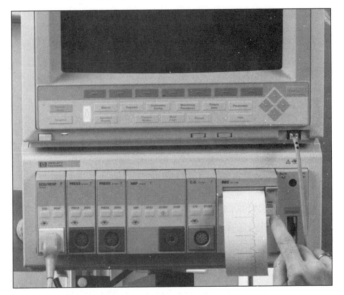

Label the rhythm strip with the patient's name, room number, date, time, and rhythm interpretation. Place the rhythm strip in the appropriate section of the patient's medical record.

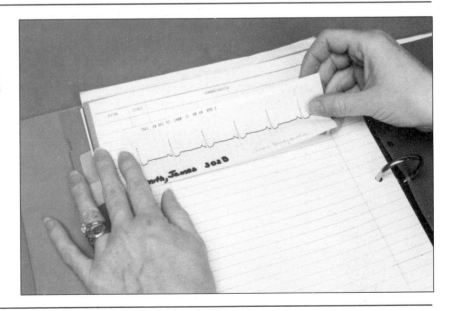

Reading rhythm strips

To help you quickly and accurately read your patient's rhythm strip, follow these steps:
• Identify the QRS complexes (which represent ventricular depolarization), and decide whether the patient's ventricular rhythm is regular or irregular.
• Count the QRS complexes within a certain interval to compute the patient's ventricular rate.
• Identify the P waves (which represent atrial depolarization) and determine whether each one precedes a QRS complex.
• Count the number of P waves within a certain time span to determine the atrial rate.
• Analyze the P wave's shape to assess atrial contraction.
• Identify the pacemaker site (the heartbeat's source).
• Measure the PR interval, the QRS complex, and the QT interval.
• Analyze the T wave's shape.
• Identify the rhythm.

To further help you interpret your patient's rhythm strip, review the ECG strips on this page. The first shows normal sinus rhythm; the rest show common arrhythmias.

Normal sinus rhythm

Impulses originate in the sinoatrial (SA) node, travel normally through the conduction system, and generate a regular rhythm of 60 to 100 beats/minute.

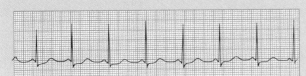

Sinus bradycardia

In this arrhythmia, impulses originate in the SA node but produce fewer than 60 beats/minute.

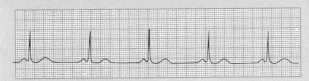

Sinus tachycardia

In this arrhythmia, impulses originate in the SA node and produce a regular rhythm of more than 100 beats/minute.

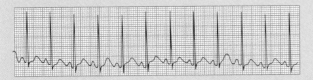

Atrial flutter

In this rhythm strip, note the rapid atrial rate, which produces 260 to 360 flutter waves/minute. The atrial rhythm is regular, but the P waves have a saw-toothed appearance. The ventricular rate is also rapid (about 150 beats/minute).

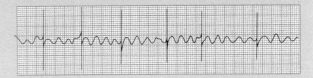

Atrial fibrillation

This rhythm strip shows classic atrial fibrillation. Multiple pacemaker sites produce between 350 and 600 fibrillation waves/minute. These waves have an abnormal, chaotic, and irregular appearance. The ventricular rate is also rapid and can be as high as 200 beats/minute.

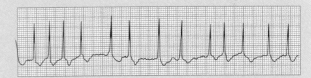

Ventricular tachycardia

In this arrhythmia, three or more premature ventricular contractions occur in succession—the rate ranges from 110 to 250 beats/minute. P waves may or may not appear.

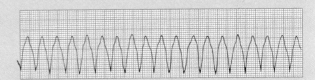

Ventricular fibrillation

On this rhythm strip, note the absence of coordinated ventricular beats. In ventricular fibrillation, the ventricles contract chaotically and irregularly from 300 to 500 times/minute.

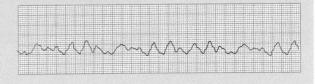

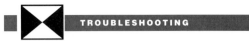

Managing cardiac monitoring problems

PROBLEM	POSSIBLE CAUSES	SOLUTIONS
False-high-rate alarm	• Monitor interpreting large T waves as QRS complexes, which doubles the rate • Skeletal muscle activity	• Reposition electrodes to lead where QRS complexes are taller than the T waves. • Place electrodes away from major muscle masses.
False-low-rate alarm	• Shift in electrical axis caused by patient movement, making QRS complexes too small to register • Low amplitude of QRS complex • Poor contact between electrodes and skin	• Reapply electrodes. Set gain so that height of complex exceeds 1 mV. • Increase gain. • Reapply electrodes.
Low amplitude	• Gain dial set too low • Poor contact between skin and electrodes; dried gel; broken or loose leadwires; poor connection between patient and monitor; malfunctioning monitor; physiologic loss of amplitude of QRS complex	• Increase gain. • Check connections on all leadwires and monitoring cable. Replace or reapply electrodes as necessary.
Wandering baseline	• Poor electrode placement or contact with skin • Thoracic movement with respirations	• Reposition or replace electrodes. • Reposition electrodes.
Artifact (waveform interference)	• Patient having seizures, chills, or anxiety • Patient movement • Electrodes applied improperly • Static electricity	• Notify doctor and treat patient as ordered. Keep patient warm and reassure him. • Help patient relax. • Check electrodes and reapply, if necessary. • Make sure cables don't have exposed connectors. Change static-causing bedclothes.
	• Electrical short circuit in leadwires or cable • Interference from decreased room humidity	• Replace broken equipment. Use stress loops when applying leadwires. • Regulate humidity to 40%.
Broken leadwires or cable	• Tension on leadwires due to repeated pulling • Cables and leadwires cleaned with alcohol or acetone, causing brittleness	• Replace leadwires and retape them, making sure to tape part of the wire into a loop. This absorbs tension that would otherwise tug at the ends of the wire. • Clean cable and leadwires with soapy water. *Do not let cable ends get wet.* Replace cable as necessary.
60-cycle interference (fuzzy baseline)	• Electrical interference from other equipment in room • Patient's bed improperly grounded	• Attach all electrical equipment to common ground. Check plugs to make sure prongs aren't loose. • Attach bed ground to the room's common ground.
Skin excoriation under electrode	• Patient allergic to electrode adhesive • Electrode remaining on skin too long	• Remove electrodes and apply nonallergenic electrodes and nonallergenic tape. • Remove electrode, clean site, and reapply electrode at new site.

PERFORMING TELEMETRY MONITORING

Battery powered and portable, telemetry provides continuous electrocardiogram (ECG) monitoring without attaching the patient directly to a hardwire monitoring system. Telemetry frees the patient from cumbersome wires and cables. This system also allows him to be comfortably mobile and safely isolated from the electrical leakage and accidental shock occasionally associated with hardwire monitoring.

Telemetry is especially useful for monitoring arrhythmias that occur during sleep, rest, exercise, or stressful situations. Unlike hardwire monitoring, telemetry can monitor only cardiac rate and rhythm.

Preparing the equipment and the patient

For telemetry, the patient wears from two to five electrodes. Aided by a small transmitter that the patient carries in a pocket or a pouch, the electrodes detect and transmit the heart's electrical activity. The transmitter sends signals to an antenna that relays the impulses to a monitor at a nursing station.

To institute telemetry monitoring, obtain a transmitter, a transmitter pouch, a telemetry battery pack, leads, and electrodes.

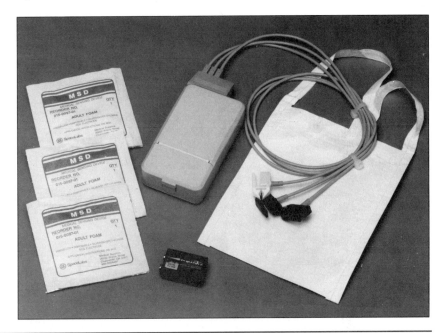

Insert a new battery into the transmitter. Be sure to match the poles on the battery with the polar markings on the transmitter case.

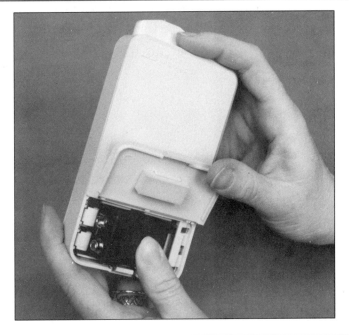

By pressing the button at the top of the unit (as shown), test the battery's charge and test the unit to ensure that the battery is operational.

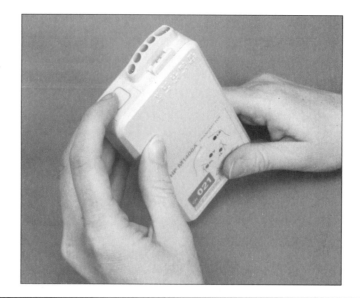

If the leadwires aren't permanently affixed to the telemetry unit, attach them securely. If leadwires must be attached individually, be sure to connect each one to the correct outlet.

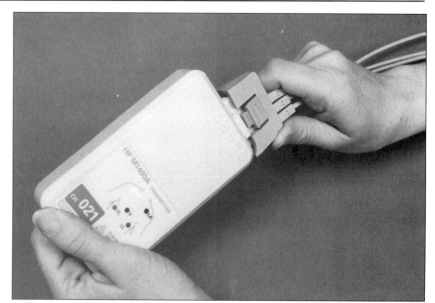

Wash your hands. Explain the procedure to the patient and provide privacy. Expose the patient's chest, and select the lead arrangement. Remove the backing from one of the gelled electrodes. Check the gel for moistness. If it's dry, discard the electrode and obtain a new one.

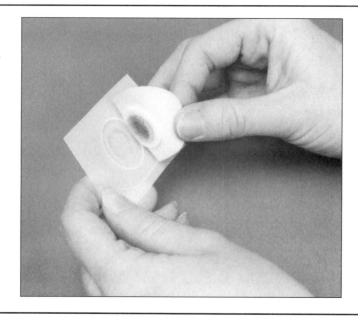

Apply the electrode to the appropriate site by pressing one side of the electrode against the patient's skin, pulling gently, and then pressing the other side against the skin. Press your fingers in a circular motion around the electrode to fix the gel and stabilize the electrode. Repeat for each electrode.

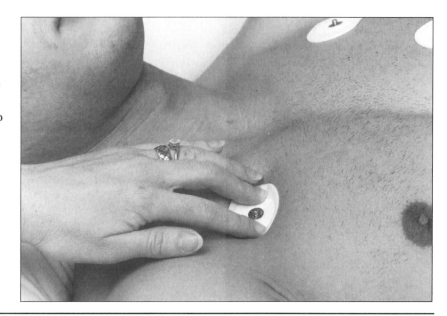

Attach an electrode to the end of each leadwire.

▶ **Clinical tip:** If you're using a clip-type electrode (as shown), attach the leadwire to the electrode after the electrode is in place on the chest. If you're using a snap-type leadwire, attach the leadwire to the electrode before you put the electrode on the chest.

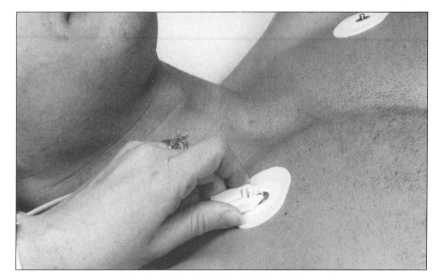

Place the transmitter in the pouch. Tie the pouch strings around the patient's neck and waist. Make sure that the pouch fits snugly without causing the patient discomfort. If no pouch is available, place the transmitter in the patient's bathrobe pocket.

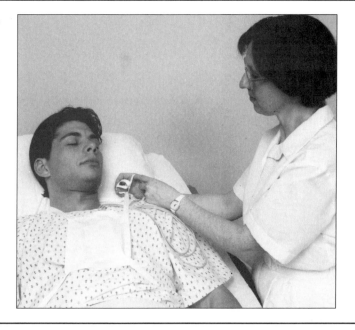

Check with the telemetry central station to ensure that the waveform transmits properly. If necessary, ask the patient to remain resting or sitting in his room while you locate his telemetry monitor at the central station. Evaluate the waveform for clarity, position, and size. Adjust the gain and baseline as needed.

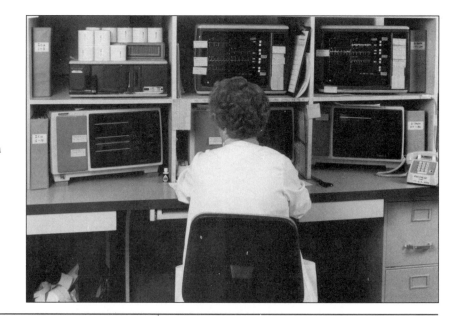

To obtain a rhythm strip, press the RECORD key at the central station. Label the rhythm strip with the patient's name, room number, date, and time. Also identify the rhythm. Place the rhythm strip in the appropriate location in the patient's chart. Document the interpretation of the rhythm on the patient record.

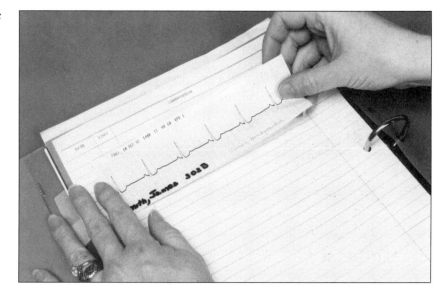

Teaching telemetry patients

To promote cooperation during telemetry monitoring, explain the procedure to the patient and allow him to ask questions. Use the following instructions as a guide.

• Show the patient the transmitter unit and explain how it works.
• Inform him that the unit won't produce sufficient electrical current to cause a shock.
• If applicable, show him the button on the transmitter that will produce a recording of his electrocardiogram at the central station. Teach him how to push the button whenever he experiences chest pain, palpitations, or related symptoms.

• Instruct the patient to remove the transmitter unit before taking a bath or shower. Stress, however, that he needs to let you know before he removes the unit.
• Explain that the telemetry unit can transmit signals only a set distance from the central station. Let the patient know how far he can move from the central station before the transmission will be interrupted.

PERFORMING ST-SEGMENT MONITORING

During a 12-lead electrocardiogram (ECG), you may detect ST-segment deviations that require special analysis. To perform this analysis, conduct continuous cardiac monitoring using a 5-lead system; such a system usually allows the best identification of the ST segment. Some bedside cardiac monitors allow ST-segment analysis during continuous monitoring.

A sensitive indicator of myocardial damage, the ST segment is normally flat or isoelectric. A depressed ST segment may result from digitalis glycosides, myocardial ischemia, or a subendocardial infarction. An elevated ST segment suggests myocardial infarction (MI).

Continuous ST-segment monitoring is especially useful for patients who have undergone thrombolytic therapy or coronary angioplasty. Although these procedures help reestablish blood flow to occluded coronary arteries, reocclusion may occur. Monitoring appropriate leads for changes in the ST segment allows early detection of reocclusion.

ST-segment monitoring is also useful for patients who've had previous episodes of cardiac ischemia without chest pain, those who have difficulty distinguishing between cardiac pain and pain from another source (such as arthritis), and those who can't communicate easily.

SELECTING THE BEST LEAD

Because ischemia typically occurs in only one portion of the heart muscle, not all ECG leads detect it; thus, you'll need to select the appropriate leads. One way is to examine ECG tracings recorded during an ischemic episode. For example, if the patient suffered an acute MI, examine both the precordial and limb leads of an ECG recorded before thrombolytic therapy. The leads showing signs of myocardial ischemia during the infarction are the same leads you'll monitor for signs of ischemia in the future.

Also, if the patient has undergone coronary angioplasty, the ECG recorded during the procedure will show you which leads to monitor. Because the balloon catheter inflated during the procedure momentarily obstructs blood flow in the affected coronary artery, ischemia results. The ECG leads that show signs of ischemia are the leads you should monitor for ST-segment changes.

When monitoring the ST segment, keep in mind that the main goal of cardiac monitoring is to detect arrhythmias. Therefore, when deciding which leads to monitor, remember that the leads most likely to reveal arrhythmias should take priority over the leads that may reveal ST-segment changes.

Preparing the equipment and the patient

Begin ST-segment monitoring by collecting the equipment you'll need: ECG electrodes, gauze pads, an ECG monitor cable, leadwires, alcohol sponges (near right), and a cardiac monitor programmed for ST-segment monitoring (such as the Hewlett-Packard Component Monitoring System shown at far right). You may also need a razor.

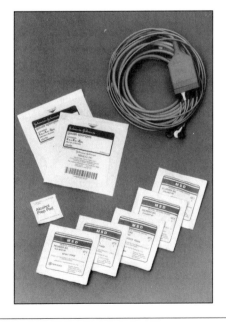 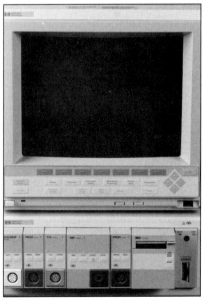

Pamela Kovach, RN, BSN, a clinical consultant for Springhouse Corporation, wrote this section. The publisher thanks *Hewlett-Packard Co.*, Waltham, Mass., and *Hill-Rom*, Batesville, Ind., for their help.

Take the equipment to the patient's bedside and explain the procedure. Then wash your hands. If your patient is not already on a monitor, turn on the device and attach the cable.

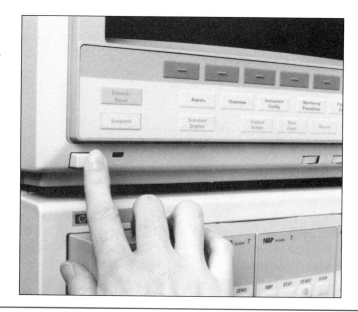

Select the sites for electrode placement according to the lead you'll be monitoring. If necessary, shave the sites. Then clean the sites with an alcohol sponge.

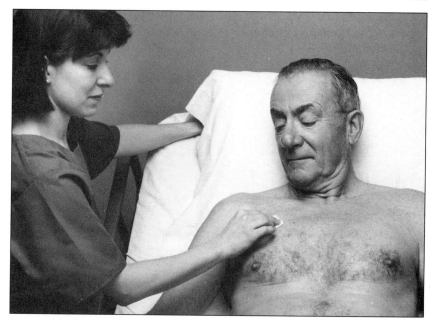

Rub the areas with a gauze pad until the patient's skin becomes red and shiny.

▷ **Clinical tip:** If the electrode has a pumice pad on the back, use it to gently abrade the patient's skin and remove dead skin cells, which will promote electrical conductivity.

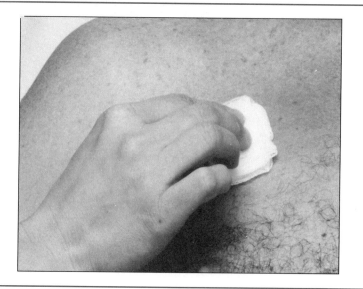

Attach the leadwires to the electrodes.

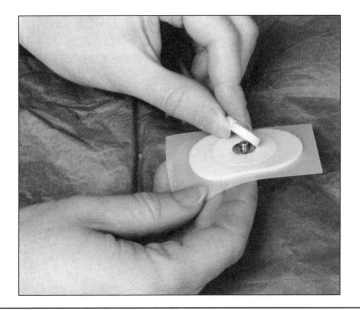

Place the electrodes on the patient's chest in the appropriate positions. For example, the leads at right are placed to record a modified chest lead (MCL$_1$).

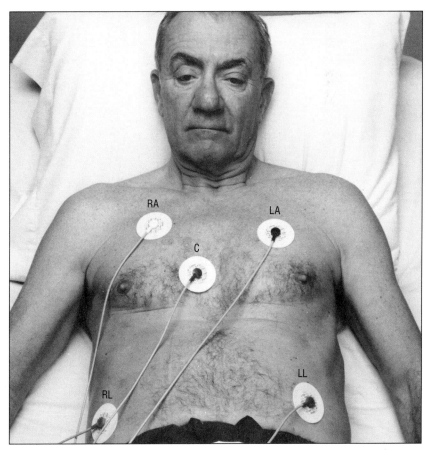

Adjusting the monitor

If necessary, activate ST-segment monitoring by pressing the MONI-TORING PROCEDURES key and then the ST key (as designated on the screen above the keys).

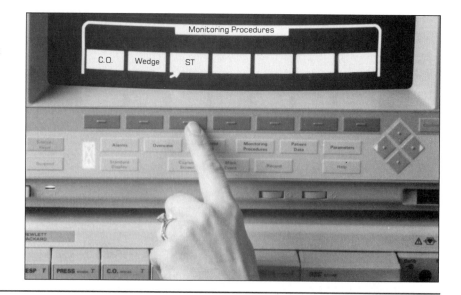

Activate individual ST parameters by pressing the ON/OFF PARAMETER key.

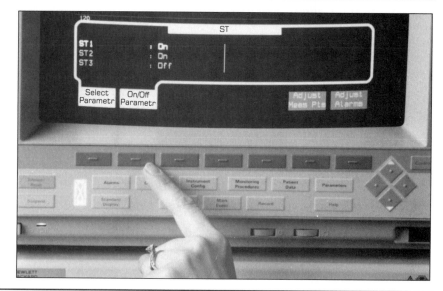

Select the appropriate ECG lead for each ST channel to be monitored by pressing the PARAMETERS key and then the key labeled ECG (as shown).

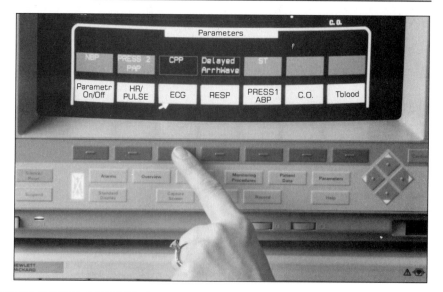

Next, press the key labeled CHANGE LEAD to select the appropriate lead. Repeat the procedure for all three channels.

▶ **Clinical tip:** If you monitor only one lead, choose the lead most likely to disclose both arrhythmias and ST-segment changes. Always give precedence, however, to the lead that best shows arrhythmias.

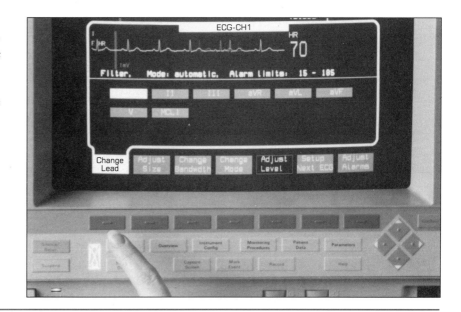

Adjust the ST-segment measurement points, if necessary. To do so, enter the ST task window by pressing the MONITORING PROCEDURES key and then ST. Then press the key labeled ADJUST MEAS PTS.

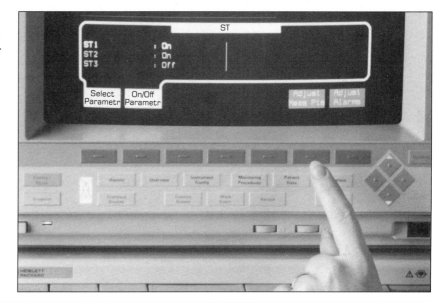

Adjust the baseline for ST-segment measurement, known as the isoelectric point. To do so, press the key marked ISO POINT to move the cursor to the PQ or TP interval (as shown).

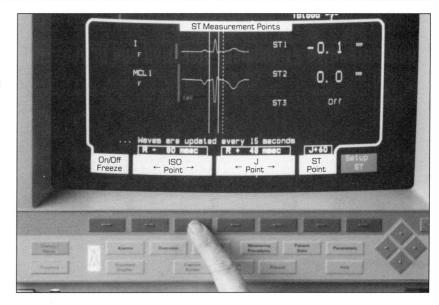

Next, adjust the J point—the transition between the QRS complex and the ST segment. To do so, press the key labeled J POINT to move the cursor to the appropriate location.

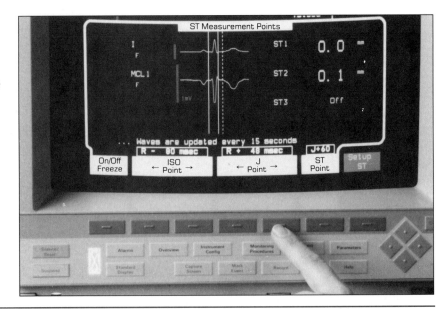

Adjust the ST point to 80 milliseconds after the J point. Do this by pressing the key labeled ST POINT and moving the cursor until the box above the key displays J + 80.

▷ *Clinical tip:* Some hospitals measure the ST point at 60 milliseconds after the J point. Check your hospital's policy before setting the ST point.

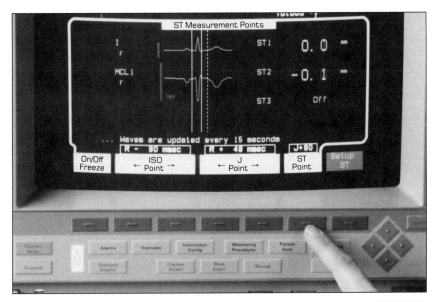

Now set the alarm limits for each ST-segment parameter. First, press the key labeled SETUP ST. Next, press the ADJUST ALARMS key. Then set the high and low limits by manipulating the high and low limit keys (as shown).

▷ *Clinical tip:* The alarms are set according to millimeters of ST-segment depression. When a limit is surpassed for more than 1 minute, both a visual and an audible alarm are activated. Check your hospital's policy, and ask the patient's doctor for alarm limit parameters.

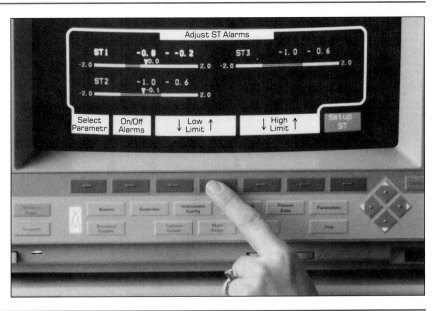

To return to the display screen, press the key labeled STANDARD DISPLAY. If the patient isn't being monitored continuously, remove the electrodes, clean his skin, and disconnect the leadwires from the electrodes.

Document the leads being monitored and the ST-segment measurement points in the patient's chart.

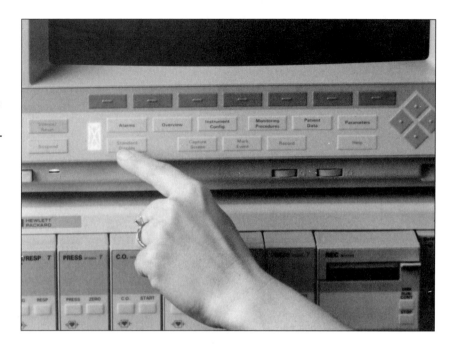

INSIGHTS AND INTERPRETATIONS

Understanding ST-segment elevation and depression

Closely monitoring the ST segment on a patient's electrocardiogram can help you detect ischemia or injury before an infarction develops.

Normal ST segment
The ST segment represents the beginning of ventricular repolarization. It immediately follows the QRS complex (the J point) and extends to the beginning of the T wave. Normally, the ST segment is isoelectric.

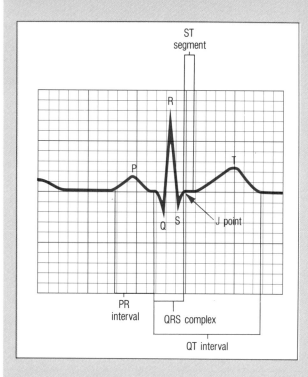

ST-segment depression
A depressed ST segment may indicate myocardial ischemia, subendocardial infarction, or digitalis toxicity. An ST segment is considered depressed when it is 0.5 mm or more from the baseline.

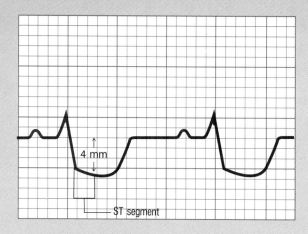

ST-segment elevation
An elevated ST segment may indicate myocardial injury. An ST segment is considered elevated when it is 1 mm or more above the baseline.

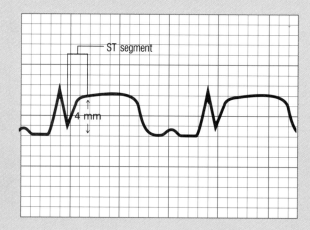

Hemodynamic Monitoring

LEARNING ABOUT HEMODYNAMIC MONITORING

Every time you take a patient's blood pressure with a sphygmomanometer, you're performing hemodynamic monitoring. Typically, though, most nurses associate hemodynamic monitoring with invasive procedures used to obtain physiologic measurements from the circulatory system. These procedures permit you to measure cardiac output, central venous pressure (CVP), and intra-arterial pressures, such as pulmonary artery pressure (PAP).

Routinely used in critical care units, invasive hemodynamic monitoring provides accurate, continuous blood pressure readings, even when your patient is in shock. To make the most of hemodynamic monitoring, you need to understand the cardiac cycle, which consists of diastole, when the heart's ventricles fill with blood, and systole, when they contract and eject the blood.

Cardiac cycle

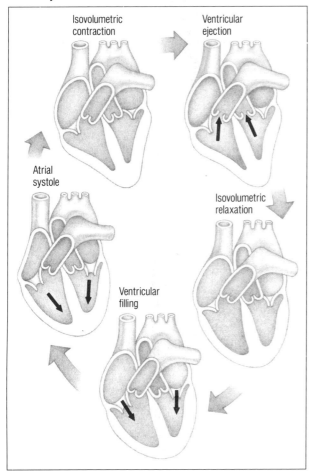

Isovolumetric contraction

Ventricular ejection

Atrial systole

Isovolumetric relaxation

Ventricular filling

This continuous cycle has no set starting point. But for the sake of clarity, assume it begins with isovolumetric contraction and proceeds sequentially through ventricular ejection, isovolumetric relaxation, ventricular filling, and atrial systole.

As depolarization spreads through the ventricles, these chambers contract. The resulting rise in pressure causes the mitral and tricuspid valves to close. Thus, all four heart valves are closed for a short time. The pulmonary and aortic valves stay closed during this phase called *isovolumetric contraction*.

In *ventricular ejection*, ventricular pressure exceeds the aortic and pulmonary arterial pressures. This forces the aortic and pulmonary valves open and permits ejection of ventricular blood.

When ventricular pressure drops below that of the aorta and pulmonary artery, the next phase—*isovolumetric relaxation*—occurs. In this phase, all four heart valves are again closed. At this time, atrial diastole occurs as blood fills the atria.

When the atrial pressure exceeds the ventricular pressure, the mitral and tricuspid valves open. This marks the *ventricular filling* phase in which blood passively enters the ventricles. About 80% of ventricular filling occurs at this time.

The last phase, *atrial systole*, coincides with late diastole, when the atria contract in response to atrial depolarization. This "atrial kick" supplies the ventricles with the remaining 20% of blood before the cycle repeats.

PRESSURE TRANSDUCER SYSTEMS

To perform invasive hemodynamic monitoring, you'll need to be familiar with a pressure transducer system. To operate this device safely and effectively, follow hospital policy and the manufacturer's directions. Keep in mind that sophisticated monitoring techniques can give a false sense of security. Monitoring is just one aspect of nursing care—an adjunct for your clinical judgment.

You'll begin invasive hemodynamic monitoring by setting up a pressure transducer system. This system converts mechanical energy (from blood pressure, for example) into electrical energy (displayed as impulses, or waveforms, on a monitor screen). You'll need this system to monitor arterial pressure, PAP, left atrial pressure, and CVP.

Jan M. Headley, RN, BS, who contributed to this section, is senior education consultant with Baxter Healthcare Corp., Edwards Critical Care Division, Irvine, Calif. The publisher thanks the following organizations for their help: *Baxter Healthcare Corp.,* Irvine, Calif.; *Doylestown (Pa.) Hospital; Hill Rom,* Batesville, Ind.; and *Marquette Electronics,* Milwaukee, Wis.

SETTING UP TRANSDUCERS

The exact type of transducer system you'll set up depends on the patient's needs and the doctor's preference. Some systems monitor pressure continuously, whereas others monitor pressure intermittently. Single-pressure transducers monitor only one type of pressure—for example, PAP. Multiple-pressure transducers can monitor two or more types of pressure, such as PAP and CVP.

Setting up a single-pressure transducer system

Gather the equipment you'll need: monitor; disposable pressure transducer; cable (to connect the pressure transducer to the monitor); preassembled pressure tubing with continuous flush device; inflatable pressure infuser bag; manifold transducer holder (if transducer will be mounted on the I.V. pole); two sterile occlusive (nonvented) caps; a carpenter's level; and a 500-ml bag of heparinized saline solution, commonly called the flush solution bag. Also obtain an I.V. pole.

▶ *Clinical tip:* Adding heparin to a flush solution is controversial. Current studies are investigating whether the system needs heparin to keep the line patent. Keeping this in mind, follow your hospital's policy. If your patient has a history of bleeding or clotting problems, use heparin with caution.

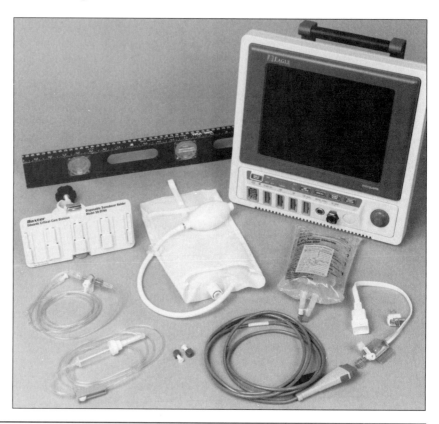

Check the label on the 500-ml bag of heparinized saline solution. Make sure that the patient's name and room number, the date and time, and the amount of added heparin are clearly and correctly labeled. If necessary, add the ordered amount of heparin to the solution—usually, 1 to 2 units of heparin/ml of solution (as shown). Then, label the bag with the appropriate information. (In many hospitals, the pharmacist prepares the flush solution.) Hang the bag that contains the continuous flush solution on the I.V. pole.

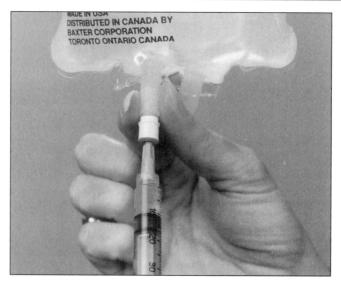

Put the pressure module into the monitor, if necessary, and connect the transducer cable to the monitor. The Marquette Eagle monitor shown here only requires the nurse to attach the transducer cable to the monitor.

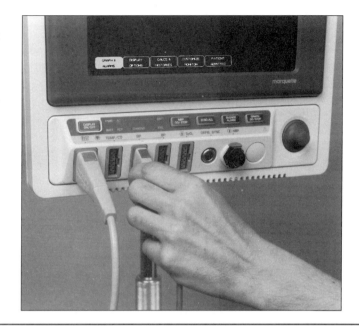

Remove the preassembled pressure tubing from the package. If necessary, connect the pressure tubing to the transducer. Tighten all tubing connections.

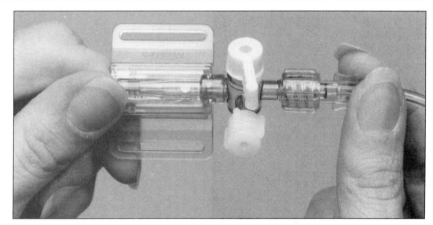

Position all stopcocks so that the flush solution flows through the entire system (near right). Then roll the tubing's flow regulator to the off position (far right).

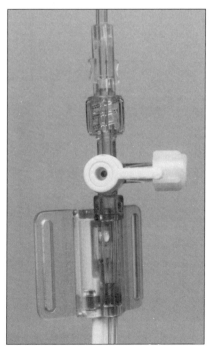 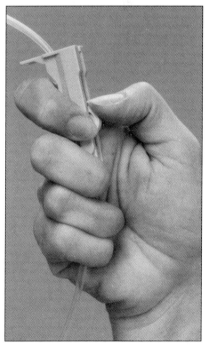

Spike the flush solution bag with the tubing, invert the bag, open the roller clamp, and squeeze all the air through the drip chamber (near right). Then, compress the tubing's drip chamber (far right), filling it no more than halfway with the flush solution.

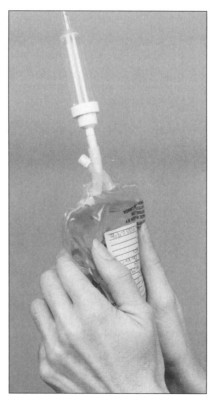 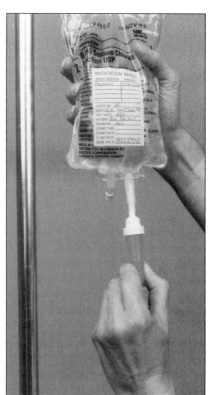

Place the flush solution bag into the pressure infuser bag. To do this, hang the pressure infuser bag on the I.V. pole and then position the flush solution bag inside the pressure infuser bag.

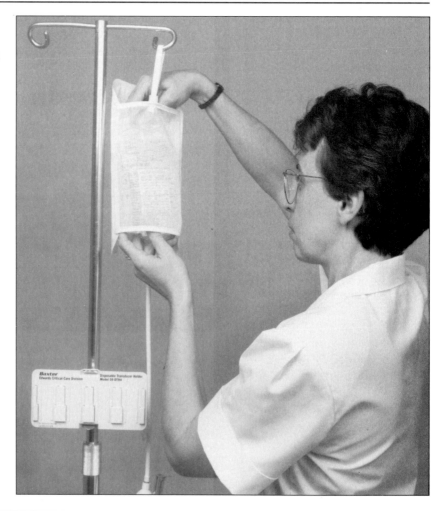

Open the tubing's flow regulator, uncoil the tube if you haven't already done so, and remove the protective cap at the end of the pressure tubing. Squeeze the continuous flush device slowly (as shown) to prime the entire system, including the stopcock ports, with the flush solution.

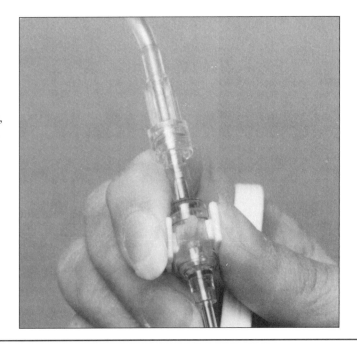

As the solution nears the disposable transducer, hold the transducer at a 45-degree angle. This forces the solution to flow upward to the transducer. In doing so, the solution forces any air out of the system.

▶ *Clinical tip:* As you prime the system, take care to remove all air bubbles—the most common cause of inaccurate pressure readings. Air bubbles may also place the patient at risk for air emboli.

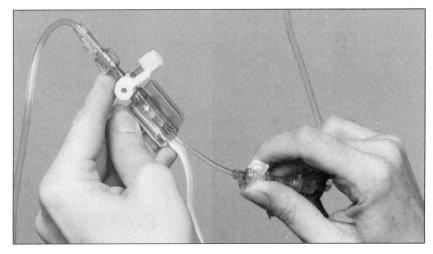

When the solution nears a stopcock, open the stopcock to air, allowing the solution to flow into the stopcock (as shown). When the stopcock fills, close it to air and turn it open to the remainder of the tubing. Do this for each stopcock.

Note: When activated, the continuous flush device allows solution to flow rapidly through the system. When you turn off the continuous flush, the solution's flow rate should be 3 to 5 ml/hour.

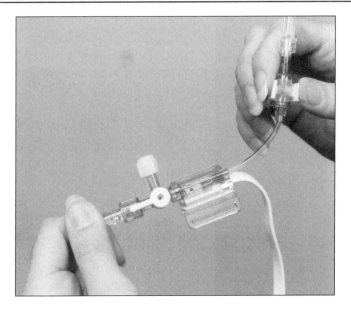

After you completely prime the system, replace the protective cap at the end of the tubing.

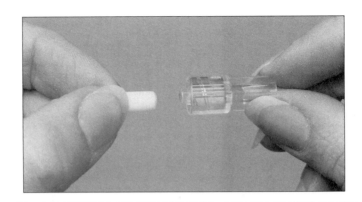

Next, inflate the pressure infuser bag to 300 mm Hg. This bag keeps the pressure in the arterial line higher than the patient's systolic pressure, thereby preventing blood backflow into the tubing and ensuring a continuous flow rate. When you inflate the pressure bag, take care that the drip chamber doesn't completely fill with fluid. Afterward, flush the system again to remove all air bubbles.

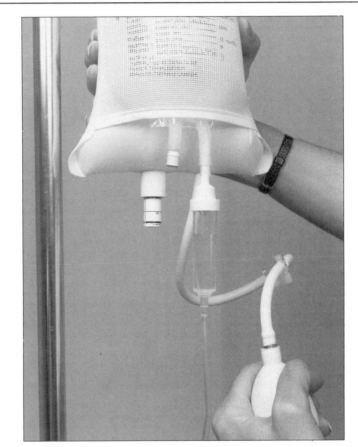

Replace the vented caps on the stopcocks with sterile nonvented caps (near right).

If you're going to mount the transducer on an I.V. pole, insert the device into its holder (far right).

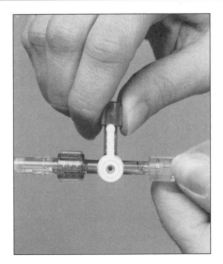
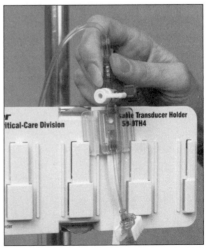

Now you're ready for a preliminary zeroing of the transducer. Zeroing adjusts the transducer so that it reads zero pressure when it's open to the atmosphere. This is important because physiologic pressures, such as arterial blood pressure, are relative to the atmospheric pressure. By zeroing the transducer, you ensure that the device accurately reads pressure within the blood vessel.

▶ **Clinical tip:** To ensure accuracy, position the patient and the transducer on the same level each time you zero the transducer or record a pressure (as shown). Typically, the patient lies flat in bed, if he can tolerate that position.

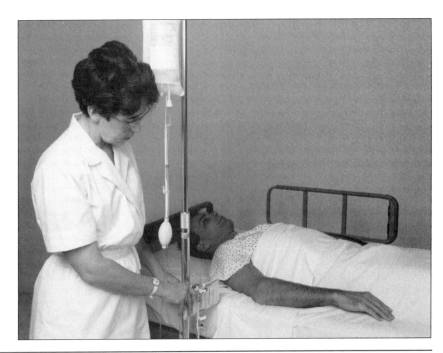

Next, use the carpenter's level to position the air-reference stopcock or the air-fluid interface of the transducer level with the phlebostatic axis (as shown at right). This is also the level of the patient's atria (midway between the posterior chest and his sternum at the fourth intercostal space, midaxillary line, as shown below).

Alternatively, you may level the air-reference stopcock or the air-fluid interface of the transducer to the same position as the catheter tip.

▶ **Clinical tip:** Experts debate the most accurate placement for the transducer. For now, use whichever placement your hospital proposes, and don't vary it.

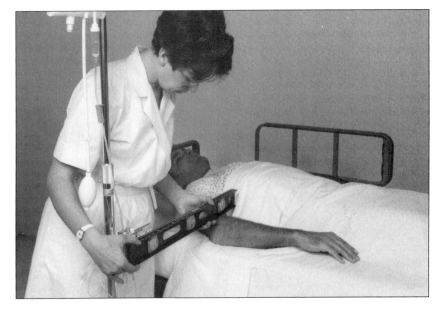

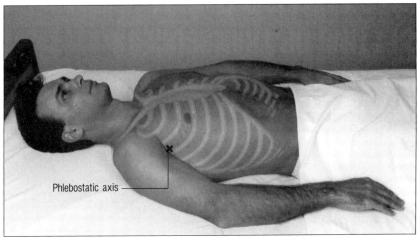

Phlebostatic axis —

After leveling the transducer, turn the stopcock next to the transducer *off* to the patient and *open* to air. Remove the cap to the stopcock port. Place the cap inside an opened sterile gauze package to prevent contamination.

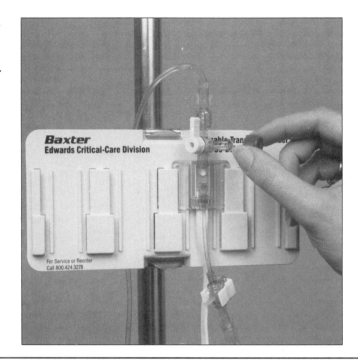

Now, zero the transducer. To do so, follow the manufacturer's direction for zeroing. If you're using the Marquette Eagle monitor shown here, press the ZERO ALL button, and immediately release it. This completes zeroing.

When you've finished zeroing, turn the stopcock on the transducer so that it's *open* to air and *open* to the patient. This is the monitoring position. Replace the cap on the stopcock. You're then ready to attach the single-pressure transducer to the patient's catheter. Document the patient's position for zeroing so that other health care team members can replicate the placement.

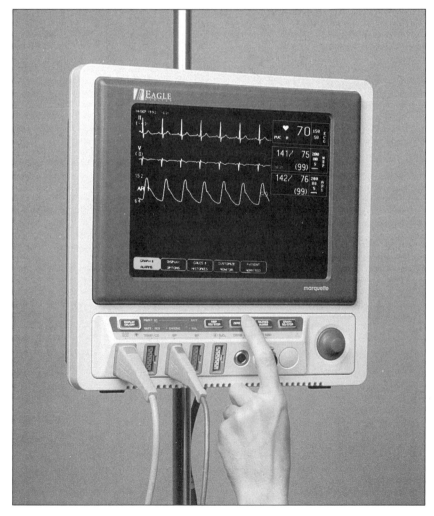

Now, you've assembled a single-pressure transducer system. The photograph at right shows how the system will look.

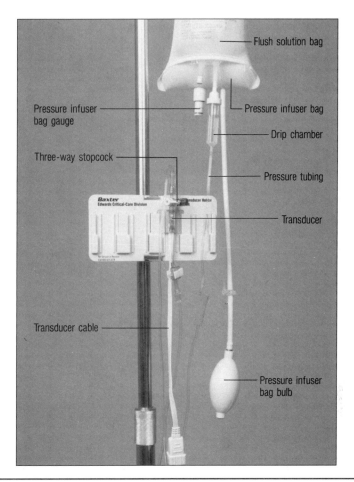

Flush solution bag

Pressure infuser bag

Pressure infuser bag gauge

Drip chamber

Three-way stopcock

Pressure tubing

Transducer

Transducer cable

Pressure infuser bag bulb

Setting up a multiple-pressure transducer system

You may use any of several methods to set up a multiple-pressure transducer system. The equipment you'll need depends on the method you select. But generally, you'll set up another single-pressure transducer system. The two setups make up the multiple-pressure transducer system.

Another way to set up a multiple-pressure transducer system is to assemble equipment as you would for a single-pressure transducer system. But you'll need another cable, and you'll substitute Y-type preassembled pressure tubing with continuous flush devices and two attached pressure transducers for the single-pressure tubing (as shown). You'll also need one more pressure-specific module (if the module isn't built into the cable).

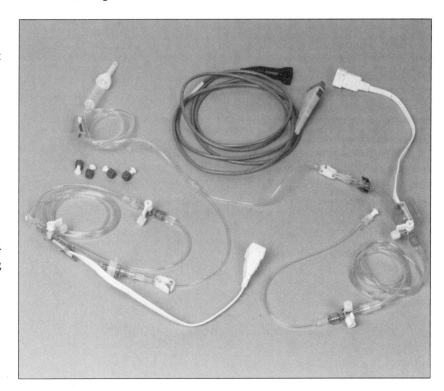

The easiest way to set up a multiple-pressure transducer is to add to the single-pressure system. You'll need another bag of heparinized saline solution in a second pressure infuser bag. Then prime the tubing, mount the second transducer, and connect an additional cable to the monitor. Finally, zero the second transducer, just as you did for the first one.

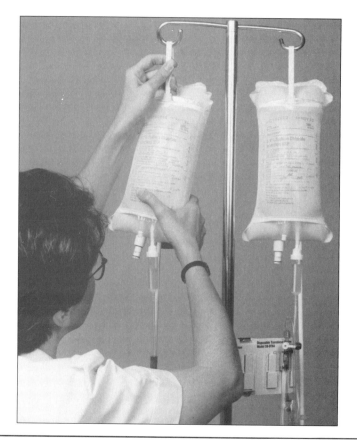

Alternatively, your hospital may use a Y-type tubing setup with two attached pressure transducers. This method requires only one bag of heparinized flush solution. To set up the system, proceed as you would for a single transducer, with this exception: First, prime one branch of the Y-type tubing and then the other. Next, attach two cables to the monitor in the modules for each pressure that you will be measuring. Finally, zero each transducer.

If you need a second pressure reading only intermittently—for example, in continuous PAP monitoring and intermittent CVP monitoring—you may vary the setup by using a transducer with a bridge.

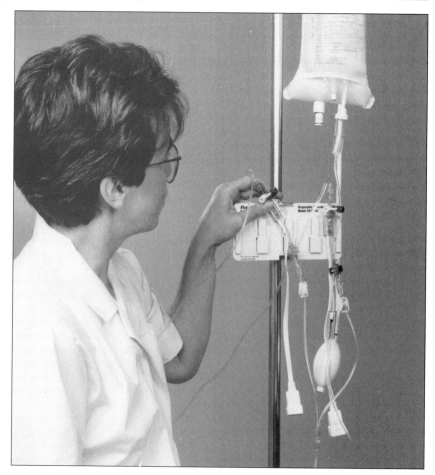

LEARNING ABOUT ARTERIAL PRESSURE MONITORING

Intra-arterial pressure monitoring is used on patients who are severely hypotensive, in shock, or receiving vasoactive medications. And because mean arterial pressure (MAP) helps determine cerebral perfusion pressure, arterial pressure monitoring may also be used when patients have increased intracranial pressure.

HOW ARTERIAL PRESSURE MONITORING WORKS

Typically, the pressure of the patient's arterial pulse wave causes fluid movement in the arterial line tubing, which is connected to a pressure transducer system. The diaphragm of the pressure transducer detects the fluid's motion and converts this mechanical energy into electrical energy.

The resultant signals create a waveform display and a digital printout of the patient's arterial pressure. (See *Understanding the arterial waveform*, below, and *Recognizing abnormal waveforms*, page 118.)

When caring for a patient who has an arterial line, monitor and record:
• systolic pressure (normal range: 100 to 140 mm Hg)
• diastolic pressure (normal range: 60 to 90 mm Hg)
• MAP (normal range: 70 to 105 mm Hg).

In general, *arterial systolic pressure* reflects the peak pressure generated by the left ventricle. It also indicates the compliance of the large arteries — the peripheral resistance.

Arterial diastolic pressure reflects the runoff velocity and the elasticity of the arterial system, particularly the arterioles.

MAP is the average pressure in the arterial system during systole and diastole. It reflects the driving, or perfusion, pressure and is determined by arterial blood volume and blood vessel elasticity and resistance.

To compute MAP, use one of these formulas:

$$\text{MAP} = \text{systolic pressure} + 2\ (\text{diastolic pressure})\ /\ 3$$
$$\text{or}$$
$$\text{MAP} = \tfrac{1}{3}\ \text{pulse pressure} + \text{diastolic pressure.}$$

Understanding the arterial waveform

Normal arterial blood pressure produces a characteristic waveform, representing ventricular systole and diastole. The waveform has five distinct components: the anacrotic limb, systolic peak, dicrotic limb, dicrotic notch, and end diastole.

The *anacrotic limb* marks the waveform's initial upstroke, which results as blood is rapidly ejected from the ventricle through the open aortic valve into the aorta. The rapid ejection causes a sharp rise in arterial pressure, which appears as the waveform's highest point. This is called the *systolic peak.*

As blood continues into the peripheral vessels, arterial pressure falls, and the waveform begins a downward trend. This part is called *the dicrotic limb.* Arterial pressure usually will continue to fall until pressure in the ventricle is less than pressure in the

aortic root. When this occurs, the aortic valve closes. The event appears as a small notch (the *dicrotic notch*) on the waveform's downside.

When the aortic valve closes, diastole begins, progressing until the aortic root pressure gradually descends to its lowest point. On the waveform, this is known as *end diastole.*

Normal arterial waveform

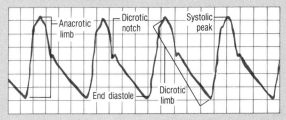

Jan M. Headley, RN, BS, a senior education consultant with Baxter Healthcare Corp., Edwards Critical Care Division, Irvine, Calif., and *Denise Salvo, RN,C, MSN,* clinical faculty member, Widener University, Chester, Pa., contributed to this section. The publisher also thanks the following organizations for their help: *Baxter Healthcare Corp., Edwards Critical Care Division,* Irvine, Calif.; *Doylestown (Pa.) Hospital; Dynatech Nevada,* Carson City, Nev.; *Hewlett Packard,* Waltham, Mass.; and *Hill Rom,* Batesville, Ind.

Recognizing abnormal waveforms

Understanding a normal arterial waveform is relatively straightforward. But an abnormal waveform isn't so easy to decipher. Abnormal patterns and markings, however, may provide important diagnostic clues to the patient's cardiovascular status, or they may simply signal trouble in the monitor. Use this chart to help you recognize and resolve waveform abnormalities.

ABNORMALITY	POSSIBLE CAUSES	NURSING INTERVENTIONS
Alternating high and low waves in a regular pattern	• Ventricular bigeminy	• Check the patient's electrocardiogram (ECG) to confirm ventricular bigeminy. The tracing should reflect premature ventricular contractions every second beat.
Flattened waveform	• Overdamped waveform or hypotensive patient	• Check the patient's blood pressure with a sphygmomanometer. If you obtain a reading, suspect overdamping. Correct the problem by trying to aspirate the arterial line. If you succeed, flush the line. If the reading is very low or absent, suspect hypotension.
Slightly rounded waveform with consistent variations in systolic height	• Patient on ventilator with positive end-expiratory pressure	• Check the patient's systolic blood pressure regularly. The difference between the highest and lowest systolic pressure reading should be less than 10 mm Hg. If the difference exceeds that amount, suspect pulsus paradoxus, possibly from cardiac tamponade.
Slow upstroke	• Aortic stenosis	• Check the patient's heart sounds for signs of aortic stenosis. Also notify the doctor, who will document suspected aortic stenosis in his notes.
Diminished amplitude on inspiration	• Pulsus paradoxus, possibly from cardiac tamponade, constrictive pericarditis, or lung disease	• Note systolic pressure during inspiration and expiration. If inspiratory pressure is at least 10 mm Hg less than expiratory pressure, call the doctor. • If you're also monitoring pulmonary artery pressure, observe for a diastolic plateau. This occurs when the mean central venous pressure (right atrial pressure), mean pulmonary artery pressure, and mean pulmonary capillary wedge pressure (pulmonary artery obstructive pressure) are within 5 mm Hg of one another.
Alteration in beat-to-beat amplitude (in otherwise normal rhythm)	• Pulsus alternans, which may indicate left ventricular failure	• Observe the patient's ECG, noting any deviation in the waveform. • Notify the doctor if this is a new and sudden abnormality.

ASSISTING WITH ARTERIAL LINE INSERTION

An arterial line—the access for invasive arterial pressure monitoring—must be inserted by a doctor. Typically, he'll advance a standard 18G to 20G over-the-needle catheter into a peripheral artery, usually the radial, brachial, or femoral artery. The radial artery is preferred. (See *Choosing an arterial catheter site.*) The line is known commonly as an "art" or "A" line.

Before accessing the radial artery, however, you'll check the patient's ulnar and radial circulation. Why? If the radial artery is blocked by a blood clot (a common complication of arterial lines), the ulnar artery alone must supply blood to the hand. A simple, reliable test of circulation can be done by performing Allen's test, which demonstrates how well both arteries supply blood to the hand.

Choosing an arterial catheter site

When your patient needs hemodynamic monitoring, the doctor will probably insert an arterial catheter in a radial or brachial artery. If these sites are unsuitable, he may insert the catheter in the femoral or dorsalis pedis artery. Here are some advantages and disadvantages to consider for each insertion site.

INSERTION SITE	ADVANTAGES	DISADVANTAGES
Radial artery	• This site is easy to locate. • The ulnar artery provides good collateral circulation to the hand. • The site is easy to observe and maintain. • The area is anatomically stable; the radius acts as a natural splint.	• The artery has a relatively small lumen, so catheter insertion may be difficult and painful. • Pressure readings may be false-high because of the site's distance from the heart.
Brachial artery	• This artery is larger than the radial artery and easily located. • The site is easy to observe and maintain. • Bleeding can usually be prevented or controlled by direct pressure. • Pressure readings may be more accurate because of the site's proximity to the heart.	• Median nerve damage is possible during catheter insertion. • Tissue damage may occur if the artery occludes because of inadequate collateral circulation to the lower arm. • To stabilize the catheter, the patient's elbow must be splinted. This may produce joint stiffness. • Thrombosis may occur if the artery is small (in children and small women) or if the patient has low cardiac output.
Femoral artery	• With its large lumen, this vessel may be the easiest artery to locate and puncture during an emergency. • The site is anatomically stable; the femur acts as a natural splint.	• Catheter insertion may damage the nearby femoral vein and major nerves. • The site poses a high risk of thrombosis. • If the artery occludes, tissue damage is possible because of inadequate collateral circulation. • The catheter is difficult to secure at this site. • Bleeding at this site is difficult to prevent or control. • The insertion site is difficult to bandage and keep clean.
Dorsalis pedis artery	• This site may be used when other sites can't be used because of burns or other injuries.	• The site poses a high risk of thrombosis.

As with other invasive hemodynamic monitoring techniques,
you'll need to set up a pressure
transducer system such as the one
shown at right. You'll also need an
I.V. pole.

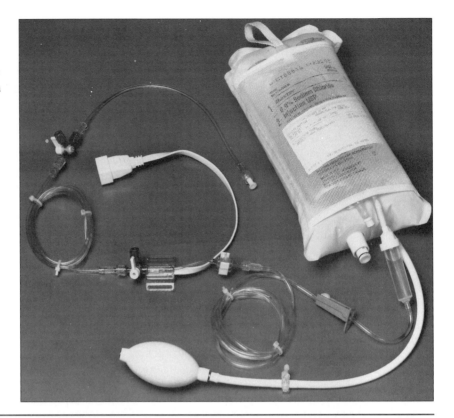

Additional supplies include sterile
gloves (two pairs: one for the doctor, one for you); a local anesthetic
(such as 1% lidocaine, as ordered
by the doctor); a 2″ 18G or 20G
over-the-needle catheter; a 3-ml
syringe with 23G needle for the
local anesthetic; povidone-iodine
solution applicator; a linen-saver
pad; nonallergenic tape; antimicrobial ointment; dry, sterile dressings for the access site, such as
3″ × 3″ or 4″ × 4″ gauze pads or
a transparent dressing, according
to hospital policy; a carpenter's
level; and an armboard. You'll also
need a monitor with arterial pressure capabilities.

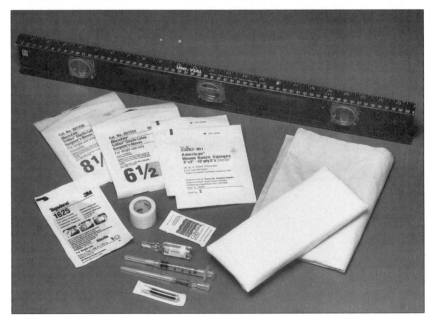

Bring the prepared pressure transducer system to the patient's room, and hang it on an I.V. pole. Insert the arterial pressure module into the monitor if it's not already in place and if you'll be using the manifold mount. Attach the mount to the I.V. pole if it's not already in place, and put the transducer into the mount. Alternatively, you can mount the transducer on the patient's arm. Next, connect the transducer cable to the monitor (as shown). Then level and zero the transducer. (See "Setting up transducers" earlier in this section.)

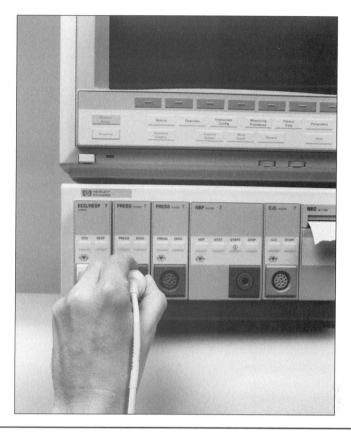

Explain the procedure to the patient. Reassure her that the doctor will use a local anesthetic to minimize discomfort. Position her comfortably, but make sure that the insertion site is level and easily accessible.

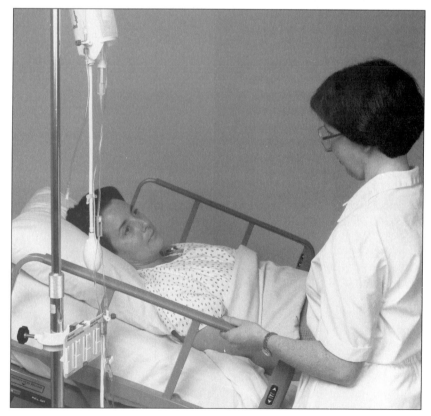

If the radial artery will be used, perform Allen's test now. Elevate the patient's hand, and have her clench and unclench this hand. Next, have her rest her arm. Then, slide a rolled towel under her wrist for support. Ask her to clench her fist while you compress her radial and ulnar arteries for about 1 minute with your fingers. Then, lower her hand.

▶ *Clinical tip:* If your patient can't clench and unclench her hand, assess collateral circulation. Get her palm to blanch by occluding both arteries, elevating her hand, and massaging her palm.

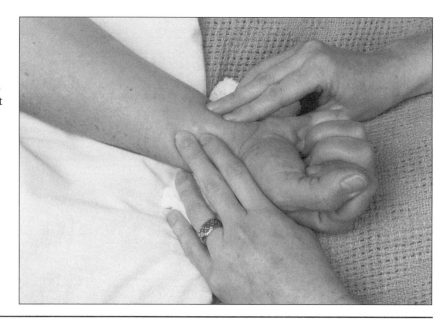

Next, lower the patient's hand. Without removing your fingers from the arteries, ask her to unclench her fist and relax her hand. The palm will appear pale because you've impaired the normal blood flow with your fingers.

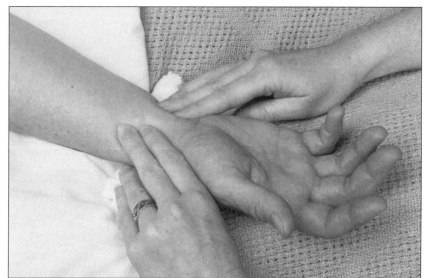

Release the pressure on the ulnar artery, but keep pressure on the radial artery. Observe the palm for a brisk return of color, which should occur within 7 seconds (showing a patent ulnar artery and adequate blood flow to the hands). If color returns in 7 to 15 seconds, blood flow is impaired; if color returns after 15 seconds, consider the flow inadequate.

If blood flow is impaired or inadequate, the radial artery shouldn't be used. At this point, proceed with Allen's test in the other hand. If neither hand colors, the doctor may insert the catheter via the brachial artery.

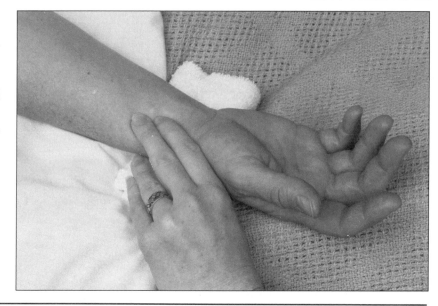

Place a linen-saver pad under the insertion site, and position the site so that it's accessible and easily visible (as shown). Put on sterile gloves and place a sterile towel over the linen-saver pad. The doctor will clean the site, using the povidone-iodine solution applicator (or an equivalent cleaning agent according to hospital policy). As needed, help the doctor prepare the site and perform the procedure.

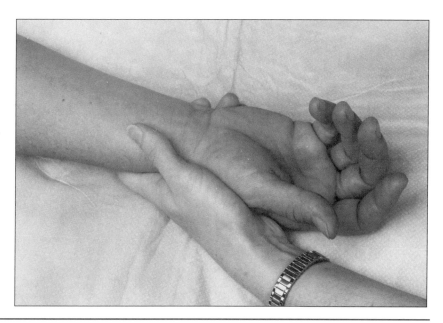

As the insertion nears completion, remove the protective cap from the end of the prepared pressure tubing.

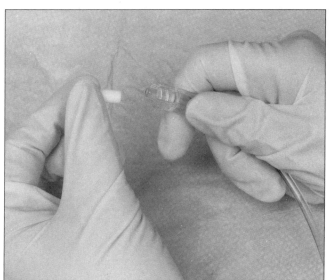

Fast-flush the tubing and, as the doctor stabilizes the catheter hub, immediately connect the tubing to the catheter hub. Fast flushing helps prevent air from entering the system when you connect the tubing to the catheter.

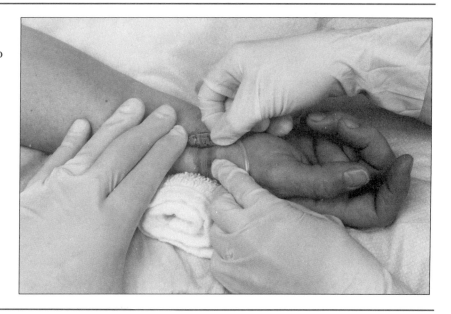

After you connect the tubing, check to make sure that the patient's arterial waveform appears on the monitor.

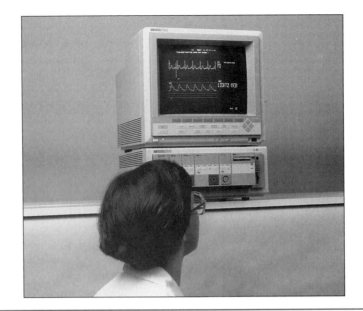

As soon as a proper waveform appears, the doctor will suture the catheter in place. Then either the doctor or nurse (in this instance, the nurse) applies an antibiotic ointment to the site and covers it with a dressing, according to hospital policy. A transparent dressing or 3″ × 3″ or 4″ × 4″ gauze pads and nonallergenic tape (shown here) may be used.

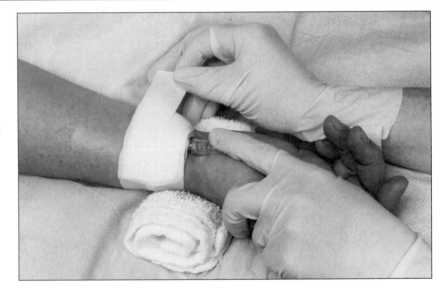

If you applied the dressing, you'll next need to level and zero the transducer. (If the doctor applies the dressing and the transducer is already mounted on the I.V. pole, you can relevel and rezero it while the doctor dresses the catheter site.) You can remove your gloves before this step, if you wish.

Now, recheck the configuration of the arterial waveform. A crisp tracing indicates accurate placement.

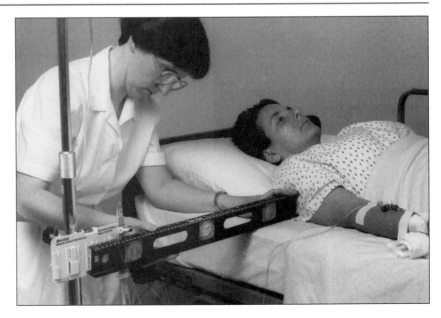

If the transducer is placed on the patient's forearm, loop the pressure tubing around the patient's thumb and attach the transducer, using the strap provided, to her forearm above the catheter insertion site.

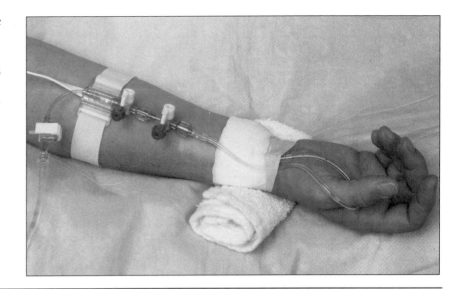

Carefully set the monitor alarms at 20 mm Hg above and below the patient's desired arterial pressure readings. Then measure and record the systolic, diastolic, and mean arterial pressures.

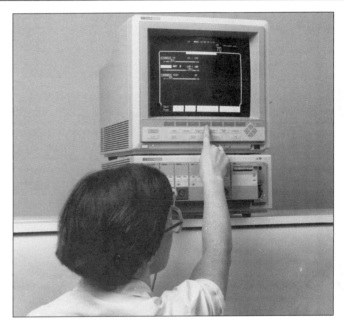

Next, secure the pressure tubing and catheter. To do this, position the patient's hand on an armboard with the palm side up. If needed, place a roll of dressing material or a rolled washcloth under the wrist.

▶ **Clinical tip:** Take care not to hyperextend or dorsiflex the wrist because this can cause neuromuscular injury to the hand or dislodge the catheter.

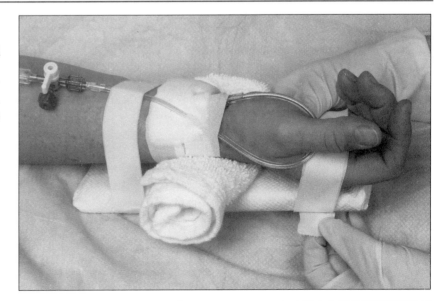

Make sure that the patient's arm is over her bed covers. Instruct her to keep her hand above the covers so that it's easily visible.

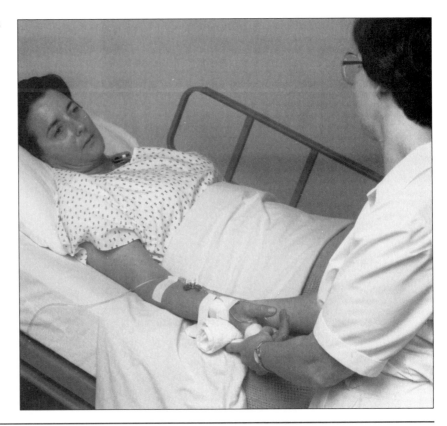

Check the circulation in the patient's hand at least once every 2 hours. Have her tell you if she has any tingling, pain, or numbness in that area. Finally, document the procedure.

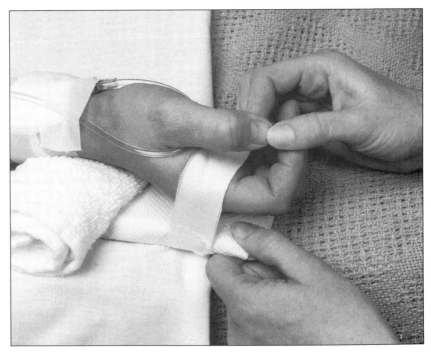

MANAGING AN ARTERIAL LINE

Once the patient's arterial line is secure and the monitor is set up, you'll need to monitor the arterial line and check the system frequently to ensure accurate pressure readings and the patient's comfort and safety. When caring for a patient's arterial line, always use sterile technique, and always observe electrical safety precautions.

Managing an arterial line consists of several patient care procedures, such as taking a cuff pressure, replacing the flush solution, changing both the flush solution and the pressure tubing, and obtaining a blood sample. The type of equipment you'll need depends on which procedure you're performing. (See *Equipment for arterial line management.*)

Equipment for arterial line management

What equipment do you need to manage your patient's arterial line? It all depends on which procedure you're doing. For the procedures noted below, you'll need the pictured items.

Assessing cuff pressure
• Blood pressure cuff and stethoscope

Changing the flush solution and pressure tubing
• Gloves and prepared pressure transducer system

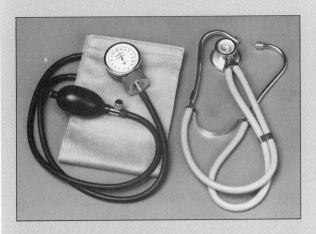

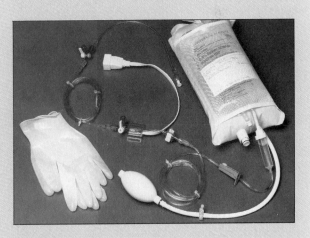

Replacing the flush solution
• A 500-ml bag of heparinized saline solution

Drawing a blood sample
• Gloves, two 5-ml syringes, 20G needle, various color-top laboratory test tubes, and several 3″ × 3″ or 4″ × 4″ sterile gauze pads

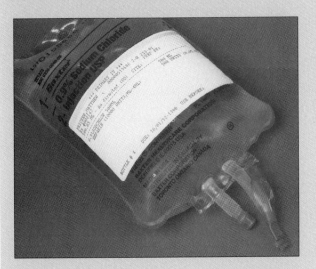

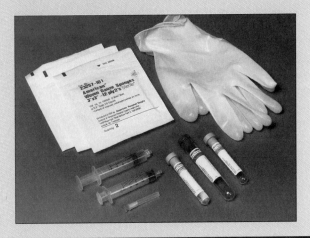

Performing routine assessment and taking a cuff pressure

Monitor the patient's arterial pressure, and assess the appearance of her arterial waveform hourly—or more often if necessary. Also, read and record the digital display of blood pressure values on the monitor, and notify the doctor of any significant changes.

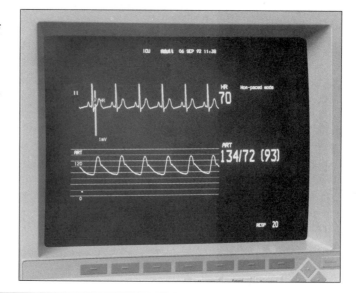

Compare the arterial line pressure with the cuff pressure as often as your hospital policy dictates, but at least once each shift. Expect the direct arterial pressure to be 5 to 15 mm Hg higher than the blood pressure cuff measurement. At the beginning of each shift and after any manipulation of the patient or the system, level and zero the system (see "Setting up transducers" earlier in this section).

▶ *Clinical tip:* Remember, a series of blood pressure measurements over time provides more reliable clinical information than a single isolated measurement.

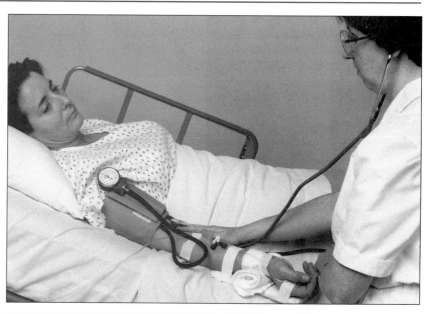

Every 2 to 4 hours, assess the patient's hand on the cannulated side, noting skin color, temperature, and circulation. Also check to ensure that the patient has sensation in the cannulated extremity distal to the insertion site. If the patient states that she's experiencing numbness or tingling (signs of neurovascular compromise), notify the doctor.

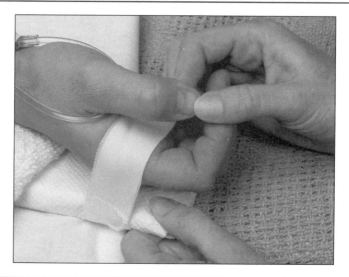

Double-check the integrity of the monitoring system. Be sure to position all stopcocks properly.

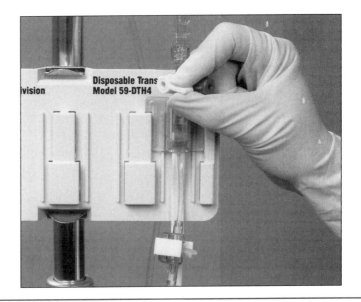

Also be sure to secure all connections (as shown). As you do this, check the waveform for damping and the pressure line to ensure that no air has entered the system.

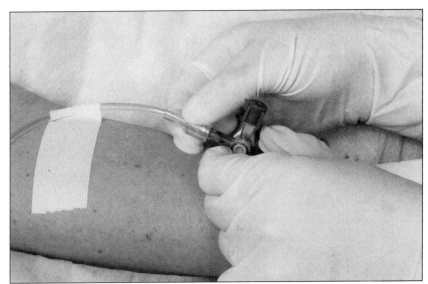

Maintain arterial line patency by flushing the line periodically. Be careful to avoid using excessive pressure, which could cause arteriospasms.

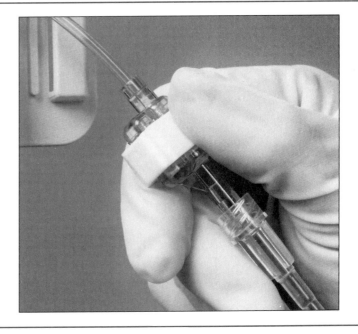

Replacing the flush solution

You may need to replace the flush solution if the flush solution bag leaks or if the I.V. tubing spike is inadvertently disconnected from the flush solution bag. Begin by turning the stopcock off to the patient. This prevents blood from flowing back into the tubing.

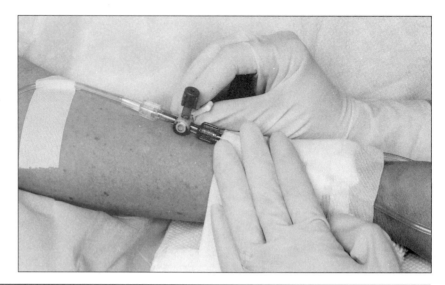

Roll the tubing's flow regulator to the off position.

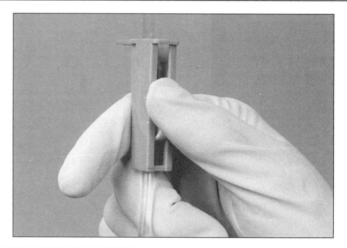

Deflate the pressure infuser bag by opening the valve near the bulb (as shown near right). Then remove the flush solution from the bag (as shown far right).

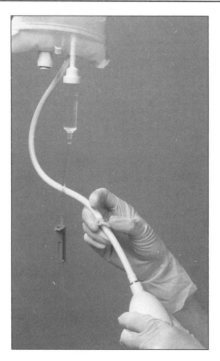
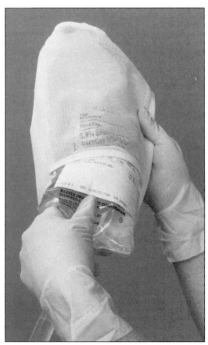

Disconnect the used heparinized flush solution bag, and attach the fresh heparinized flush solution bag to the pressure tubing. Then invert the bag and squeeze it. This forces any air in the bag out through the tubing. Throughout the procedure, take care not to introduce air into the system.

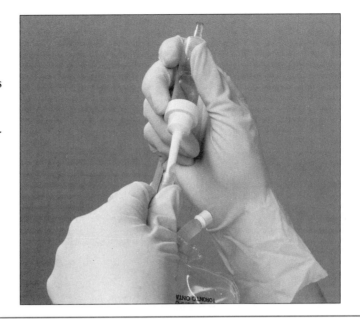

Compress the drip chamber on the new bag until the chamber fills halfway with the flush solution (as shown near right). Then put the bag into the pressure infuser bag, hang the bag on the I.V. pole, and inflate the pressure infuser bag to 300 mm Hg (as shown far right).

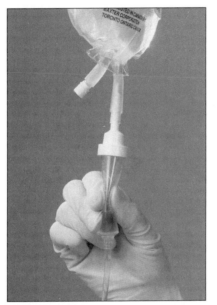
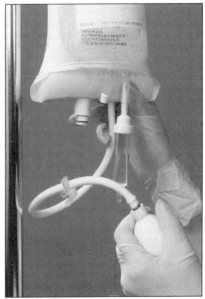

Next, open the pressure tubing's flow regulator and flush the tubing with the new solution. Hold a sterile gauze pad under each stopcock port to catch the expelled solution.

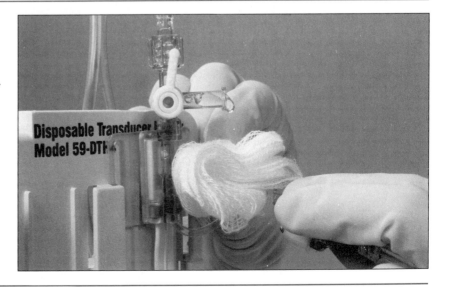

After you've removed all the air, turn each stopcock so that the system is open to the patient (as shown). Replace the occlusive caps on the stopcock ports. If necessary, flush any blood from the tubing.

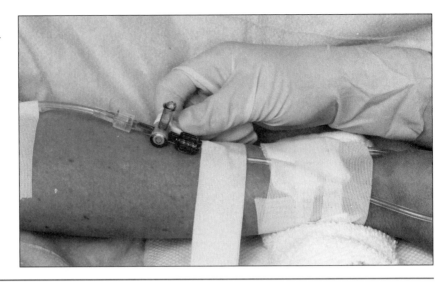

Changing the flush solution and the pressure tubing

As directed by your hospital policy, you'll need to change both the flush solution and the pressure tubing periodically, usually every 48 hours. First, prepare a new pressure transducer system (as described in "Setting up transducers" earlier in this section). Then place a linen-saver pad under the patient's forearm, and put on gloves.

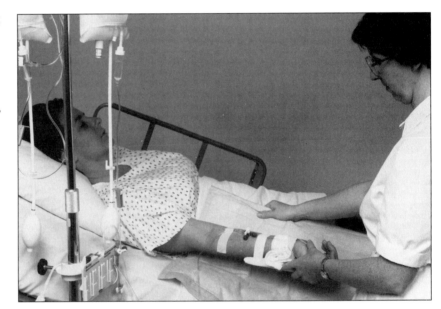

Remove the dressings over the site and examine the site. Next, flush the old system. Then, as you apply pressure to the artery, disconnect the old tubing and quickly screw the new tubing into the catheter hub (as shown). You may want someone to assist by stabilizing the catheter hub as you connect the new tubing. Tighten all connections and redress the site.

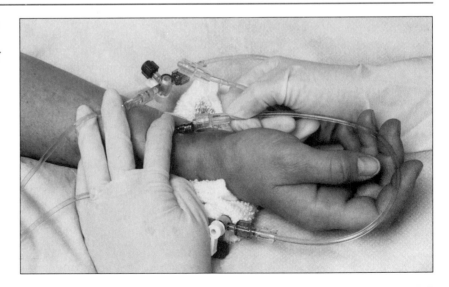

Flush the new system, and attach the transducer cable to the new transducer.

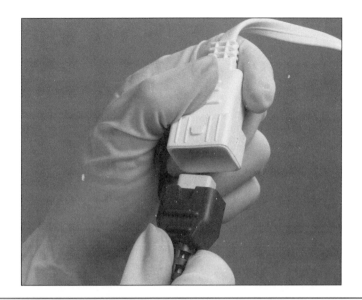

Finally, level and zero the new transducer. Watch for the waveform to appear on the monitor.

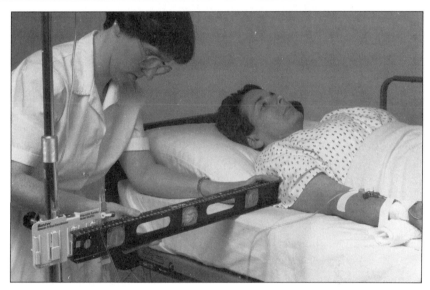

Obtaining a blood sample from an arterial line

Assemble your equipment, wash your hands, and put on gloves. Next, turn off the alarms. Remove the occlusive cap from the stopcock closest to the patient and place it on a 3″ × 3″ or 4″ × 4″ sterile gauze pad. Then insert a 5-ml syringe into the stopcock. Turn the stopcock off to the flush solution and open to the sampling port. Slowly withdraw 3 to 5 ml of blood from the line.

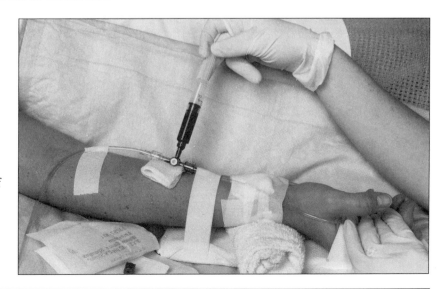

Turn the stopcock halfway back so that it's open to the patient. (This will close the system in all directions.) Finally, remove the syringe and discard this blood according to hospital policy.

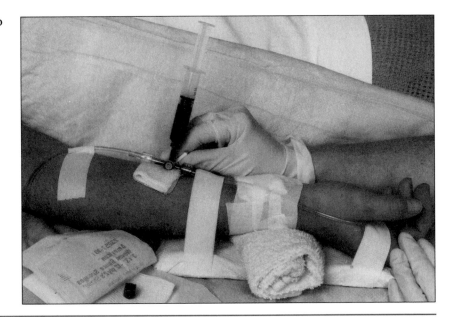

Attach a fresh, sterile 5-ml syringe to the stopcock. Turn the stopcock so that it's open to the sampling port, and draw blood into the syringe. Again, turn the stopcock to the halfway position. Remove the syringe. Attach a 20G needle, and inject the blood into the appropriate color-top tube for the ordered test (as shown).

Then turn the stopcock off to the patient and open to the sampling port. Flush the line. Hold a gauze pad under the port to collect the expelled solution.

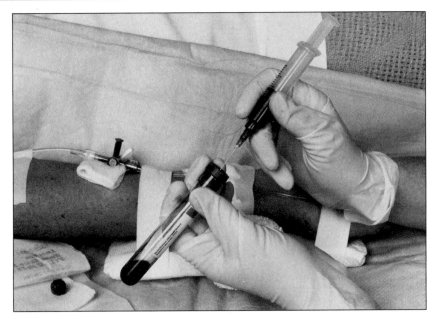

After clearing the port, turn the stopcock off to the port and open to the patient. Reapply the cap to the stopcock port, and flush the entire system. Check to make sure that the waveform is correct, and turn on the alarms. Finally, document the procedure.

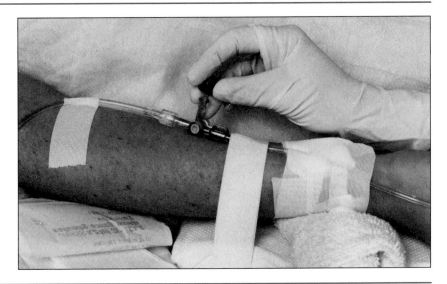

Dealing with problems of arterial lines

When you care for a patient with an arterial line, several problems may interfere with proper functioning of the setup or your ability to interpret a waveform. This chart outlines causes and solutions to some of the most common problems.

PROBLEM	CAUSE	SOLUTION
Damped waveform Appearing as a small waveform with a slow rise in the anacrotic limb and a reduced or nonexistent dicrotic notch, a damped waveform may result from interference with transmission of the physiologic signal to the transducer.	• Air in the system	• Check the system for air, paying particular attention to the tubing and the transducer's diaphragm. If you find air, aspirate it or force it from the system through a stopcock port. Never flush any fluid containing air bubbles into the patient.
	• Loose connection	• Check and tighten all connections.
	• Clotted catheter tip	• Attempt to aspirate the clot. If you're successful, flush the line. If you're not successful, avoid flushing the line; you could dislodge the clot.
	• Catheter tip resting against the arterial wall	• Reposition the catheter insertion area—usually the wrist—and flush the catheter. Or reposition the catheter by carefully rotating it or pulling it back slightly.
	• Kinked tubing	• Unkink the tubing.
	• Inadequately inflated pressure infuser bag	• Inflate the pressure infuser bag to 300 mm Hg.
Drifting waveform Waveform floats above and below the baseline.	• Temperature change in the flush solution	• Allow the temperature of the flush solution to stabilize before infusing it.
	• Kinked or compressed monitor cable	• Check the cable and relieve the kink or compression.
Inability to flush the arterial line or to withdraw blood Activating the continuous flush device fails to move the flush solution, and blood can't be withdrawn from the stopcock.	• Incorrectly positioned stopcocks	• Properly reposition the stopcocks.
	• Kinked tubing	• Unkink the tubing.
	• Inadequately inflated pressure infuser bag	• Inflate the pressure infuser bag to 300 mm Hg.
	• Clotted catheter tip	• Attempt to aspirate the clot. If you're successful, flush the line. If you're not successful, avoid flushing the line; you could dislodge the clot.
	• Catheter tip resting against the arterial wall	• Reposition the catheter insertion area, and flush the catheter. Or reposition the catheter by carefully rotating it or pulling it back slightly.
	• Position of the insertion area	• Check the position of the insertion area, and change it as indicated. For radial and brachial arterial lines, use an armboard to immobilize the area. With a femoral arterial line, keep the head of the bed at a 45-degree angle or less to prevent catheter kinking.
Artifact Waveform tracings follow an erratic pattern or fail to appear as a recognizable diagnostic pattern.	• Electrical interference	• Check electrical equipment in the room.
	• Patient movement	• Ask the patient to lie quietly while you try to read the monitor.
	• Catheter whip or fling (excessive catheter tip movement)	• Shorten the tubing, if possible.

(continued)

Dealing with problems of arterial lines *(continued)*

PROBLEM	CAUSE	SOLUTION
False-high pressure reading Arterial pressure exceeds the patient's normal pressure without a significant change in baseline clinical findings. Before responding to this high pressure, recheck the system to make sure that the reading is accurate.	• Improper calibration	• Recalibrate the system.
	• Transducer positioned below the phlebostatic axis or as indicated	• Relevel the transducer with the phlebostatic axis or as indicated.
	• Catheter kinked	• Unkink the catheter.
	• Clotted catheter tip	• Attempt to aspirate the clot. If you're successful, flush the line. If you're not successful, avoid flushing the line; you could dislodge the clot.
	• Catheter tip resting against the arterial line	• Flush the catheter, or reposition it by carefully rotating it or pulling it back slightly.
	• I.V. tubing too long	• Shorten the tubing by removing extension tubing (if used), or replace the administration set with a set that has shorter tubing.
	• Small air bubbles in tubing close to patient	• Remove air bubbles.
False-low pressure reading Arterial pressure drops below the patient's normal pressure without a significant change in baseline clinical findings. Before responding to this low pressure, recheck the system to ensure that the reading is accurate.	• Improper calibration	• Recalibrate the system.
	• Transducer positioned above the level of the phlebostatic axis or as indicated	• Relevel the transducer with the phlebostatic axis or as indicated.
	• Loose connections	• Check and tighten all connections.
	• Catheter kinked	• Unkink the catheter.
	• Clotted catheter tip	• Attempt to aspirate the clot. If you're successful, flush the line. If you're not successful, avoid flushing the line; you could dislodge the clot.
	• Catheter tip resting against the arterial line	• Reposition the catheter insertion area, and flush the catheter. Or reposition the catheter by carefully rotating it or pulling it back slightly.
	• I.V. tubing too long	• Shorten the tubing by removing the extension tubing (if used), or replace the administration set with a set having shorter tubing.
	• Large air bubble close to the transducer	• Reprime the transducer.
No waveform No waveform appears on the monitor.	• No power supply	• Turn on the power.
	• Loose connections	• Check and tighten all connections.
	• Stopcocks turned off to the patient	• Position the stopcocks properly. Make sure that the transducer is open to the catheter.
	• Transducer disconnected from the monitor module	• Reconnect the transducer to the monitor module.
	• Occluded catheter tip	• Attempt to aspirate the clot. If you're successful, flush the line. If you're not successful, avoid flushing the line; you could dislodge the clot.
	• Catheter tip resting against the arterial wall	• Flush the catheter, or reposition it by carefully rotating it or pulling it back slightly.

Minimizing risks of arterial lines

For most critically ill patients, the advantages of arterial lines overcome the disadvantages. However, because any invasive hemodynamic monitoring procedure poses some risk, you'll need to watch your patient for complications that may result from an arterial line. This summary of major complications covers causes, effective responses, and tips for prevention.

COMPLICATIONS AND SIGNS AND SYMPTOMS	POSSIBLE CAUSES	NURSING INTERVENTIONS	PREVENTION
Thrombosis • Loss or weakening of pulse below arterial line insertion site • Loss of warmth, sensation, and mobility in limb below insertion site • Damped or straight waveform on monitor display or printout	• Arterial damage during or after insertion • Sluggish flush solution flow rate • Failure to heparinize flush solution adequately • Failure to flush catheter routinely and after withdrawing blood samples • Irrigation of clotted catheter with a syringe	• Notify the doctor. He may remove the line. • Document the complication and record your interventions.	• Check the patient's pulse rate immediately after catheter insertion, then once hourly. • Reduce injury to the artery by splinting the limb holding the line and by taping the catheter securely. • Check the flush solution's flow rate hourly; maintain the rate at 3 to 4 ml/hour. • Heparinize the flush solution according to hospital policy. • Flush the catheter once hourly and after withdrawing blood samples. • Never irrigate an arterial catheter. You may flush a blood clot into the bloodstream.
Blood loss • Bloody dressing; blood flowing from disconnected line	• Dislodged catheter • Disconnected line	• Stop the bleeding. • Check the patient's vital signs. • Notify the doctor if blood loss is great or if the patient's vital signs change. • If the line is disconnected, avoid reconnecting it. Instead, immediately replace contaminated equipment. • If the catheter is pulled out of the vein, remove it and apply direct pressure to the site; then notify the doctor. • When the bleeding stops, check the patient's pulse and the insertion site frequently for signs of thrombosis or hematoma. • Document the complication and your interventions.	• Check the line connections and insertion site frequently. • Tape the catheter securely and splint the patient's limb.
Air embolism or thromboembolism • Drop in blood pressure • Rise in central venous pressure • Weak, rapid pulse • Cyanosis • Loss of consciousness • Damped waveform	• Air in tubing • Loose connections	• Place the patient on his left side and in Trendelenburg's position. If air has entered the heart chambers, this position may keep the air on the heart's right side. The pulmonary artery can then absorb the small air bubbles. • Check the arterial line for leaks. • Notify the doctor immediately, and check the patient's vital signs. • Administer oxygen, if ordered. • Document the complication and your interventions.	• Expel all air from the line before connecting it to the patient. • Make sure that all connections are secure; then check connections routinely. • Change the flush solution bag before it empties. • Prevent thromboembolism by keeping the arterial line patent with heparinized flush solution.

(continued)

Minimizing risks of arterial lines (continued)

COMPLICATIONS AND SIGNS AND SYMPTOMS	POSSIBLE CAUSES	NURSING INTERVENTIONS	PREVENTION
Systemic infection • Sudden rise in temperature and pulse rate • Chills and shaking • Blood pressure changes	• Poor aseptic technique • Equipment contaminated during manufacture, storage, or use • Irrigation of clotted catheter	• Look for other sources of infection first. Obtain urine, sputum, and blood specimens for cultures and other analyses, as ordered. • Notify the doctor. He may discontinue the line and send the equipment to the laboratory for study. • Document the complication and record your interventions.	• Review care procedures and ensure aseptic technique. • Take care not to contaminate the arterial line insertion site when bathing the patient. • If any part of the line disconnects accidentally, don't rejoin it. Instead, replace the parts with sterile equipment. • Change system components as recommended: I.V. flush solution and pressure tubing every 48 hours, transparent dressing every 7 days, nontransparent dressing every 24 to 48 hours, and catheter every 72 hours.
Arterial spasm • Intermittent loss or weakening of pulse below insertion site • Irregular waveform on monitor screen or printout	• Trauma to vessel during catheter insertion • Artery irritated by catheter after insertion	• Notify the doctor. • Prepare lidocaine, which the doctor may inject directly into the arterial catheter to relieve the spasm. *Caution:* Make sure that the lidocaine doesn't contain epinephrine, which could cause further arterial constriction. • Document the complication as well as your interventions.	• Tape the catheter securely to prevent it from moving in the artery. • Splint the patient's limb to stabilize the catheter.
Hematoma • Swelling at insertion site and generalized swelling of limb holding the arterial line • Bleeding at site	• Blood leakage around the catheter (resulting from weakened or damaged artery) • Failure to maintain pressure at site after removing catheter	• Stop the bleeding. • If the hematoma appears while the catheter is in place, notify the doctor. • If the hematoma appears within 30 minutes after you remove the catheter, apply ice to the site. Otherwise, apply warm, moist compresses to help speed the hematoma's absorption. • Document the complication and record your interventions.	• Tape the catheter securely and splint the insertion area to prevent damage to the artery. • After the catheter is removed, apply firm, manual pressure over the site for about 10 minutes or until bleeding stops. Then apply a pressure bandage.
Inaccurate pressure readings • Patient's clinical appearance inconsistent with pressure values	*False-high values* • Transducer positioned too low • Small air bubbles in arterial line *False-low values* • Transducer positioned too high • Large air bubble in arterial line	• Relevel and rezero the transducer system. • Remove air bubbles. • Relevel and rezero the transducer system. • Remove air bubble. • Document the complication and record your interventions.	• Be sure to zero and calibrate the transducer system precisely. • Properly level the transducer at the level of the patient's right atrium (the phlebostatic axis). • Keep air from entering the pressure tubing or system. • Check the arterial waveform configuration for abnormalities.

What to do about a displaced arterial line

Your patient is in danger of hypovolemic shock from blood loss if his arterial line is pulled out or otherwise displaced. Follow these steps to avert serious complications.

What to do first
• Immediately apply direct pressure at the insertion site, and have someone summon the doctor. Because arterial blood flows under high intravascular pressure, be certain to maintain firm, direct pressure for 5 to 10 minutes to encourage clot formation at the insertion site.
• Check the patient's I.V. line and, if ordered, increase the flow rate temporarily to compensate for blood loss.

After the bleeding stops
• Apply a sterile pressure dressing.
• Reassess the patient's level of consciousness (LOC) and orientation, and offer reassurance.
• Estimate the amount of blood loss from your observations of the blood and from the changes in the patient's blood pressure and heart rate.
• Assist the doctor as he reinserts the catheter. Ensure that the patient's arm is immobilized and that the tubing and catheter are secure.
• Withdraw blood for a complete blood count and arterial blood gas analysis, as ordered.

Ongoing care
• Frequently assess the patient's vital signs, LOC, skin color and temperature, and circulation at the insertion site and beyond.
• Watch for further bleeding or hematoma formation at the insertion site.
• Once the patient's condition stabilizes, reduce the I.V. flow rate to the previous keep-vein-open level.

REMOVING AN ARTERIAL LINE

As a nurse, you're usually responsible for removing an arterial catheter and applying a dressing. Both procedures require sterile technique. After you remove the catheter, keep pressure on the site until bleeding stops completely—otherwise, hemorrhage could result. Then, before applying the pressure dressing, inspect the site again to ensure against recurrent bleeding.

To begin, you'll need sterile gloves (two pairs); a sterile suture set; 3″ × 3″ or 4″ × 4″ sterile gauze pads; and 2″ nonallergenic tape or a large, cloth adhesive bandage.

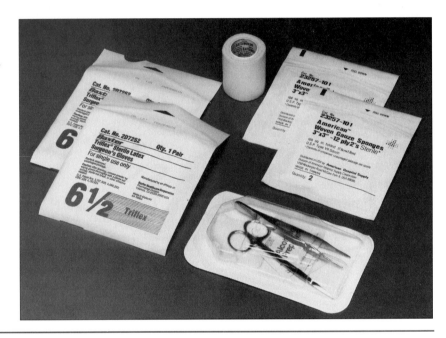

Explain the procedure to the patient. Turn off the arterial line monitor alarms but not the electrocardiogram monitor or other alarms.

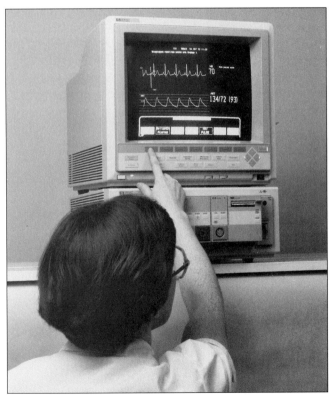

Put on the first pair of gloves. Turn the stopcock closest to the patient to the off position.

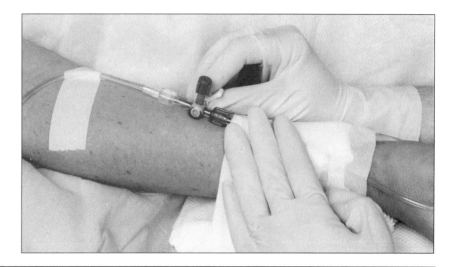

Remove the dressing, and cut and remove the sutures.

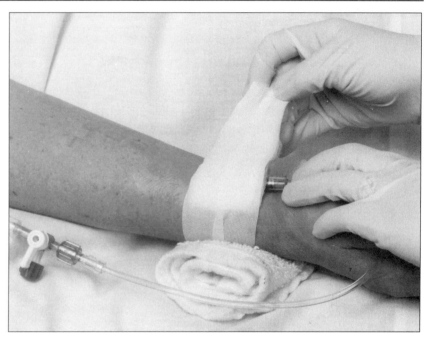

After removing the sutures, gently and quickly pull out the arterial catheter with one hand. At the same time, use the other hand to apply direct pressure to the insertion site with a 3″ × 3″ or 4″ × 4″ sterile gauze pad.

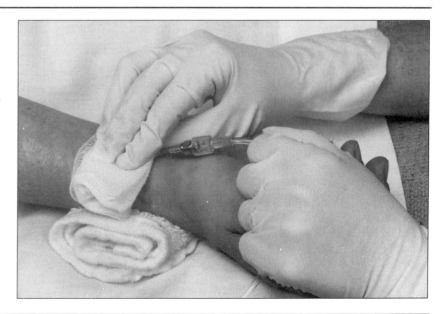

Press firmly on the site for 5 to 10 minutes or until the bleeding stops. If bleeding persists for longer than 15 minutes, notify the doctor.

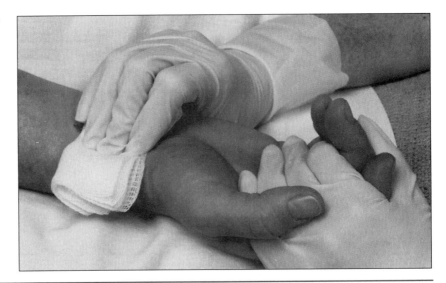

Once the bleeding stops, put on a new pair of sterile gloves. Apply a small, sterile pressure dressing to the site. Be sure to place the tape no more than three quarters of the way around the arm (as shown). Assess perfusion at the insertion site and beyond, as well as the dressing's integrity. Then dispose of the equipment according to hospital policy, and document the procedure.

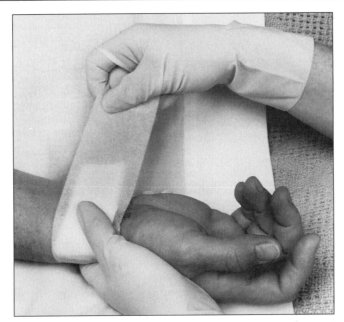

Place the patient's arm above the bed covers (as shown), and instruct the patient to keep the site above the bed covers and in clear view for at least 1 hour to ensure prompt detection of bleeding. Check the site frequently for bleeding, which may recur if the seal over the puncture site breaks.

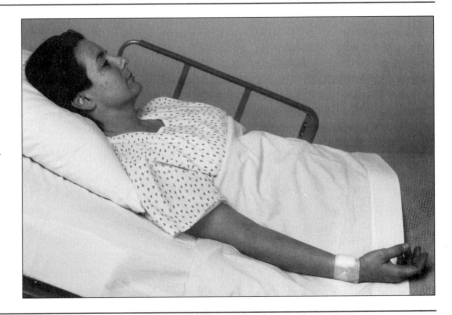

LEARNING ABOUT PULMONARY ARTERY CATHETERIZATION

Pulmonary artery catheterization can help you learn about a patient's cardiovascular and pulmonary status, obtain blood samples, and infuse solutions. With a basic pulmonary artery catheter, you can measure intracardiac pressure, pulmonary artery pressure (PAP), and cardiac output. This kind of catheter has two lumens, a balloon-inflation valve, and a thermistor.

The *distal lumen* opens into the pulmonary artery. When attached to a transducer, it allows you to measure pulmonary artery wedge pressure (PAWP) — also called pulmonary capillary wedge pressure or, sometimes, pulmonary artery obstructive pressure. The distal lumen hub is usually yellow or marked PA DISTAL.

The *proximal lumen* opens into the right atrium or the vena cava, depending on the size of the patient's heart. This lumen measures the pressure in the right atrium. It also delivers the bolus of injectate used to measure cardiac output and functions as a route for fluid infusion. The hub is usually blue or marked INJECTATE or PROXIMAL.

The *balloon-inflation valve* functions as the access point for inflating the balloon at the distal tip of the catheter for PAWP measurement.

The *thermistor*, which lies about 4 cm from the distal tip of the catheter, measures core body temperature. When connected to a cardiac output monitor, the thermistor measures temperature changes related to cardiac output.

With more sophisticated multilumen catheters, you can continuously monitor mixed venous oxygen saturation levels, intermittently measure the right ventricular volume and ejection fractions, and initiate atrial, ventricular, or atrioventricular sequential pacings.

Inserted by the doctor in the internal jugular, subclavian, femoral, or brachial vein, the catheter has a balloon tip and is flow directed, allowing venous circulation to carry it through the right atrium and ventricle to the pulmonary artery. (See *Insertion sites for a pulmonary artery catheter.*) To evaluate catheter placement, you'll set up a monitoring system and evaluate the waveforms.

Insertion sites for a pulmonary artery catheter

The most common sites for percutaneous insertion of a pulmonary artery catheter are the right internal jugular, the subclavian, and the femoral veins. The doctor may also insert a pulmonary artery catheter into the brachial vein, but this approach requires incising the vein in a cutdown procedure.

The right internal jugular is considered the safest insertion site. Although the subclavian vein is easily accessed, its use carries certain risks. The most significant risk is pneumothorax, resulting from puncturing the lung at a level above the clavicle during catheter insertion. Additionally, using the subclavian vein may cause the catheter or the introducer to bend or kink during insertion.

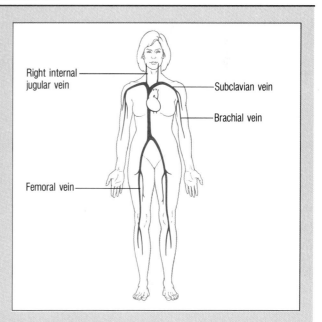

Right internal jugular vein

Subclavian vein

Brachial vein

Femoral vein

Jan M. Headley, RN, BS, who contributed to this section, is a senior education consultant with Baxter Healthcare Corp., Edwards Critical-Care Division, Irvine, Calif. The publisher thanks the following organizations for their help: *Baxter Healthcare Corp.,* Irvine, Calif.; *Doylestown (Pa.) Hospital; Dynatech Nevada Inc.,* Carson City, Nev.; *Hewlett-Packard Co.,* Waltham, Mass.; and *Hill-Rom,* Batesville, Ind.

PREPARING FOR CATHETER INSERTION

Begin by checking the doctor's order, which indicates why the patient needs catheterization. This information will help you select the appropriate catheter, such as the basic thermodilution pulmonary artery catheter. Choose a catheter of the proper size (for most adults, a #7.5 French). Next, make sure that the sterilization date on the catheter package hasn't expired. If the doctor will insert the catheter percutaneously, you'll also need to obtain an introducer.

▶ **Clinical tip:** Check the manufacturer's recommendations when choosing an introducer. Typically, it will be a half size larger than the catheter. This guards against damaging the balloon tip during insertion. However, if you expect to infuse a large volume of fluid through the catheter's side port, select an introducer that's a full size larger than the catheter. The additional space between the catheter and introducer allows for easier fluid infusion.

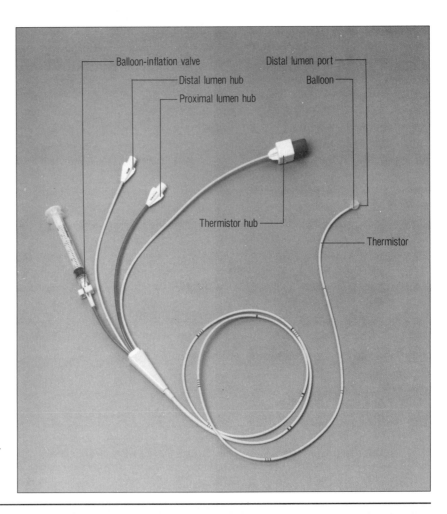

You'll also need a sterile introducer kit that contains a sterile contamination sheath. In addition, gather a sterile basin, sterile water or 0.9% sodium chloride solution, sterile and clean gloves, a face shield (or eye goggles and mask), one or more sterile gowns (depending on hospital policy), sterile drapes, povidone-iodine swabs, sutures, povidone-iodine ointment, sterile 3″ × 3″ and 4″ × 4″ gauze pads, hypoallergenic tape, a marking pen, a carpenter's level or ruler, a clean towel (optional), and lidocaine (optional).

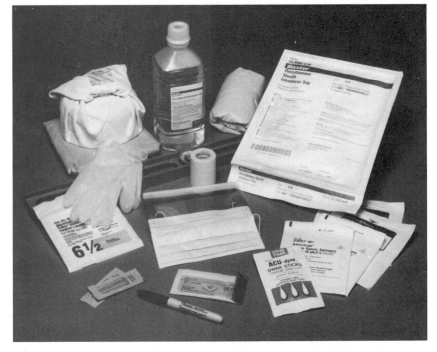

After you assemble the equipment for placing the catheter, set up the system for monitoring arterial pressures once the catheter is inserted. To monitor pulmonary artery and intermittent right atrial pressures, you'll need at least one pressure transducer and flush system (as shown). However, to continuously monitor right atrial pressure (or central venous pressure), add a second transducer and flush system to the original setup. If you think you'll need an extra pair of clean gloves, obtain them now.

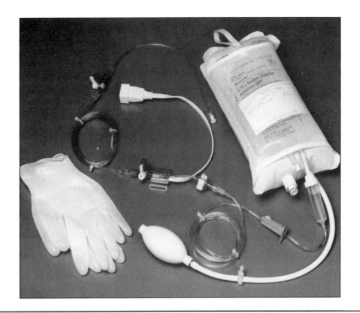

Place the crash cart close to the patient's bed in case of an emergency.

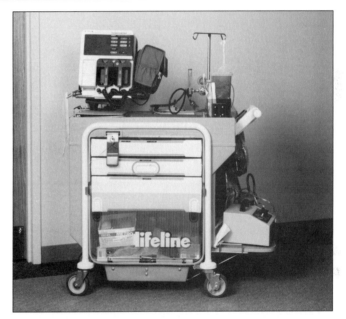

Turn on the patient's bedside monitor to give it time to warm up enough to display the waveforms accurately. (Check the manufacturer's instructions; some monitors require up to 20 minutes.) Also make sure that the monitor has the number of pressure modules needed to monitor the pressures required.

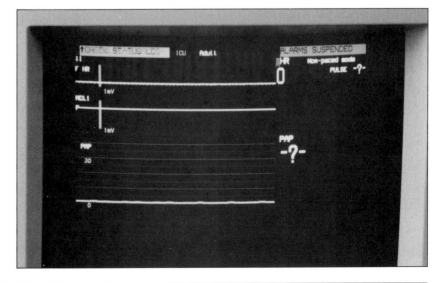

Explain the procedure to the patient and his family, and check that the patient has given informed consent for the procedure. Then take the patient's vital signs and assess cardiac rhythm.

Caution: Although pulmonary artery catheter insertion has no contraindications, patients who have a left bundle-branch block risk developing a right bundle-branch block. In such a situation, be prepared to assist with emergency pacing.

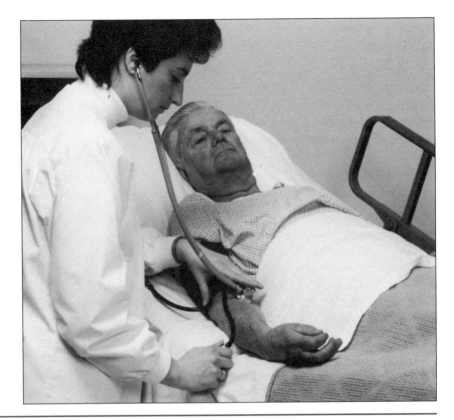

Before catheter insertion, ensure accurate pressure readings by positioning the transducer at the phlebostatic axis—the patient's fourth intercostal space and the midpoint between the anterior and posterior chest wall. (Because PAPs indirectly reflect left atrial pressures, the zero point should be level with the left atrium.) Position the transducer's air-fluid interface (located at the vent, or zero, port of the transducer's stopcock) level with this point (as shown). The head of the patient's bed may be flat or elevated.

▷ *Clinical tip:* Take care to position the transducer precisely. If the vent port is too low, pressure readings will be falsely elevated. Conversely, if the vent port is too high, pressure readings will be falsely low.

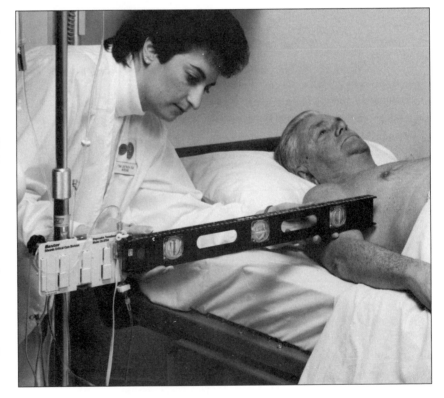

Put a piece of tape on the patient's chest, and use a marking pen to pinpoint the phlebostatic axis on the tape or the patient's chest. This marking allows every nurse to use the same reference point when obtaining pressure readings.

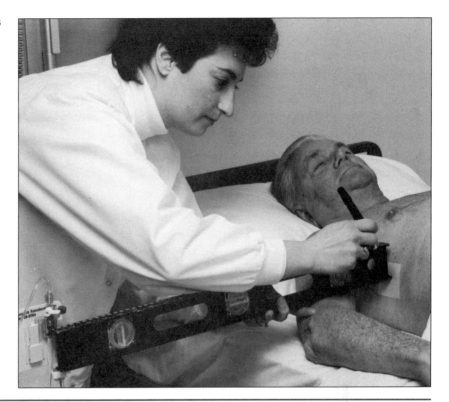

Next, remove the cap from the vent port. Then turn the stopcock off to the patient, thereby opening the transducer to air.

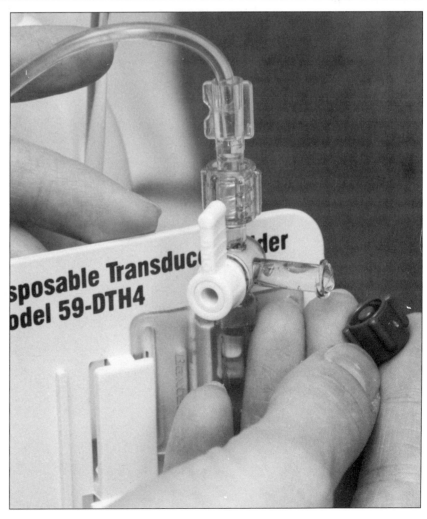

Press the ZERO button on the monitor. Then press the CALIBRATE button according to the directions supplied by the manufacturer. Keep in mind that some monitors require manipulation of a calibration button or knob and some monitors calibrate automatically.

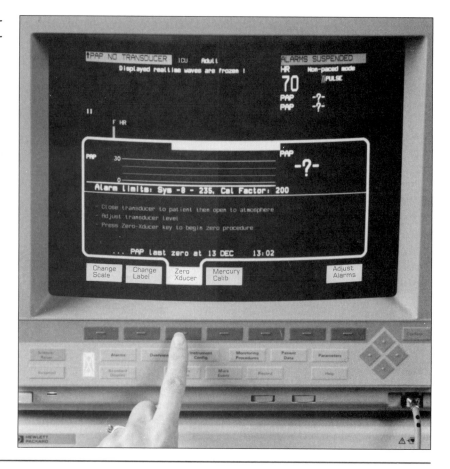

Following the manufacturer's instructions, select the appropriate mode and scale—for example, a mean pressure mode and a scale of 0 to 30 or 0 to 60 mm Hg. Keep in mind that larger scales may produce small waveforms that are difficult to read.

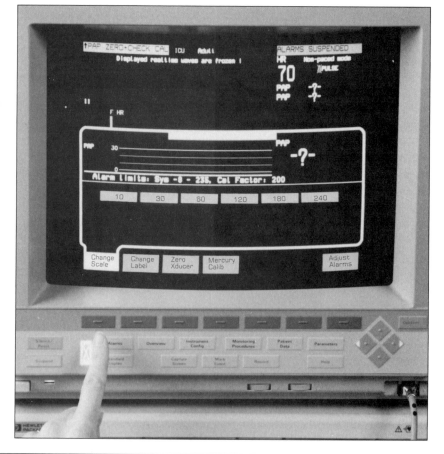

ASSISTING WITH CATHETER INSERTION

Roll an overbed table to the same side of the bed as the insertion site. Use this area to create a sterile field. Bring all of the equipment you assembled for insertion to this area.

Note: Insertion procedures may remain constant even with different insertion sites. The following steps focus on insertion through the subclavian vein.

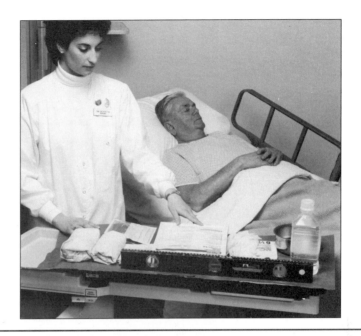

Have the patient lie on his back without a pillow. Adjust the bed to the desired height, and place the patient in a slight Trendelenburg's position. If necessary to help the doctor locate the insertion site, place a rolled towel under the patient's scapula.

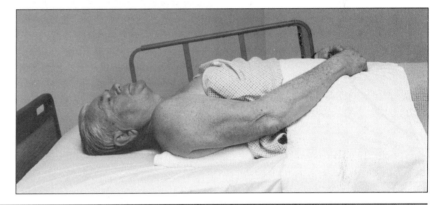

While the doctor puts on a face shield (or goggles and mask), sterile gown, and sterile gloves, you'll need to put on a face shield (or goggles and mask), a gown, and clean gloves. Throughout the procedure, observe universal precautions.

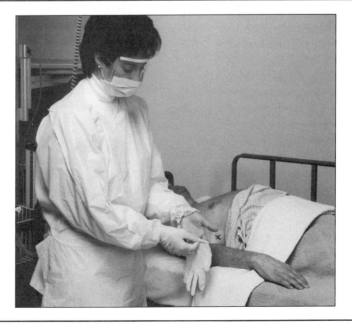

As the doctor cleans the insertion site with povidone-iodine swabs (or ointment) and drapes the insertion area, position the patient's face away from the insertion site. This keeps the patient from breathing on and contaminating the site. It also facilitates insertion of the catheter.

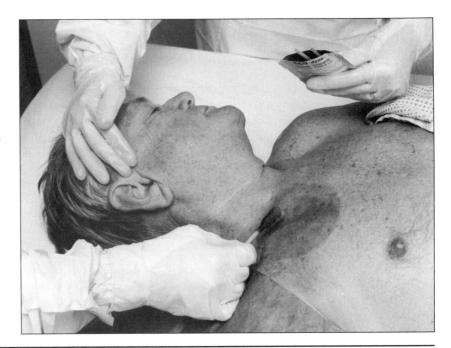

Maintaining sterile technique, assist with opening the prepackaged introducer and with its insertion. Continuing to maintain sterile technique, open the outer wrapping of the pulmonary artery catheter, positioning it so that the doctor can remove the inner sterile package. After the doctor opens the inner wrapping, prepares the catheter insertion tray, and applies the contamination sheath, he'll hand you the lumen hubs. Be sure to touch only the hubs of the catheter.

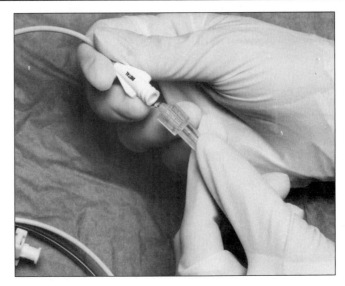

Continuing to use sterile technique, connect the pressure tubing to the distal catheter lumens. Using the pressure tubing fast-flush device, flush the lumen. (You may use a syringe containing sterile heparinized flush solution or a sterile I.V. setup to flush the proximal lumen before connecting the pressure tubing.)

Note: If you're using multiple-pressure lines, make sure that the distal lumen is attached to the line that will reflect pressure on the monitor screen. If it isn't, you won't obtain the correct waveform.

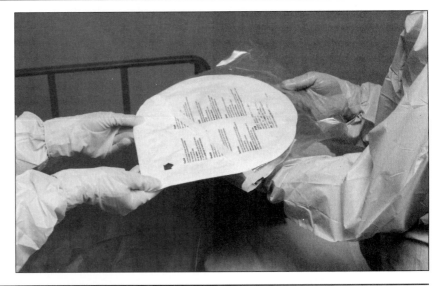

Before inserting the catheter, the doctor will inflate the balloon with air to ensure its integrity. Inspect the inflated balloon for symmetrical shape. Pour sterile water or 0.9% sodium chloride solution into a small sterile basin so that the doctor can submerge the balloon to check for bubbles indicating a leak.

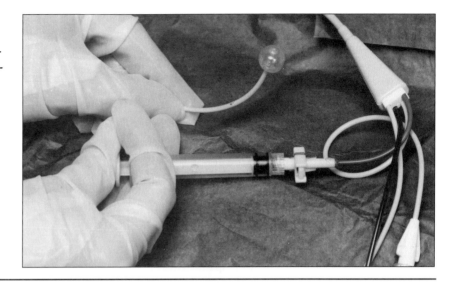

After deflating the balloon, the doctor will insert the catheter through the introducer and gently advance the catheter 15 to 20 cm to a point marked on the catheter by two black bands. At this distance, the catheter should have exited the end of the introducer sheath and be near the junction of the superior vena cava and right atrium. The monitor should display oscillations consistent with the patient's respirations. If the patient is awake, have him cough or take some deep breaths to enhance the oscillations.

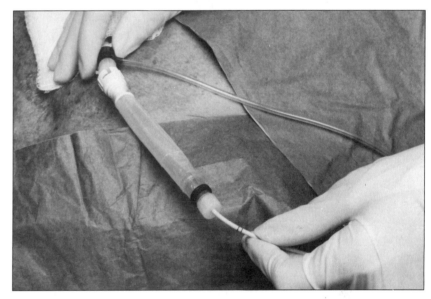

As ordered, use the volume-limited 3-cc syringe in the pulmonary artery catheter package to inflate the balloon. Verify the maximum balloon inflation volume printed on the shaft of the catheter. Typically, you'll use 1.5 cc of air for a #7.5 French catheter. Avoid overinflating the balloon, which causes the balloon to lose elasticity or to rupture.

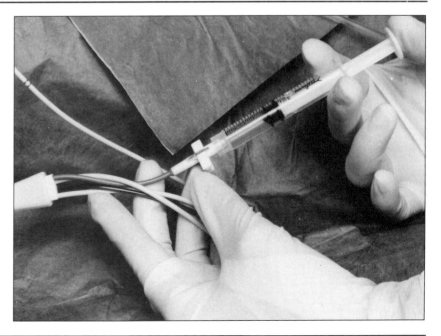

To keep the balloon inflated, close the red gate valve (or the appropriate stopcock) on the catheter (as shown).

Note: Insertion is the only time you'll use this valve or stopcock to keep the balloon inflated.

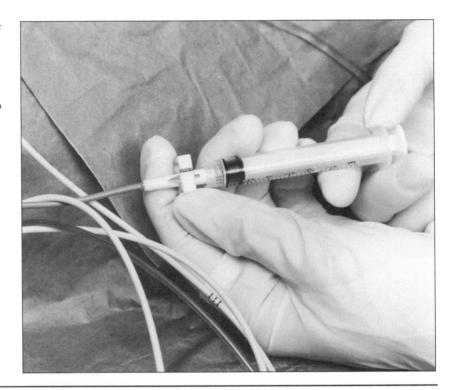

As the doctor advances the catheter, monitor waveforms, pressure values (which provide evidence of the catheter's location), and electrocardiogram tracings. If possible, obtain printed waveforms for each chamber. Watch closely for the waveform indicating that the catheter has advanced between 20 and 25 cm to the right atrium (as shown). Typically, you'll see two small waves for each PQRST complex. You should also observe a normal mean pressure ranging between 2 and 6 mm Hg.

Note: Pressure ranges cited in this section reflect standards accepted by the American Association of Critical-Care Nurses (AACN) and published in the AACN's 1991 *Core Curriculum for Critical Care Nursing.*

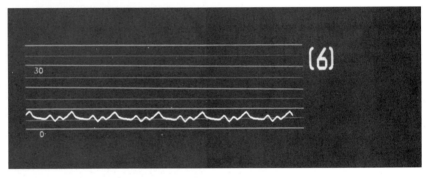

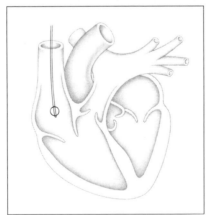

When the catheter advances 30 to 35 cm, its tip should enter the right ventricle. Watch for a right ventricular waveform, such as the one shown at right. Also keep track of pressure values. Normal systolic pressure ranges from 20 to 30 mm Hg; normal diastolic pressure, from 0 to 5 mm Hg. Pay particular attention to the diastolic pressure. An increase indicates that the catheter has advanced into the pulmonary artery.

▶ *Clinical tip:* Keep a bolus of lidocaine handy and remain alert for ventricular ectopy when the catheter enters the right ventricle. Usually, ventricular irritability subsides when the catheter tip reaches the pulmonary artery. If not, the doctor may withdraw the catheter or order lidocaine.

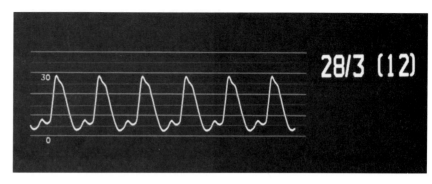

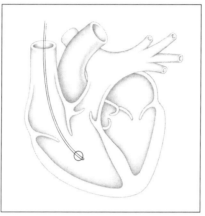

Continue watching the monitor for a waveform showing that the catheter has advanced 35 to 40 cm into the pulmonary artery. You should see a smooth upstroke (reflecting systole) and a downstroke (representing diastole) and a dicrotic notch resulting from the pulmonic valve closing. The closed valve also accounts for the higher diastolic pressure ranges. Normally, PAPs range as follows: systolic, 20 to 30 mm Hg; diastolic, 10 to 20 mm Hg; and mean, 10 to 15 mm Hg.

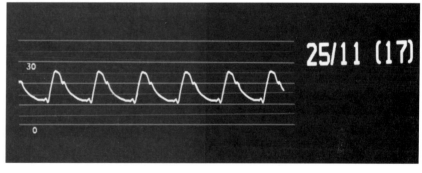

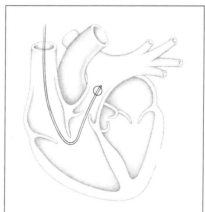

Seeing catheter markings between 40 and 50 cm at the insertion site indicates that the circulation has carried the catheter tip to a distal branch of the pulmonary artery. Now, you can assess the PAWP, derived from the inflated balloon wedged in this area. Because the balloon occludes blood flow from the pulmonary artery and the right side of the heart, the waveform and pressure values reflect pressure in the left atrium. At this point, the normal mean pressure ranges between 6 and 12 mm Hg.

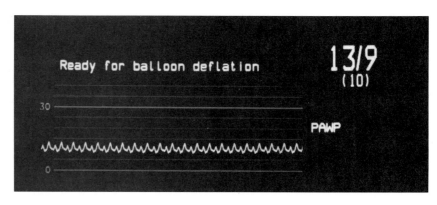

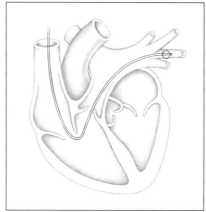

After noting this pressure, unlock the gate valve and detach the syringe. This allows the balloon to deflate passively. Never aspirate air to deflate the balloon. Doing so could cause the balloon to lose elasticity.

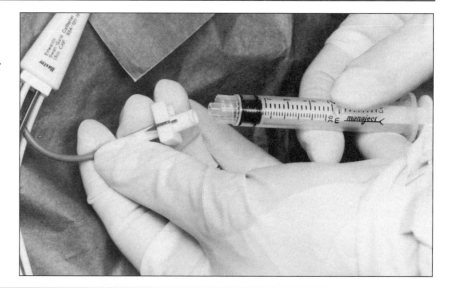

To ensure that the balloon has deflated, observe the monitor for the return of the PAP waveform (as shown).

Caution: Leaving the balloon inflated for a prolonged time could result in a pulmonary infarction.

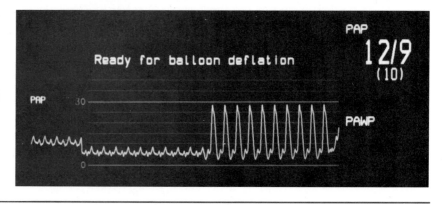

Next, the doctor will withdraw the catheter between 1 and 2 cm to remove any loop that may have formed in the right ventricle, decreasing the chance for catheter migration.

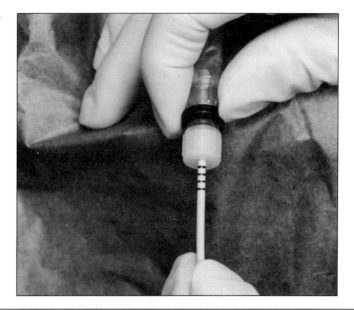

Slowly reinflate the balloon until you again obtain a PAWP waveform. Note the amount of air required to obtain the tracing; it should still be 1.5 cc.

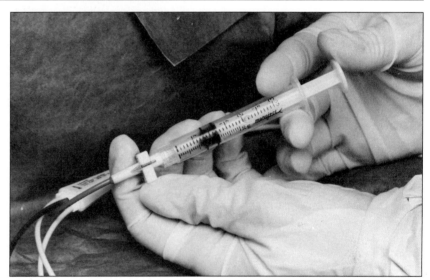

Once you're sure that the catheter is properly positioned, remove the syringe and allow the balloon to deflate passively. Again check the monitor for resumption of the PAP waveform. If the doctor hasn't already sutured the introducer in place, he usually does so now.

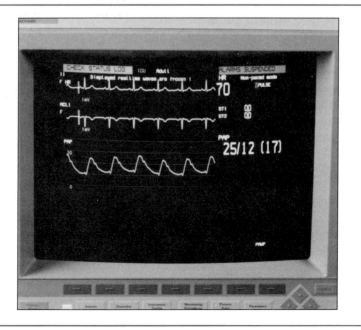

Take off your clean gloves, and put on sterile gloves to apply a sterile, occlusive dressing over the insertion site. Arrange for a bedside chest X-ray to verify correct catheter placement.

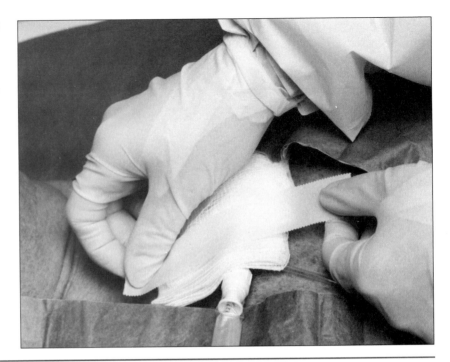

Document the procedure, noting the date and time, the insertion site, the doctor who inserted the catheter, the type of dressing applied, the concentration of the heparinized flush solution, and the patient's tolerance of the procedure. Also document the pressures and waveforms obtained for each heart chamber during insertion. Record whether any arrhythmias occurred during or after insertion, and note the volume of air required to obtain a PAWP tracing.

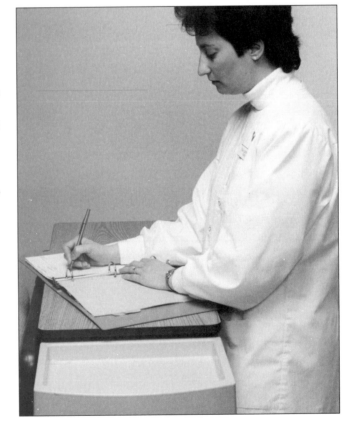

MANAGING A PULMONARY ARTERY LINE

When your patient has a pulmonary artery line, your responsibilities include caring for the catheter insertion site and the catheter as well as monitoring pulmonary artery pressure (PAP), right atrial pressure (RAP), and pulmonary artery wedge pressure (PAWP).

You'll change the dressing according to hospital policy (usually every 24 hours), observe the site for infection and catheter slippage or kinking, and document these procedures.

How often you'll need to obtain pressure readings will vary with the patient's condition. For example, routine orders may require you to note PAP and PAWP every 1 to 4 hours. If the patient's condition is unstable or if you need to evaluate certain treatment effects, you'll take readings more often. However, you'll need to limit the frequency of PAWP measurements in patients who are elderly, who have pulmonary hypertension, or who are otherwise at high risk for pulmonary artery rupture.

Pulmonary artery rupture is a rare but life-threatening risk for any patient undergoing PAWP measurement. That's why some hospitals allow only doctors or specially trained nurses to perform the procedure.

Measuring PAP and other pressures

PAP, RAP, and PAWP are the pressures you'll measure. To monitor PAP, place the patient in a supine position (as shown). If he can't tolerate being completely flat, raise the head of the bed slightly. Then level, zero, and balance the transducer system, as described in "Assisting with catheter insertion" earlier in this section.

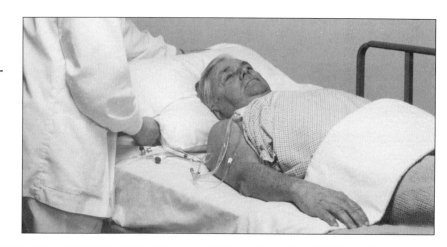

Note and record the systolic and diastolic PAP values. To obtain an accurate PAP reading, record the value at end-expiration in the respiratory cycle. *Never* remove the patient from a ventilator to obtain a measurement. If rapid or irregular respirations interfere with identifying the end-expiration period, average the measurements through an entire respiratory cycle.

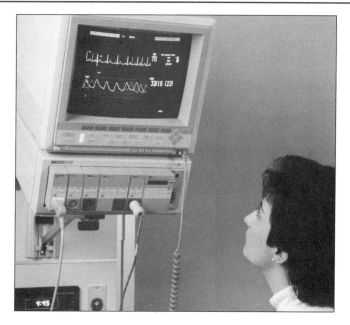

If the patient's monitoring system continuously measures PAP and only intermittently measures RAP, turn the stopcock on the transducer in the appropriate direction: off to the distal lumen for PAP and on to the proximal lumen for RAP.

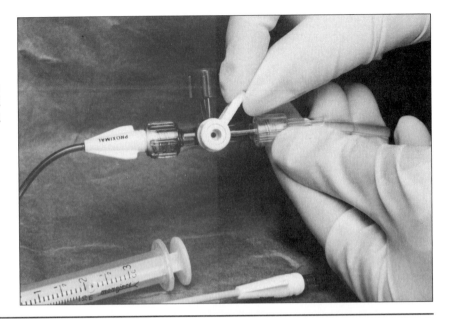

Check the monitor to observe the waveform change from PAP to RAP (as shown). Record the measured pressure. Then return the stopcock to the position for PAP. Recheck the monitor to make sure that it again displays the PAP waveform.

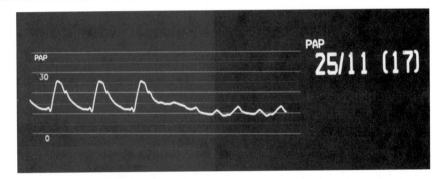

If you're continuously monitoring the patient's RAP, observe the monitor screen for the RAP value. Then record your findings.

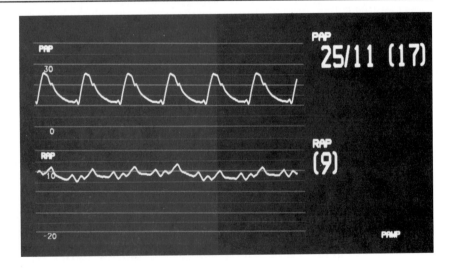

To obtain the PAWP value, first adjust the monitor to the mean mode. Then check the transducer to ensure that it's still properly leveled. Your next step will be to wedge the catheter in a more distal branch of the pulmonary artery to help evaluate left ventricular pressure and function. To do so, remove the volume-limited syringe from the balloon-inflation valve that comes with the pulmonary artery catheter.

Note: Gloves are optional, depending on the situation.

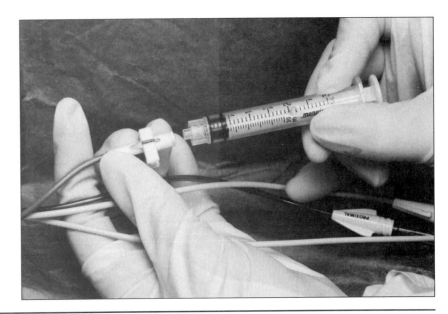

Pull back the plunger of the syringe until it stops, which should be at 1.5 cc.

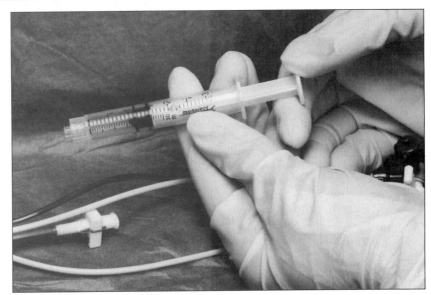

Reattach the syringe to the balloon-inflation valve.

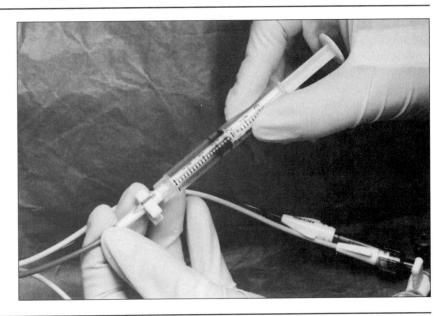

Slowly depress the plunger to inflate the balloon. You should feel *slight* resistance. If you feel marked resistance or no resistance at all, stop inflating the balloon immediately.

Caution: Lack of resistance suggests a ruptured balloon.

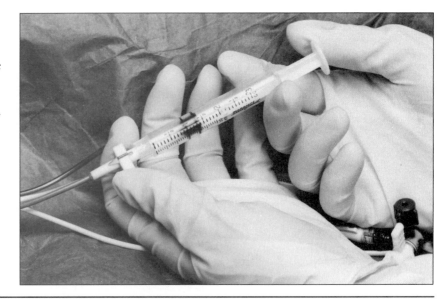

As you inflate the balloon, look for a PAWP waveform on the monitor (as shown). As soon as this tracing pattern appears, stop inflating the balloon. Never inject more air than the minimum required to obtain a wedge tracing, and never inject more than 1.5 cc. Quickly read the pressure.

▶ *Clinical tip:* Keep careful track of the pressure needed to inflate the balloon. If a wedge tracing appears after injecting less than 1.25 cc of air, then the catheter has migrated to a more distal portion of the pulmonary artery.

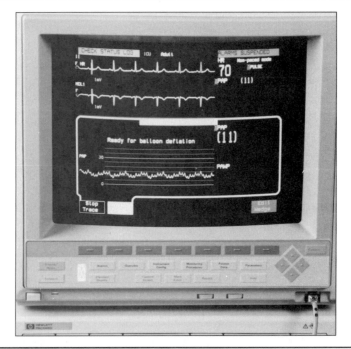

Next, detach the syringe from the pulmonary artery catheter so that the balloon deflates passively. Never leave the balloon inflated over more than two respiratory cycles, or 10 to 15 seconds. Doing so could induce a pulmonary infarction.

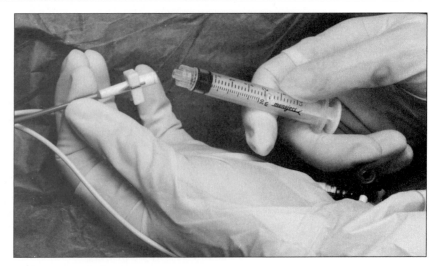

Maintaining a pulmonary artery catheter

Ensure that the patient's bedside monitor continuously displays the PAP waveform. This way, you'll immediately recognize waveform changes signifying problems with the pulmonary artery catheter, such as a migrating tip that lodges, rather than floats, in the vessel. Arrange for daily chest X-rays, as ordered, to verify proper catheter placement.

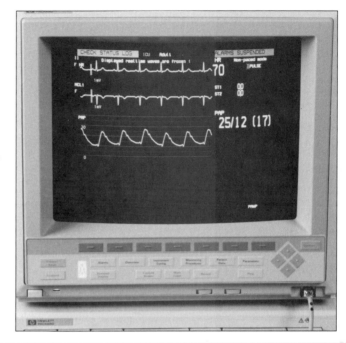

Ensure a constant flush rate of 3 ml/hour. To do this, continuously monitor the pressure bag portion of the flush system (as shown). This apparatus should stay inflated at 300 mm Hg—the pressure needed to maintain the flush rate.

▶ **Clinical tip:** Always watch the PAP waveform. As long as you see a clear waveform with clear dicrotic notches, you won't need to flush the system manually. Also make sure that the flush solution is the only agent infused through the distal port. Don't use this port for any other fluids or drugs.

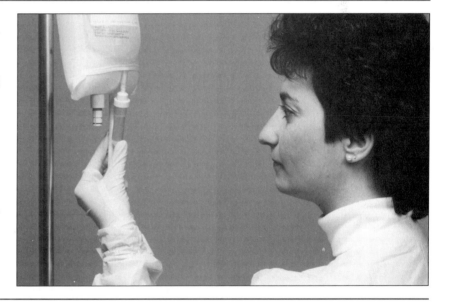

Then check the right atrial (RA) lumen. If you're monitoring RAP—either continuously or intermittently—this lumen should have a flush system attached (as shown) to keep it patent. If you're using the RA lumen only for instilling injectate to assess cardiac output, you can maintain patency with an I.V. drip. In such a case, make sure that the solution infuses at a minimum rate of 10 ml/hour.

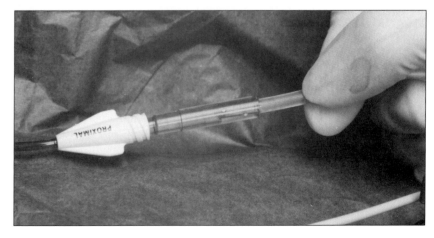

Responding to abnormal waveforms and pressures

When your patient has a pulmonary artery catheter, do you know how to respond to an uncharacteristic waveform on the monitor? For example, what action should you take for an erratic waveform? How should you respond to a concurrent arrhythmia on the electrocardiogram (ECG)? How can you deal with an obviously inaccurate pressure reading? Use the following to help you recognize and resolve common problems.

No waveform on monitor

A waveform may fail to appear on the monitor for several reasons—for example, the transducer is not open to the catheter, the transducer or monitor has been set up improperly, or a catheter is clotted.

Corrective measures include checking the stopcock, calibration, or scale mechanisms; tightening connections; rezeroing the setup; or replacing the transducer.

Overdamped waveform

If air bubbles, blood clots, or a catheter tip lodged in the vessel wall causes an overdamped waveform to appear on the patient's monitor, you may correct the problem in several ways.

Try removing any air bubbles observed in the catheter tubing and transducer. Try restoring patency to a clotted catheter by aspirating the clot with a syringe. (*Never* irrigate the line as a first step.) Or try moving a lodged catheter by repositioning the patient or by having him cough and breathe deeply. If you need to move the catheter itself, do so only according to hospital policy.

Changed waveform configuration

Noisy or erratic tracings may result from an incorrectly positioned catheter, loose connections in the setup, or faulty electrical circuitry.

Respond to this problem by repositioning the patient (or the catheter, if necessary), arranging for a chest X-ray to verify catheter location, or checking and tightening connections in the catheter and transducer apparatus.

Catheter fling

An erratic waveform may also result from catheter fling, which reflects excessive catheter movement (possibly caused by an arrhythmia or excessive respiratory effort). In such a case, you may need to reposition the catheter according to hospital policy.

False pressure readings

If the monitor records pressures that are inaccurately too high or too low, try repositioning the transducer (level with the phlebostatic axis) or rezeroing the monitor setup.

Ventricular irritability

An ECG tracing indicating an arrhythmia may result from the catheter irritating the ventricular endocardium or the heart valves.

After confirming this arrhythmia on the patient's ECG, notify the doctor and administer antiarrhythmic drugs, as ordered.

Note: The doctor may prevent this problem during insertion by keeping the balloon inflated when advancing the catheter through the heart.

Right ventricular waveform

A pulmonary artery catheter migrating into the right ventricle will produce a ventricular tracing.

In this situation, inflate the balloon with 1.5 cc of air to move the catheter back to the pulmonary artery. If this measure fails, notify the doctor immediately so that he can reposition the catheter.

Continuous PAWP waveform

In obtaining the pulmonary artery wedge pressure (PAWP) to evaluate ventricular function, the catheter may migrate or the balloon may remain inflated. Either situation may cause a continuous PAWP waveform to appear.

To correct this, reposition the patient or have him cough and breathe deeply. Keep the balloon inflated no longer than two respiratory cycles or 15 seconds.

Missing PAWP waveform

The monitor may fail to record a PAWP waveform—possibly from a malpositioned catheter, insufficient air in the balloon tip, or even a ruptured balloon.

To intervene:
• reposition the patient (don't aspirate the balloon)
• reinflate the balloon adequately (remove the syringe from the balloon lumen, wait for the balloon to deflate passively, and then instill the correct volume of air)
• assess the balloon's competence (note resistance during inflation, feel how the syringe's plunger springs back after the balloon inflates, and check for blood leaking from the balloon lumen).

If the balloon has ruptured, turn the patient onto his left side, tape the balloon-inflation port, and notify the doctor.

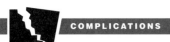

Dealing with hazards of pulmonary artery lines

Any patient who has a pulmonary artery catheter in place is at risk for several complications. Besides observing the patient's electrocardiogram, waveform pattern, and pressure values on the bedside monitor, watch for the following signs and symptoms of complications. Implement appropriate care measures to resolve or prevent them. Keep in mind that these procedures vary according to each state's nurse practice act.

Bacteremia
If your patient has an elevated temperature, chills, warm skin, headache, and malaise, he's showing signs and symptoms of an infection, such as bacteremia. Administer antibiotic medications as ordered. To prevent such an infection, maintain sterile technique. Also be sure to maintain and change the monitoring setup according to hospital policy.

Bleedback
Caused by leaks in the pulmonary artery catheter apparatus or a pressure bag that's inflated below 300 mm Hg, bleedback is easily seen in the pressure tubing. To intervene early, be sure to tighten connections in the monitoring setup. Preventive measures include returning stopcocks to their proper position after use and keeping the pressure bag adequately inflated.

Bleeding at the insertion site
If the patient has prolonged oozing or frank bleeding at the insertion site after catheter withdrawal, apply firm pressure until the bleeding stops. To prevent this problem, maintain pressure on the site during catheter withdrawal and for at least 10 minutes afterward, and apply a pressure dressing over the site. At a femoral site, apply a sandbag for 1 to 2 hours. (Also be sure to assess distal circulation routinely to ensure that a hematoma isn't obstructing blood flow.)

Pulmonary embolism
A thrombus that migrates from the catheter into pulmonary circulation or a catheter tip clotted from inadequate flushing may cause a pulmonary embolism. To prevent this, administer anticoagulants as ordered, and use a continuous flush system.

If prevention fails and your patient shows signs and symptoms of pulmonary embolism, such as sharp and stabbing chest pain, anxiety, cyanosis, dyspnea, tachypnea, and diaphoresis, try to aspirate blood (don't irrigate if you suspect an embolus). If you can't aspirate blood, a pulmonary embolus may be obstructing the line. Notify the doctor at once.

Ruptured pulmonary artery
In pulmonary artery rupture (from pulmonary hypertension, thrombus, catheter migration into the peripheral branch of the artery, or improper inflation or prolonged wedging of the catheter's balloon), the patient will experience restlessness, tachycardia, hypotension, hemoptysis, and dyspnea. In such a situation, notify the doctor immediately.

Keep in mind several preventive measures:
• Slowly inflate the balloon only until the PAWP waveform appears on the monitor, and then let the balloon deflate passively.
• Never overinflate the balloon.
• Reposition a migrating catheter (if permitted).

Pulmonary infarction
Chest pain, hemoptysis, fever, pleural friction rub, and low arterial oxygen levels point to pulmonary infarction, possibly from the catheter migrating into a wedged position in the blood vessel. Don't flush the catheter if you suspect that it has migrated. Do monitor pulmonary artery pressure continuously and notify the doctor.

Never allow the balloon to be inflated for more than two respiratory cycles or 15 seconds.

REMOVING A PULMONARY ARTERY CATHETER

Typically, a pulmonary artery catheter stays in place no longer than 3 days. In most states, pulmonary artery catheter removal is not considered within the nurse's domain. In other states, advanced collaborative standards of practice allow skilled nurses to perform this procedure. Before attempting to remove a pulmonary artery catheter, however, check with your hospital administrator about practice requirements and legal responsibilities in your locality.

To remove a pulmonary artery catheter, you'll need a suture removal kit, sterile 3″ × 3″ or 4″ × 4″ gauze pads, sterile gloves, antimicrobial swabs, and hypoallergenic tape. You'll also need equipment for observing universal precautions. Gather a face shield (or goggles and mask), a gown, and gloves.

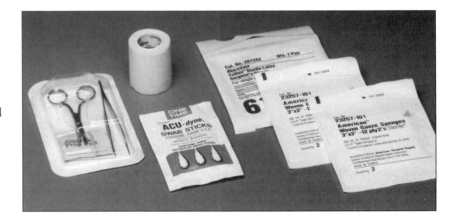

Explain the procedure to the patient as you take his vital signs and note the electrocardiogram (ECG) pattern. As ordered, obtain a chest X-ray to check for kinks or knots in the catheter.

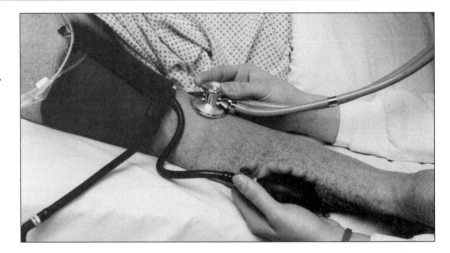

If possible, place the patient in a supine position.

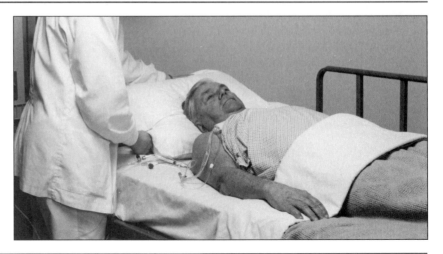

If you're removing the catheter from the subclavian or internal jugular vein, turn the patient's face away from the site.

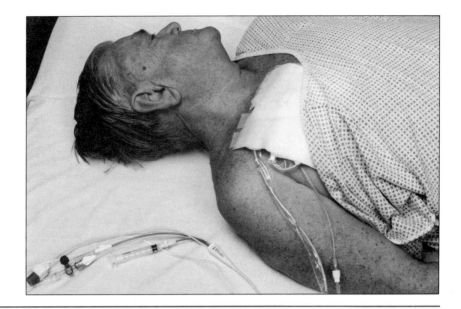

Put on gloves, gown, and face shield, and gently remove the dressing from the catheter site. Assist the doctor as he takes out the sutures. If you're removing the catheter, take out the sutures yourself. If the introducer will remain in place, leave the sutures securing the introducer intact. Then dispose of the dressing and remove your gloves.

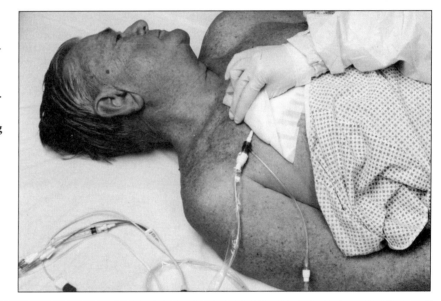

Turn all stopcocks off to the patient.

Caution: To observe the waveforms during removal, leave the stopcocks turned on to the distal port. Keep in mind that an air embolism may result, so exercise extreme caution when doing so.

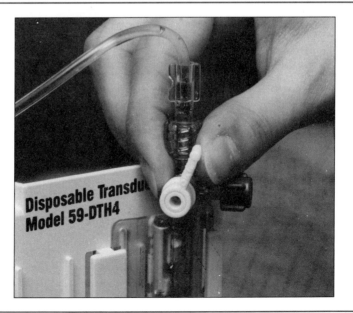

Next, make sure that the balloon is deflated.

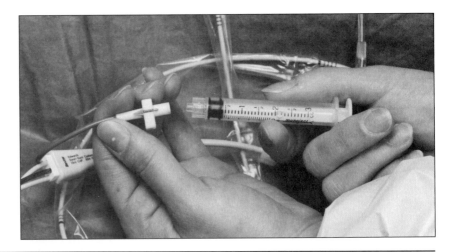

If you'll be removing the catheter, put on sterile gloves.

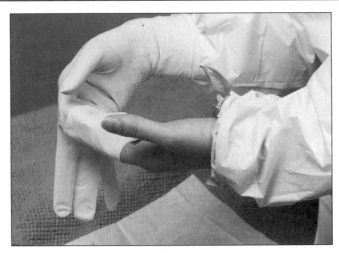

Slowly and smoothly withdraw the catheter (near right); at the same time watch the monitor for arrhythmias.

Caution: If you feel any resistance, stop immediately and notify the doctor.

If you remove both the catheter and the introducer, apply pressure to the site using the sterile gauze pads. If the introducer will remain in place, observe the introducer's diaphragm for a bleedback. If you observe no bleedback, assume that the hemostatic valve within the introducer is intact. Next, clean the site with antimicrobial swabs before covering it with a sterile occlusive dressing (far right). Then document the date and time of catheter removal and the patient's tolerance of the procedure. Include a current description of the insertion site.

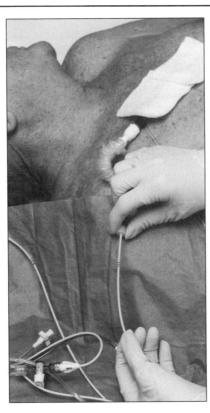

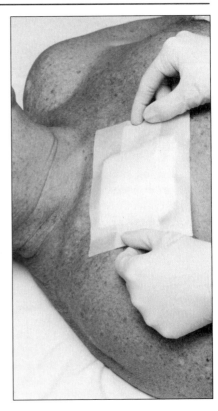

LEARNING ABOUT C.V.P. MONITORING

Central venous pressure (CVP) is monitored with either a pressure transducer system or a water manometer. Both kinds of equipment accommodate intermittent or continuous CVP monitoring. The monitor is connected to a catheter that has been threaded through the subclavian or jugular vein (or the basilic, cephalic, or saphenous veins) to a position in or near the right atrium.

In a critically ill patient, a central venous line allows you to obtain pressure readings, blood for laboratory samples, and access to a large vessel for rapid administration of large amounts of fluid.

When the left ventricle is functioning normally, CVP monitoring helps evaluate the patient's cardiac status and response to fluid administration. CVP values assist you in evaluating venous return to the heart and in indirectly determining how well the heart is pumping.

CORRELATING C.V.P. WITH CARDIAC FUNCTION

Essentially, CVP measurements reflect events in the cardiac cycle and, in so doing, depict cardiac function. During ventricular diastole, the atrioventricular (AV) valves open. As diastole ends, each open valve creates what amounts to a common heart chamber. The pressure created by blood volume in the ventricles now extends back into the atria so that pressure measured in the right atrium indirectly mirrors the volume status of the right ventricle (called preload). During systole, the AV valves close and the semilunar valves open. Now the pressure measured in the atria indicates atrial filling.

FACTORS AFFECTING C.V.P.

Anything that affects the patient's hydration status can affect CVP. For example, an increase in circulating volume is reflected as an increase in venous return to the heart and will cause CVP to rise. (See *What causes CVP changes?*)

Certain mechanical factors can also affect CVP. For example, if your patient is on a ventilator, his intrathoracic pressure will be higher on inspiration and lower on expiration—the opposite of normal respirations. When monitoring CVP in such a case, take the reading at end-expiration.

 INSIGHTS AND INTERPRETATIONS

What causes CVP changes?

Although most experts consider 3.7 to 7.4 mm Hg (5 to 10 cm H_2O) a normal range for central venous pressure (CVP), this range may vary slightly (for example, 1.5 to 5.9 mm Hg [2 to 8 cm H_2O]). The factors that may cause changes include conditions that alter venous return, circulating blood volume, or cardiac performance.

Note CVP changes that indicate a trend: The trend may be more significant than the individual values. For example, patients with chronic pulmonary problems, such as cor pulmonale, may have high CVP values without acute heart failure.

To interpret pressure readings correctly, establish the patient's baseline CVP; then measure CVP at 15-, 30-, and 60-minute intervals. Report fluctuations of more than 1.5 mm Hg (2 cm H_2O), which may indicate a change in the patient's status.

What increases CVP?
• Increased venous return from conditions that cause hypervolemic states, such as volume overload or hepatic disease
• Depressed cardiac function
• Vasoconstriction
• Cardiac tamponade
• Chronic or acute pulmonary hypertension
• Positive end-expiratory pressure administered with mechanical ventilation

What decreases CVP?
• Decreased venous return and hypovolemia from hemorrhage or dehydration
• Loss of vascular tone caused by vasodilation (for example, from sepsis), which contributes to venous pooling and reduced blood return to the heart

Contributors to this section are *Jan M. Headley, RN, BS*, a senior education consultant at Baxter Healthcare Corp., Edwards Critical-Care Division, Irvine, Calif.; and *Paulette Dorney, RN, MSN, CCRN*, a critical care staff development instructor at North Penn Hospital, Lansdale, Pa. The publisher thanks the following organizations for their help: *Baxter Healthcare Corp., Edwards Critical-Care Division*, Irvine, Calif.; *Hewlett-Packard Co.*, Waltham, Mass.; and *Hill-Rom*, Batesville, Ind.

MONITORING C.V.P. WITH A PRESSURE TRANSDUCER

If you're attaching the central venous catheter to a computerized pressure transducer monitoring system, such as the one described on these pages, you can use either the proximal lumen of a pulmonary artery catheter or a single-lumen central venous catheter. If the catheter has several lumens, one lumen can be used for continuous central venous pressure (CVP) monitoring and the others for fluid administration.

Although you'll care for and maintain the catheter in this system as you would any catheter, you'll obtain the pressure values in a different way. This monitoring system communicates pressure values in digital form on the monitor screen. A CVP waveform display is another feature of this system.

Gather a prepared pressure transducer setup and a carpenter's level. Take them to the patient's bedside. You'll also need tape and a marking pen.

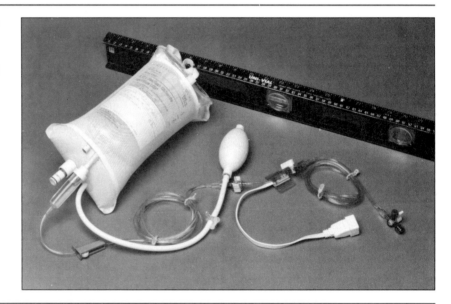

Explain the procedure to the patient, answer his questions, and reassure him. Wash your hands. Place the patient in a supine position if he can tolerate it. If not, use semi-Fowler's position. Make sure that you note the patient's position on his chart.

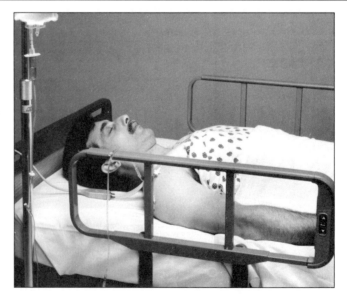

If the pressure transducer cable isn't already attached to the pressure module of the monitor, attach it now. *(Note:* If your hospital policy requires you to wear gloves or if you think leakage may occur, put on gloves.)

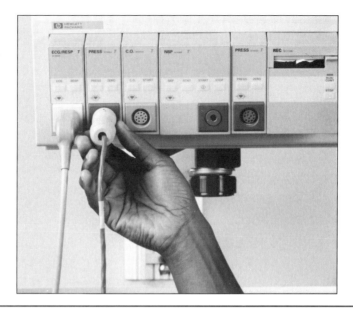

Then, if the prepared pressure transducer setup isn't attached to the appropriate lumen of the pulmonary artery catheter or the central venous catheter, attach it (as shown).

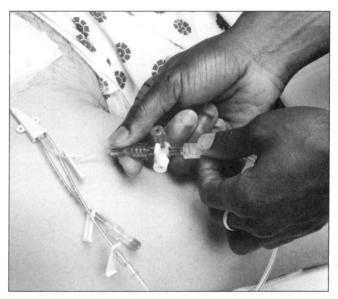

Locate the patient's phlebostatic axis by mentally bisecting the fourth intercostal space at the midpoint of the anteroposterior chest wall. (You can also use the midaxillary line, but doing so may produce less accurate pressure readings than using the midpoint landmark.) Then put a piece of tape on the patient's side, and use a marking pen to pinpoint the phlebostatic axis, which is level with the right atrium. Position the transducer level with the mark.

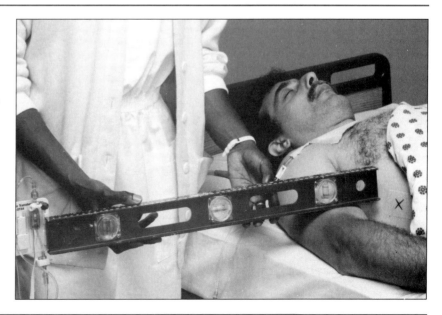

Turn the stopcock so that it's closed to the patient and open to air.

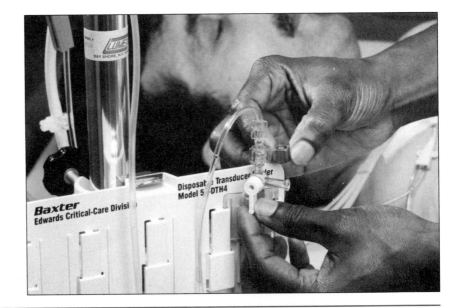

Next, zero the monitor by pressing the ZERO XDUCER key (as shown).

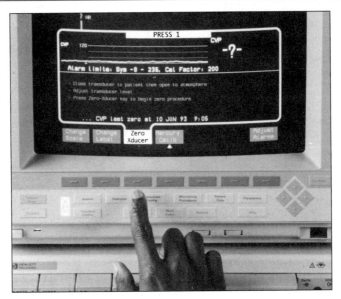

Afterward, position the stopcock so that it's closed to air and open to the patient. Then watch for CVP waveforms to appear on the monitor.

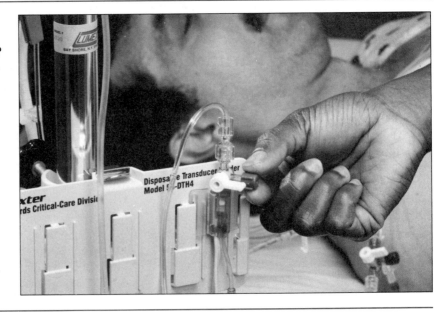

Check the monitor scale. If it's incorrect, select the proper scale by pressing the designated monitor key. (Consult the manufacturer's directions.)

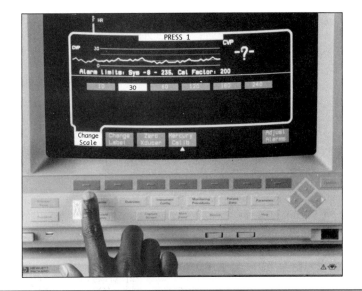

The amplitude of the CVP waveform reflects the phase of the respiratory cycle. Observe the CVP waveform for alterations resulting from unusual respiratory variations. Note the pressure value at end-expiration, and document this value on the patient's chart.

▶ *Clinical tip:* You may want to obtain a printout of the CVP tracing for reference when the waveform shows several respiratory variations.

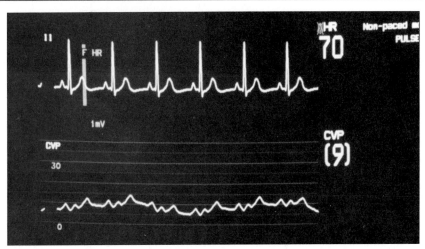

Converting pressure values

Although the water manometer—the first device developed for monitoring central venous pressure at the bedside—is still in use today, the pressure transducer system is used in most hospitals. Both methods measure right atrial pressure—the pressure transducer in millimeters of mercury (mm Hg) and the water manometer in centimeters of water (cm H_2O). If your hospital uses both pressure transducers and water manometers, you may have to convert pressure values.

Use this formula to convert cm H_2O to mm Hg:

$$cm\ H_2O \div 1.36 = mm\ Hg$$

Conversely, use this formula to change mm Hg to cm H_2O:

$$mm\ Hg \times 1.36 = cm\ H_2O$$

Understanding the CVP waveform

When the CVP catheter is attached to a pressure monitoring system, the bedside monitor can usually display digital pressure values, CVP waveforms, and electrocardiogram (ECG) tracings. Synchronizing the CVP waveform with the ECG helps you identify components of the tracing. Keep in mind that cardiac electrical activity precedes the mechanical activities of systole and diastole.

Normal waveforms

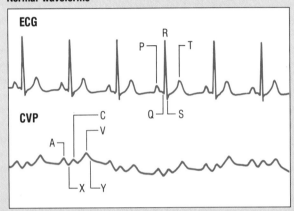

Comparing electrical activity

The P wave on the ECG reflects atrial depolarization, which is then followed by atrial contraction and increased atrial pressure. Corresponding to the PR interval on the ECG, the A wave sequence on the CVP waveform represents atrial contraction.

The X descent on the CVP waveform represents atrial relaxation and declining pressure after systole, when the atrium expels blood into the ventricle.

As the cardiac cycle progresses, the tricuspid valve closes, producing a small backward bulge known as the C wave.

The atrium filling with venous blood during diastole produces another rise in pressure and a V wave, which corresponds to the T wave of the ECG.

After atrial filling, the tricuspid valve opens. Most of the blood in the right atrium passively empties into the right ventricle, causing atrial pressure to fall. On the CVP waveform, this decline appears as the Y descent.

The A and V waves are almost the same height, indicating that atrial systole and atrial diastole produce about the same amount of pressure. Consequently, right atrial pressures are recorded as mean values because they're almost the same.

What causes rising waves?

Conditions that cause increased resistance to ventricular filling, such as heart failure or tricuspid stenosis, generate elevated A waves.

Elevated V waves result from regurgitant flow—for example, from tricuspid insufficiency or from inadequate closure of the tricuspid valve due to heart failure. Although the V wave may be elevated in tricuspid insufficiency, its height doesn't correspond to the amount of regurgitant flow.

Elevations in the A and V waves may result from cardiac tamponade, constrictive pericardial disease, or heart failure. Increased resistance to ventricular filling causes the elevated A wave; functional regurgitation causes the elevated V wave.

What causes descending waves?

Cardiac tamponade causes a smaller Y descent than an X descent. This results partly from an increase in heart rate and the right atrium's inability to empty efficiently because of the blood backflow that occurs with tamponade.

If the patient has a disorder causing constrictive pericardial disease, the Y descent exceeds the X descent. In such cases, ventricular filling occurs rapidly, producing the exaggerated Y deflection.

LEARNING ABOUT CARDIAC OUTPUT MONITORING

Measuring cardiac output—the volume of blood ejected from the heart over 1 minute—helps evaluate cardiac function. Normally, cardiac output ranges from 4 to 8 liters/minute. Values below this range result from:
• decreased myocardial contractility caused by myocardial infarction, drug effects, acidosis, or hypoxia
• decreased left ventricular filling pressure resulting from hypovolemia
• increased systemic vascular resistance related to arteriosclerosis or hypertension
• decreased ventricular flow related to valvular heart disease.

High cardiac output can occur with some arteriovenous shunts and from decreased vascular resistance (as in septic shock). In some cases, an unusually high cardiac output can be normal (for example, in well-conditioned athletes).

Cardiac output values along with mean arterial pressure, right atrial pressure, mean pulmonary artery pressure, and pulmonary artery wedge pressure can also provide further information about cardiovascular function—for example, stroke volume and vascular resistance.

REVIEWING MEASURING METHODS

Indirect methods of measuring cardiac output include the Fick method, the indicator-dilution method, and the thermodilution method. The Fick and indicator-dilution methods are performed mostly in cardiac catheterization laboratories or in research projects.

Fick method

Effective for detecting low cardiac output, the Fick method calculates cardiac output (CO) by measuring oxygen levels in the blood before and after the blood passes through the lungs and, using a spirometer, by measuring oxygen consumption—the amount of air entering the lungs each minute, as follows:

$$\text{CO (liter/min)} = \frac{\text{oxygen consumption (cc/min)}}{\text{arterial oxygen content (ml/min)} - \text{venous oxygen content (ml/min)}}$$

A drawback to this procedure is that the patient must be in a steady physiologic state. Most patients requiring cardiac output determinations are critically ill, which is frequently defined as an "unsteady state." This technique also requires simultaneous expired air and blood samples, controlled inspired oxygen content values, and arterial blood samples.

Indicator-dilution method

This method uses a computer to evaluate cardiac output. Computations involve measuring the volume and concentration of an injected dye indicator as it passes from the pulmonary artery to the brachial artery over a certain time. The results are plotted as a time and dilution-concentration curve.

The drawback of this technique is that it requires complex equipment skills to obtain accurate results and, therefore, is not a clinically practical method.

Thermodilution method

Used at bedside, the thermodilution method applies indicator-dilution principles, using temperature changes in the pulmonary artery blood as the indicator. The procedure requires the addition of a thermistor (a temperature sensor) onto the pulmonary artery catheter. Thermodilution monitoring is relatively easy, rapid (values can be computed approximately every minute), and clean (no blood sampling is required).

CALCULATING THE CARDIAC INDEX

Because it takes into account the patient's size, the cardiac index is a more accurate indicator of cardiac output. To calculate the cardiac index, divide the cardiac output value by the patient's body surface area (BSA). Normally, the cardiac index ranges from 2.5 to 4 liters/minute/m² (of BSA).

You can obtain the patient's BSA by plotting his height and weight on the Du Bois BSA nomogram. This chart consists of three columns. Mark the patient's height on the scale in column one and his weight in column three. Then draw a line linking these two points. The point at which your line intercepts column two indicates the patient's estimated BSA.

Jan Headley, RN, BS, and *Loraine Hopkins Pepe, RN, MSN, CCRN, CS,* contributed to this section. Ms. Headley is a senior education consultant for Baxter Healthcare Corp., Edwards Critical-Care Division, Irvine, Calif. Ms. Pepe is a staff nurse in the medical-surgical intensive care unit at Chestnut Hill Hospital, Philadelphia. The publisher thanks the following organizations for their help: *Baxter Healthcare Corp., Edwards Critical-Care Division,* Irvine, Calif.; *Doylestown (Pa.) Hospital; Hewlett-Packard Co.,* Waltham, Mass.; and *Hill-Rom,* Batesville, Ind.

Another method used to calculate BSA is the Boyd method. This method uses a formula to calculate BSA for children and for adults with a large body mass. The DuBois and Boyd methods generally have similar results except when BSA is very large. Although these two methods are popular, several other methods for calculating BSA exist. Many bedside computers can also calculate the patient's BSA when you enter the patient's height and weight. Check your hospital's policy to determine which method to use.

UNDERSTANDING THERMODILUTION MONITORING

In thermodilution monitoring, a balloon-tipped, flow-directed catheter is inserted into a large vein, advanced to the right side of the heart, and positioned in the pulmonary artery. You'll inject a specific amount of solution called an injectate (at a specific temperature) into the proximal port of the pulmonary artery catheter. (Depending on your equipment, you can also use the right atrium—or the lumen marked RA.)

As the injectate mixes with the surrounding blood and flows into the pulmonary artery, a thermistor embedded in the catheter senses the temperature change and a bedside computer plots the change. This plotting, known as a time-temperature (thermodilution) curve, contains the information needed to calculate the cardiac output. Once the computer processes the data, results appear on the monitor. Some monitors display the actual thermodilution curve.

Several factors must be considered during thermodilution monitoring: the injectate type and temperature, the correct selection of a computation constant, and the type of delivery system.

Injectate: Type and temperature

Dextrose 5% in water (D_5W) is the recommended I.V. solution because the computation constant is based in part on this solution's specific gravity and temperature response. Using 0.9% sodium chloride solution instead produces a 2% decrease in the cardiac output value.

The injectate may be room temperature or iced. Because researchers show conflicting results when comparing room-temperature and iced injectates and their impact on cardiac output readings, follow your hospital's policy when preparing the injectate for your patient.

Computation constant

The computation constant accounts for the gain of heat from the catheter tubing as injectate travels through the catheter into the blood. Its selection is based on such variables as the volume and temperature of the injectate as well as the size and type of catheter you plan to use. Usually the catheter manufacturer supplies the computation constant values (sometimes in chart form). Verify this number any time you change one of the variables. Most bedside computers require you to alter the computation constant manually, although some have sensing capabilities that can detect changes in the variables.

Keep in mind that an inaccurate computation constant can produce an error of up to 100% in the cardiac output value. Also, if you change the injectate volume from 5 to 10 ml without changing the computation constant, the resulting cardiac output value may differ significantly from the true value.

Delivery systems

Besides having a choice of injectates and temperatures when using the thermodilution method, you'll also have a choice of delivery systems: closed and open. Each system works with room-temperature or iced injectate.

PERFORMING CLOSED THERMODILUTION MONITORING

If you select the closed system, you'll use one syringe to feed injectate into the bloodstream via the catheter in a closed-loop system. The closed system reduces the risk of contamination inherent in the open system by eliminating the need for multiple entry into a sterile system.

You'll need a bolus injectate system (such as the Baxter CO-Set shown here, which includes a cooling container, coiled tubing, and an insulated 10-ml syringe), injectate (a 500-ml bag of D_5W or 0.9% sodium chloride solution), a thermistor, connecting cables, and a stopcock. If you're using iced injectate, obtain the ice and water.

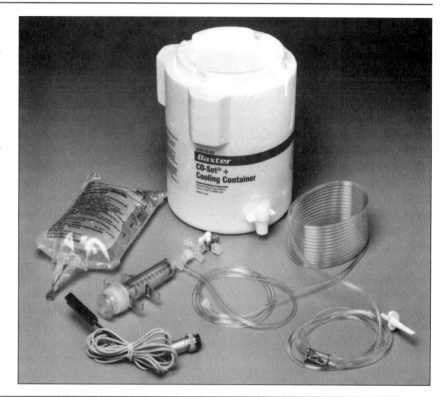

You'll also need a cardiac output computer or a module for the bedside monitor.

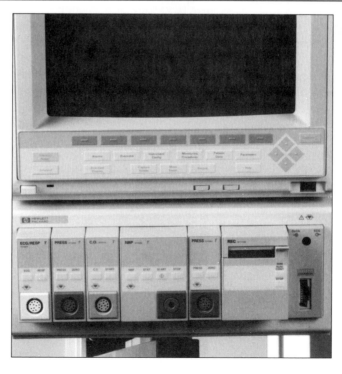

Take the equipment to the patient's bedside. Explain the procedure and wash your hands. Plug the connecting cable into the cardiac output module.

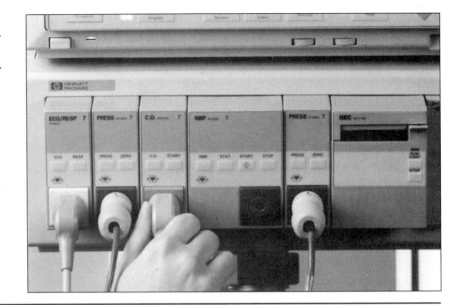

Then plug the catheter connector into the thermistor connector of the pulmonary artery (PA) catheter.

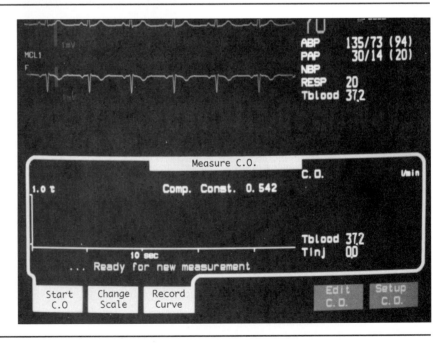

Press the module's CARDIAC OUTPUT key. A computation constant number will appear on the display screen (as shown). Consult the manufacturer's instructions to make sure that this number is appropriate for the injectate, its temperature range, and the type of catheter you're using.

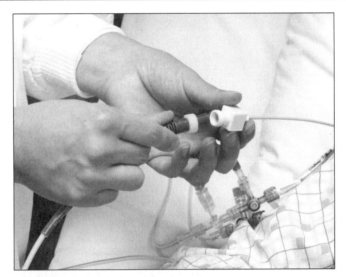

Check to see that two stopcocks are in place on the catheter's proximal lumen. If they're not, attach two now. Both stopcocks should be turned off to the capped end (as shown).

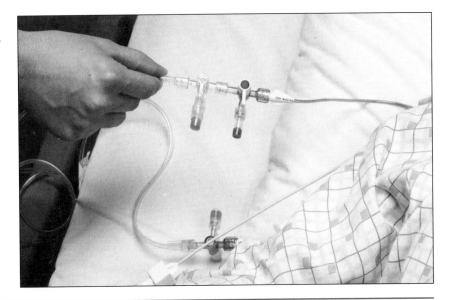

Next, observe the pulmonary artery pressure (PAP) waveform on the monitor to verify that the PA catheter is properly positioned with the balloon tip deflated. An improperly positioned catheter may produce inaccurate cardiac output values.

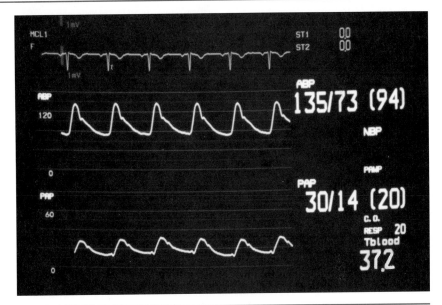

Though some hospital policies require the patient to lie flat, your hospital may permit the patient to lie supine with his head slightly elevated (but no more than 30 degrees). Document the patient's exact position on his chart so that he lies in the same position for future cardiac output measurements.

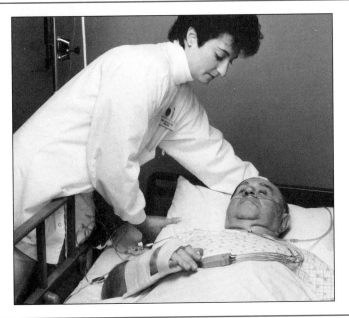

Attach the I.V. solution bag to the injectate delivery system. To prime the system, unclamp the snap clamp on the I.V. tubing and allow the solution to flow through the tubing. Slowly pull the syringe plunger out and then push it in (as shown) to remove any air. Repeat this procedure five to six times to ensure that the system is free of air. Then place the cooling container on the I.V. pole.

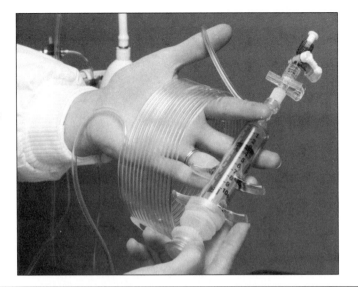

Close the clamp once you've primed the tubing. Place the coiled portion of the tubing into the cooling container (as shown). If you're cooling the injectate, make sure that the iced solution surrounds the coil. If you're using room-temperature injectate, don't place the coiled tubing in the cooling container.

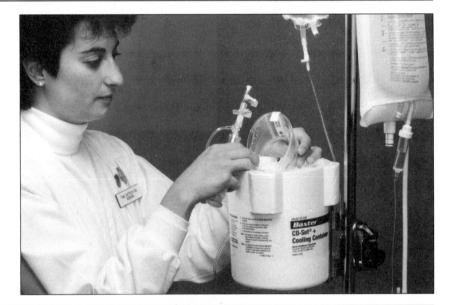

Next, put on gloves and attach the system to the stopcock closest to the catheter's proximal lumen.

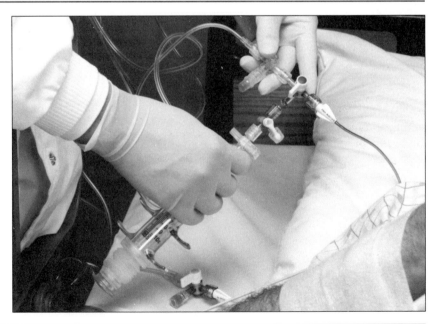

Attach the in-line temperature probe to the hub on the closed system set.

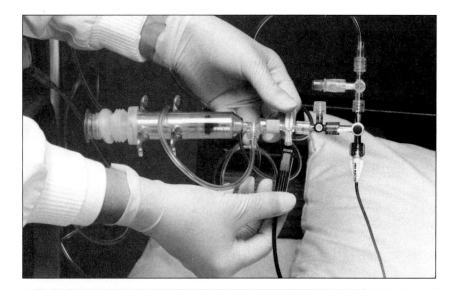

Make sure that the stopcock closest to the catheter's proximal lumen is closed (as shown).

Depending on your hospital's policy, the proximal lumen may be reserved for cardiac output measurements. However, it may need a continuous-drip infusion line if medications will be administered to the patient intermittently through it. If this is the case, attach a prepared continuous-drip infusion line to the second stopcock and close this stopcock to the pressure side of the proximal lumen (to suspend any concurrent pressure waveform measurements).

▶ *Clinical tip:* If the proximal lumen isn't reserved for cardiac output measurement, avoid using this site to infuse vasoactive agents or other medications that can't be discontinued temporarily.

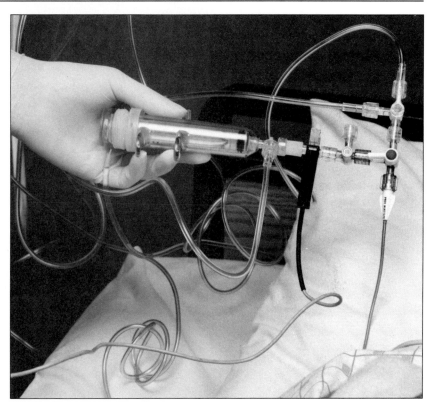

Open the snap clamp on the I.V. solution tubing.

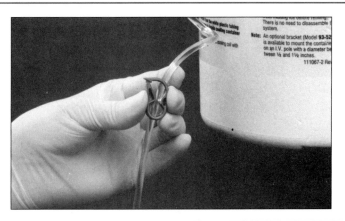

Carefully withdraw exactly 10 ml of injectate into the insulated syringe attached to the proximal lumen. Be aware that an error in the injectate volume can produce an error in the cardiac output value. (For example, injecting 11 ml instead of 10 ml can produce a 10% error.)

▶ *Clinical tip:* If you're using an uninsulated syringe barrel, avoid excessive handling, which may warm a room-temperature injectate 1° C (1.8° F) in 28 seconds and an iced injectate 1° C in 13 seconds. A 1° C change in the delivered injectate temperature can produce an error of 2.8% or more in the cardiac output value.

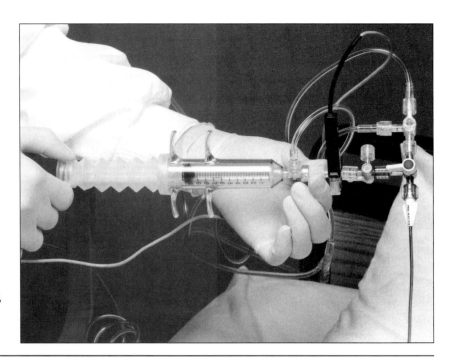

Press the START key on the monitor module. When the monitor indicates that it's ready, observe the patient's breathing (as shown) and instill the injectate rapidly and smoothly during the end-expiratory phase of the respiratory cycle. The injection should take no more than 4 seconds to complete. If your monitor displays the thermodilution curve, look for a smooth and sharp rise in the curve.

Be sure to instill the injectate during the end-expiratory phase each time you perform the procedure to ensure reliable and consistent results.

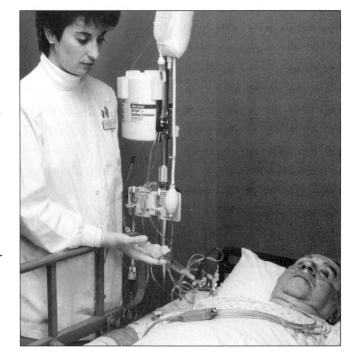

Check the injectate's temperature on the monitor during or immediately after injection. Iced injectate should measure between 6° and 12° C (42.8° and 53.6° F). Room-temperature injectate should measure between 18° and 25° C (64.4° and 77° F), or at least 10° C (18° F) below the patient's blood temperature.

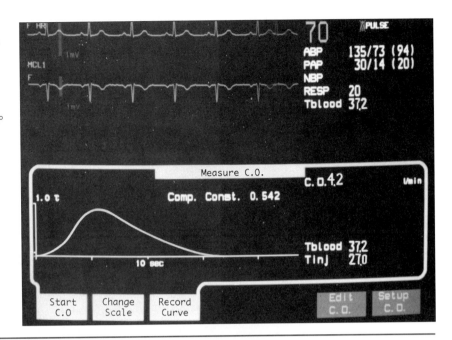

Repeat the injection procedure at least three times—more if necessary—to obtain a mean cardiac output value. Discard any reading that isn't within 10% of the other readings.

When you finish the procedure, close the snap clamp on the injectate solution line.

▶ *Clinical tip:* Be sure to close the snap clamp. If you forget to do so and then hang the injectate bag on an I.V. pole, gravity will force the solution into the syringe; this will result in inconsistent injectate temperatures, requiring you to repeat the procedure from the beginning.

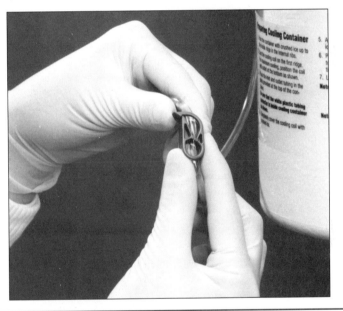

Turn the stopcock to the open position so that the pressure flush from the I.V. solution will keep the line patent. If the lumen you were using to measure cardiac output was also being used to monitor right atrial pressure (RAP), observe the monitor for the return of an RAP waveform. Then reposition the patient if necessary to make him more comfortable.

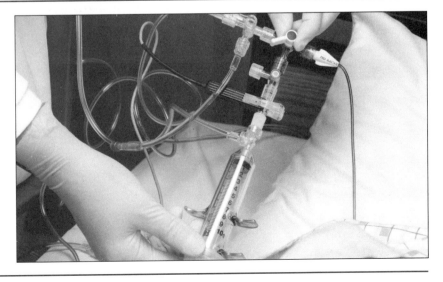

Average the readings to obtain the mean cardiac output value. Typically, an individual reading within 10% of the other readings is considered acceptable and representative of the patient's condition.

If you repeatedly obtain individual values that deviate by more than 10% from the others, you may have to reassess the patient's condition, double-check your technique, and repeat the procedure.

Record the mean cardiac output value on the patient's chart. Be sure to describe how the patient tolerated the procedure.

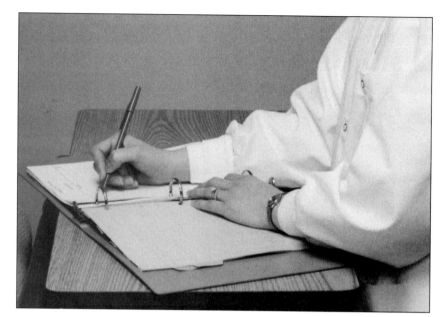

PERFORMING OPEN THERMODILUTION MONITORING

If you select the open system of thermodilution monitoring, you'll use several prefilled syringes, attaching a new syringe to the catheter lumen each time you instill injectate.

You'll need an injectate temperature sensor or cable, the injectate (a 250-ml or 500-ml bag of D₅W or 0.9% sodium chloride solution), a stopcock, five 10-ml syringes with 1″ or 1½″ 20G needles, an insulated container, a plastic bag, and an alcohol pad. If you're using iced injectate, obtain the ice and water.

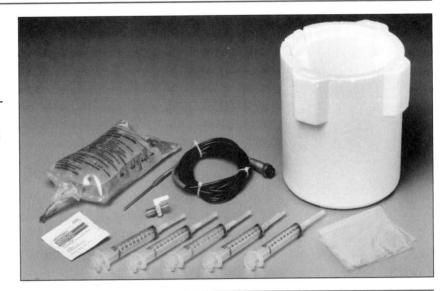

You'll also need a cardiac output computer or a module for the bedside monitor.

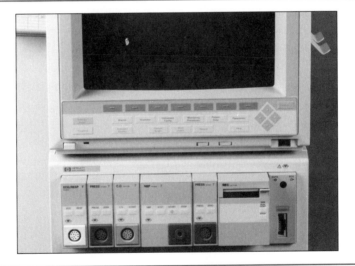

Take the necessary equipment to the patient's bedside. Explain the procedure and wash your hands. Plug the connecting cable into the cardiac output module. Then plug the catheter connector into the thermistor connector of the PA catheter (as shown).

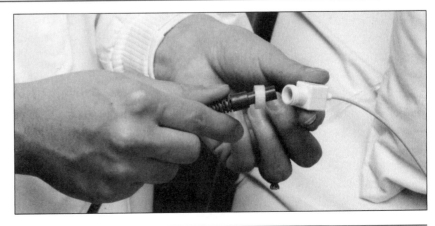

Press the module's CARDIAC OUT-
PUT key. A computation constant
number will appear on the display
screen. Verify that the computation constant is correct for the
catheter type and for the volume
and temperature of the injectate
you'll be using. Reset the computation constant if necessary.

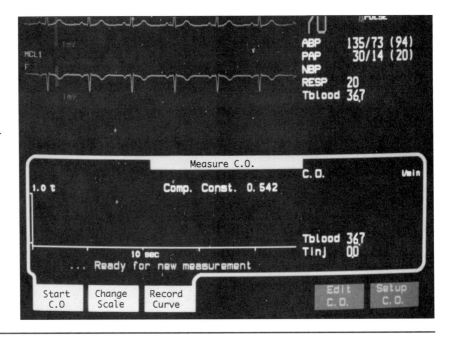

Don gloves. If a stopcock isn't already in place on the catheter's
proximal lumen, quickly attach
one now. Don't allow air to enter
the catheter.

▶ *Clinical tip:* Be sure to avoid
infusing medications (especially vasoactive drugs) through
the RA lumen before instilling the
injectate. Doing so could alter the
cardiac output reading.

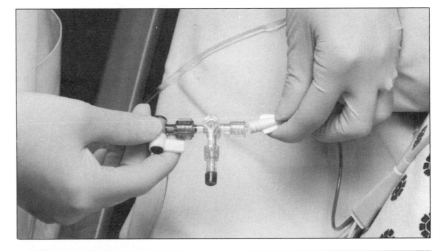

Observe the pulmonary artery
pressure (PAP) waveform on the
monitor to verify that the catheter
is correctly positioned and that
the balloon tip is deflated. An improperly positioned catheter may
produce inaccurate cardiac output
values.

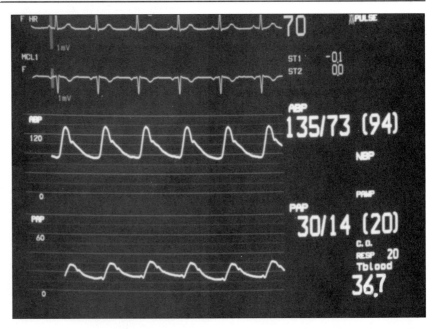

Place the patient in a supine position. Depending on your hospital's policy, you may elevate the head of the bed up to 30 degrees for patient comfort. Record the patient's exact position on her chart to serve as a reference for future cardiac output measurements.

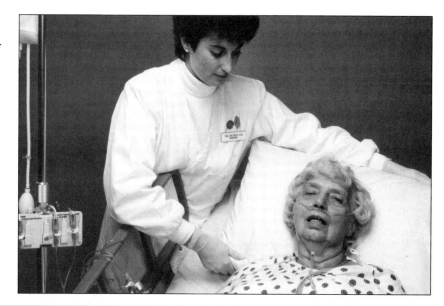

If you're using iced injectate, fill an insulated container with ice and water.

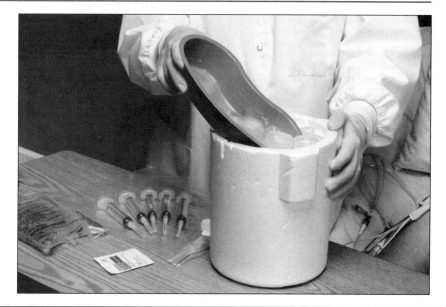

Wipe the injection port of the I.V. bag with an alcohol pad. Then draw exactly 10 ml of injectate from the I.V. bag into each of the five 10-ml syringes.

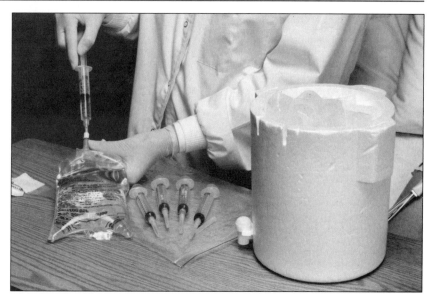

Remove the plunger from one of the syringes. Place the injectate temperature sensor inside the syringe as you put the syringe in the ice solution.

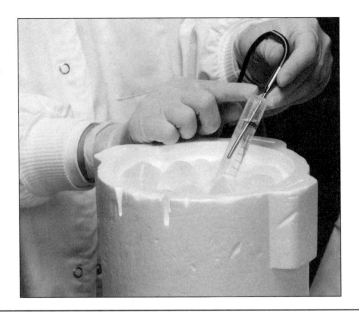

Put the remaining four syringes in the plastic bag.

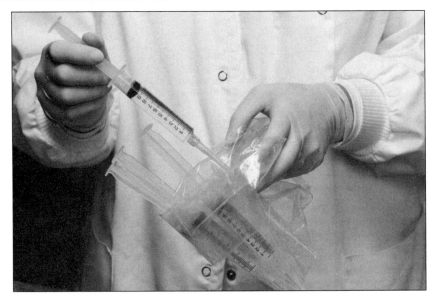

Then place the bag of syringes in the ice solution. The bag will protect the injectate from possible contamination from the ice. During the procedure, the syringe with the sensor will monitor the temperature of the injectate in all the syringes. After the procedure, you'll discard this syringe.

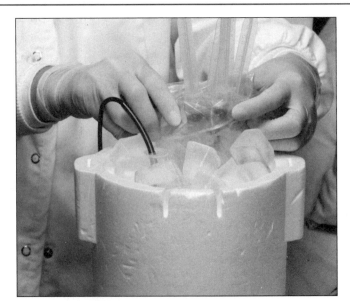

Allow the syringes to chill. Then observe the monitor to ensure that the injectate temperature remains steady at 6° to 12° C (42.8° to 53.6° F).

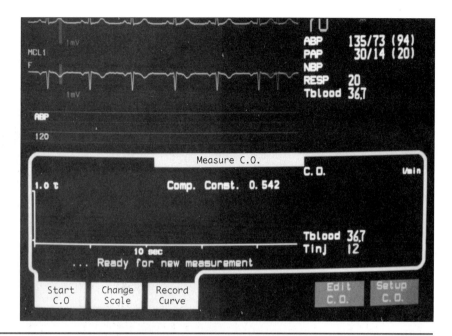

If you're using room-temperature injectate, make sure that the injectate temperature remains between 18° and 25° C (64.4° and 77° F) or at least 10° C (18° F) below blood temperature. Remove the plunger from one of the filled syringes and place the temperature sensor inside. (This syringe will be discarded after the procedure.) Observe the temperature on the monitor.

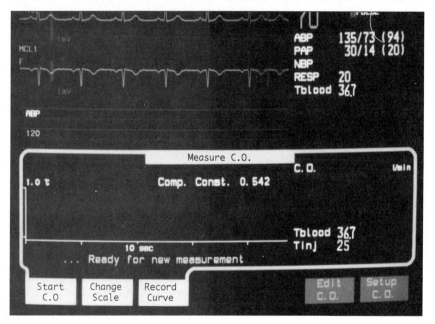

Attach one of the prefilled syringes to the stopcock on the proximal lumen. Turn the stopcock so that it's closed to the I.V. infusion or pressure flush and open to the catheter.

▶ *Clinical tip:* Avoid prolonged handling of the syringe because this may warm the injectate and alter the cardiac output values.

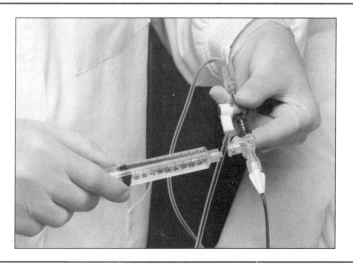

Press the module's START key. When the monitor indicates that it's ready, rapidly and smoothly instill the injectate within 4 seconds during the end-expiratory phase of the respiratory cycle.

▶ **Clinical tip:** Because blood flow varies during the respiratory cycle, instill the injectate during the same phase of the cycle each time you perform the procedure to ensure consistent and accurate results.

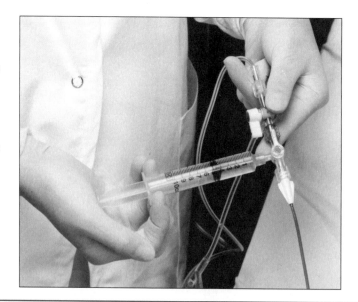

If your monitor displays a thermodilution curve, watch for a smooth and sharp rise initiating the curve. Continue to observe the curve as you repeat the injection procedure at least three times. Discard any reading that isn't within 10% of the other readings.

You'll need at least three readings to obtain a reliable mean value—four or more if you have to discard a reading outside the acceptable 10% range. If you repeatedly obtain individual values that vary by more than 10%, reassess the patient's condition, double-check your technique, and repeat the procedure.

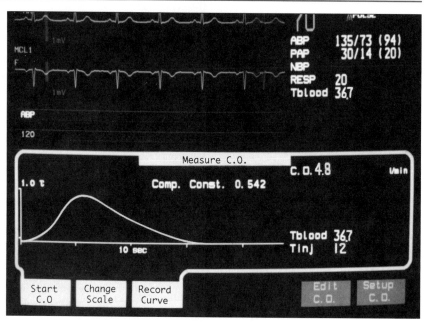

When the procedure is complete, turn the stopcock so that it's open to the I.V. infusion or pressure flush. If the lumen you were using was also being used to monitor the right atrium, observe the monitor for the return of a right atrial pressure waveform. Then place the patient in a comfortable position.

Average the readings to obtain a mean cardiac output value. Document this value and the patient's tolerance of the procedure.

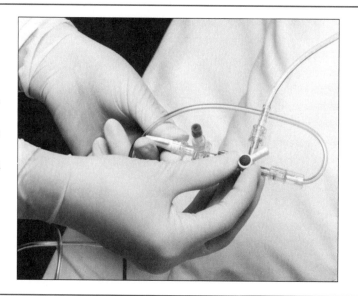

Measuring cardiac functions

To measure various aspects of cardiac function, combine cardiac output values with other key values obtainable when the patient has a pulmonary artery line and a separate arterial line. These values include mean arterial pressure, right atrial pressure, mean pulmonary artery pressure, and pulmonary artery wedge pressure. Then calculate stroke volume, stroke volume index, systemic vascular resistance, or pulmonary vascular resistance using the formulas below. For continuity, the same values for cardiac output (CO), heart rate (HR), and stroke volume (SV) will be used throughout the equations.

Keep in mind that some monitoring systems compute these values automatically.

Stroke volume

To determine SV—the volume of blood pumped by the ventricle in one contraction—multiply the CO by 1,000 and divide by the HR. Normal SV ranges between 60 and 100 ml/beat. Use this equation:

$$SV = \frac{CO \times 1,000}{HR}$$

Example: Here the patient's CO is 5.5 liters/minute and his HR is 80 beats/minute.

$$SV = \frac{5.5 \times 1,000}{80} = \frac{5,500}{80} = 68.75 \text{ ml/beat}$$

Stroke volume index

To assess whether the patient's SV is adequate for his body size, compute the stroke volume index (SVI). Do this either by dividing the SV by the patient's body surface area (BSA) or by dividing his cardiac index (CI) by his HR. Normally, the SVI ranges between 33 and 47 ml/beat/m² of BSA. Use either of these equations:

$$SVI = \frac{SV}{BSA} \text{ or } \frac{CI}{HR}$$

Example: As we determined in the example above, the patient's SV is 68.75 ml/beat. His BSA is 1.64 m² and his CI (calculated by dividing his CO by his BSA) is 3.35 liters/min/m².

$$SVI = \frac{SV}{BSA} = \frac{68.75}{1.64} = 42 \text{ ml/beat/m}^2$$

or

$$SVI = \frac{CI}{HR} = \frac{3.35}{80} = 0.042 \text{ liters/beat/m}^2$$

Systemic vascular resistance

To assess systemic vascular resistance (SVR)—the degree of left ventricular resistance known as afterload—deduct right atrial pressure (RAP) from mean arterial pressure (MAP). Then multiply by a rounded conversion factor of 80 to commute the value into units of force (dynes/sec/cm⁻⁵). Divide this value by the CO value.

Many hospitals consider a range of 800 to 1,200 dynes/sec/cm⁻⁵ to be a normal SVR value; however, the American Association of Critical-Care Nurses (AACN) accepts 900 to 1,400 dynes/sec/cm⁻⁵ as a normal range. To do your own calculations, use this equation:

$$SVR = \frac{(MAP - RAP) \times 80}{CO}$$

Example: Here the patient's MAP is 93 and his RAP is 6; CO remains 5.5. Note that 80 is the conversion factor.

$$SVR = \frac{(93 - 6) \times 80}{5.5} = \frac{6,960}{5.5} = 1,265 \text{ dynes/sec/cm}^{-5}$$

Pulmonary vascular resistance

To measure pulmonary vascular resistance (PVR)—or right ventricular afterload—deduct pulmonary artery wedge pressure (PAWP) from mean pulmonary artery pressure (MPAP). To commute the value into units of force (dynes/sec/cm⁻⁵), multiply the result by a rounded conversion factor of 80. Then divide the product by the CO value.

According to the AACN, the normal range for PVR is 155 to 255 dynes/sec/cm⁻⁵. To calculate your patient's PVR, use this equation:

$$PVR = \frac{(MPAP - PAWP) \times 80}{CO}$$

Example: Here the patient's MPAP is 20 and his PAWP is 5; his CO remains 5.5. Again the conversion factor is 80.

$$PVR = \frac{(20 - 5) \times 80}{5.5} = \frac{1,200}{5.5} = 218 \text{ dynes/sec/cm}^{-5}$$

Analyzing thermodilution curves

The thermodilution curve provides valuable information about cardiac output, injection technique, and equipment problems. When studying the curve, keep in mind that the area under the curve is inversely proportional to cardiac output: The smaller the area under the curve, the higher the cardiac output; the larger the area under the curve, the lower the cardiac output.

Besides providing a record of cardiac output, the curve may indicate problems related to technique, such as erratic or slow injectate instillations, or other problems, such as respiratory variations or electrical interference. The curves below correspond to those typically seen in clinical practice.

Normal thermodilution curve

With an accurate monitoring system and a patient who has adequate cardiac output, the thermodilution curve begins with a smooth, rapid upstroke and is followed by a smooth, gradual downslope. The curve shown below indicates that the injectate instillation time was within the recommended 4 seconds and that the temperature curve returned to baseline blood temperature.

The height of the curve will vary, depending on whether you use a room-temperature or an iced injectate. Room-temperature injectate produces an upstroke of lower amplitude.

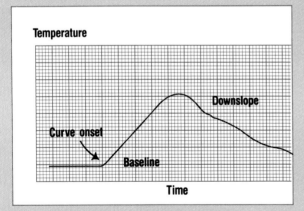

Low-cardiac-output curve

A thermodilution curve representing low cardiac output shows a rapid, smooth upstroke (from proper injection technique). But because the heart is ejecting blood less efficiently from the ventricles, the injectate warms slowly and takes longer to be ejected from the ventricle. Consequently, the curve takes longer to return to baseline. This slow return produces a larger area under the curve, corresponding to low cardiac output.

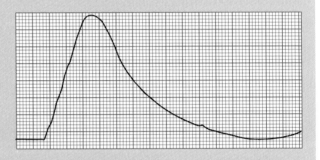

High-cardiac-output curve

Again, the curve has a rapid, smooth upstroke from proper injection technique. But because the ventricles are ejecting blood too forcefully, the injectate moves through the heart quickly and the curve returns to baseline more rapidly. The smaller area under the curve suggests higher cardiac output.

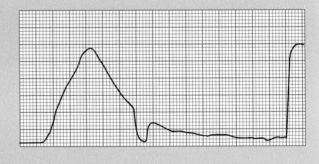

Analyzing thermodilution curves *(continued)*

Curve reflecting poor technique
This curve results from an uneven and too slow (taking more than 4 seconds) administration of injectate. The uneven and slower-than-normal upstroke and the larger area under the curve erroneously indicate low cardiac output. A kinked catheter, unsteady hands during the injection, or improper placement of the injectate lumen in the introducer sheath may also cause this type of curve.

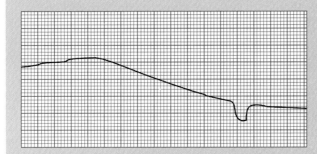

Curve associated with respiratory variations
To obtain a reliable cardiac output measurement, you need a steady baseline pulmonary artery blood temperature. If the patient has rapid or labored respirations, or if he's receiving mechanical ventilation, the thermodilution curve may reflect inaccurate cardiac output values. The curve below from a patient receiving mechanical ventilation reflects fluctuating pulmonary artery blood temperatures. The thermistor interprets the unsteady temperature as a return to baseline. The result is a curve erroneously showing high cardiac output (small area under the curve).

Note: In some cases, the equipment senses no return to baseline at all and produces a sinelike curve recorded by the computer as 0.00.

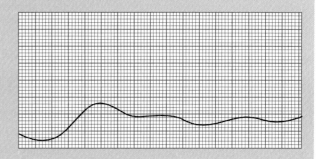

Correcting problems of cardiac output monitoring

PROBLEM	CAUSES	INTERVENTIONS
Cardiac output values lower than expected	Injectate volume greater than indicated for computation constant	• Be sure to instill only the injectate volume that's appropriate for the computation constant.
	Erroneous computation constant (set too low)	• Before injection, verify that the computation constant setting and the injectate volume are compatible. • To avoid repeating the injection procedure, correct the cardiac output (CO) value and the computation constant (CC) setting. To do so, use this formula: CO wrong × CC right ÷ CC wrong = CO right. Then reset the monitor for the next serial injection, using the correct computation constant.
	Injectate lumen exits in right ventricle	• Confirm proper placement of the injectate lumen by observing the monitor for right atrial waveforms.
Cardiac output values higher than expected	Injectate volume smaller than indicated for computation constant	• Before injection, verify that the injectate volume is correct for the determined computation constant. • Look for and expel air bubbles from the injectate syringe.
	Erroneous computation constant (set too high)	• Before injection, verify that the computation constant setting and the injectate volume are compatible. • To avoid repeating the injection procedure, correct the cardiac output (CO) value and the computation constant (CC) setting. To do so, use this formula: CO wrong × CC right ÷ CC wrong = CO right. Then reset the monitor for the next serial injection, using the correct computation constant.
	Catheter tip too far into pulmonary artery	• Check catheter placement by obtaining a pulmonary artery wedge pressure (PAWP) tracing. If the catheter is placed correctly, 1.25 to 1.5 cc of air will be necessary to obtain a PAWP tracing. • Reposition the catheter if necessary.
	Left to right ventricular septal defect	• Observe the PAWP tracing. A giant "V" wave indicates a ventricular septal defect and resultant incorrect cardiac output values. • Prepare to use another cardiac output monitoring method, such as the Fick method.
Cardiac output values deviating at least 10% from the mean (no pattern)	Arrhythmias, such as premature ventricular contractions and atrial fibrillation	• Observe the electrocardiogram monitor while monitoring cardiac output, and try to instill injectate during a period without arrhythmias. • Increase the number of serial injections to five or six, and average the values. • If the arrhythmias continue, notify the doctor.
	Catheter whip (turbulent, erratic waveform resulting from turbulence of blood circulating around intrusive catheter)	• Observe the waveforms, and reposition the catheter if necessary. • If catheter whip doesn't decrease spontaneously after the catheter is inserted or repositioned, increase the number of serial cardiac output determinations.
	Varying pulmonary artery baseline temperature (which causes drift during respiration)	• Obtain cardiac output values when respirations are steadier and less labored. • Minimize temperature variations by administering injectate during the same phase of the respiratory cycle each time you measure cardiac output. • Increase the number of serial injections.
	Variations in venous return (for example, from rapid bolus administration of drugs or fluids or from the patient's shivering, coughing, or restlessness)	• Avoid giving bolus injections of drugs or fluids just before measuring cardiac output. • If shivering accompanies a fever, notify the doctor. • Avoid measuring cardiac output until coughing or restlessness subsides.
	Inadequate signal-to-noise ratio	• To strengthen the signal, increase the injectate volume or lower the injectate temperature (for example, by using iced injectate for patients with hypothermia).
	Poor injection technique	• Observe the upstroke on the thermodilution curve to detect an error in injection technique. • Use two hands to deliver a bolus injection quickly and evenly.

MONITORING CARDIAC OUTPUT AND SvO$_2$ CONTINUOUSLY

Performed together, continuous cardiac output and mixed venous oxygen (SvO$_2$) monitoring supplies up-to-the-minute information about your patient. It uses a specially modified pulmonary artery (PA) catheter, which measures cardiac output by a thermal filament located near the proximal injection port.

Once positioned in the right ventricle, the filament heats the blood in a pulsating pattern. Then a thermistor on the catheter's end measures the temperature changes created by heat "pulses" as blood flows through the heart into the pulmonary artery. These temperature changes are detected and recorded by a computer that correlates them with the pattern of heat pulsations. The result is a thermodilution curve, with cardiac output computed from the area under the curve.

For measuring SvO$_2$, the instrument uses a spectrophotometric technique and light-emitting diodes to measure oxygen levels in venous blood.

Advantages

Because this kind of continuous monitoring doesn't rely on an injectate to produce thermal changes, it eliminates the danger of incorrectly preparing or connecting the temperature sensors needed when using an injectate. Also, older thermodilution methods provided data at only one point in time; continuous monitoring produces information at all times. This allows you to evaluate treatment effectiveness and to detect changes in the patient's condition before they might otherwise be recognized. Updated every 30 seconds, readings reflect an average of the last 3 to 5 minutes of data.

Gathering the equipment

To initiate continuous cardiac output and SvO$_2$ monitoring, assemble all the equipment you'll need for inserting a PA catheter and a small bedside monitor console with the necessary cables, such as the Vigilance monitor (manufactured by Baxter Healthcare Corp.) shown here.

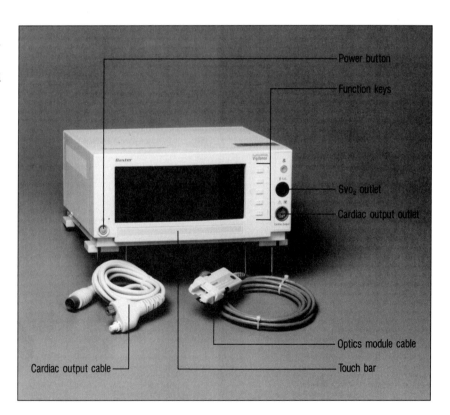

Power button

Function keys

SvO$_2$ outlet

Cardiac output outlet

Optics module cable

Touch bar

Cardiac output cable

Karen E. Michael, RN, MSN, a case manager with Greater Atlantic Health Service in Philadelphia, contributed to this section. The publisher thanks *Hill-Rom,* Batesville, Ind., and *Baxter Healthcare Corp.,* Irvine, Calif., for their help.

You'll also need a PA catheter such as the CCOmbo catheter shown here (also manufactured by Baxter for use with the Vigilance system). The seven lumens of this catheter are color-coded for their various functions.

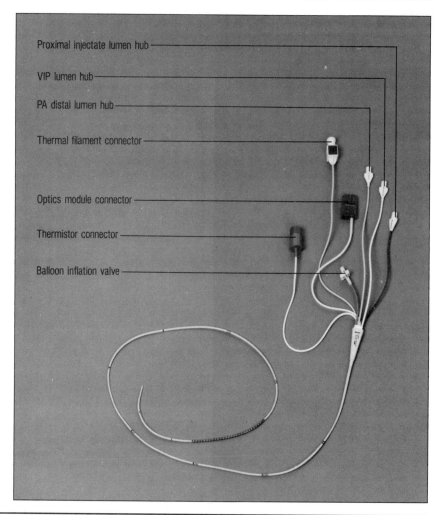

Proximal injectate lumen hub

VIP lumen hub

PA distal lumen hub

Thermal filament connector

Optics module connector

Thermistor connector

Balloon inflation valve

Place the monitor at the patient's bedside, and explain the procedure. To prepare the monitor for use, first plug it into an electrical outlet. Then plug the cardiac output cable and the optics module cable into the monitor (as shown), if they're not already in place.

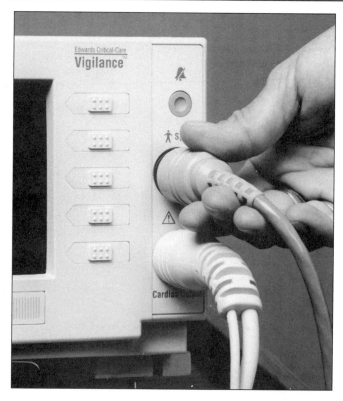

Press the power button to turn on the monitor. Watch for the trend screen to appear on the monitor's display screen.

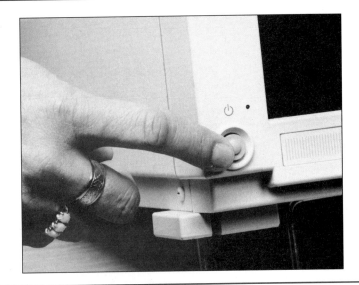

Setting up for continuous cardiac output monitoring

To the right of the display screen are five keys whose functions are identified on the screen itself. (This allows the functions to change with the programs—or menus—on the display screen while the keys remain stationary.) Beneath the screen is a touch-sensitive bar.

    Press the function key for PA-TIENT DATA (as shown), and watch for the patient data screen to appear.

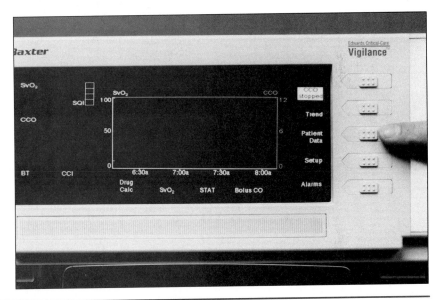

To enter the patient's height and weight, press the EDIT key on the patient data screen and watch for the edit data screen to appear.

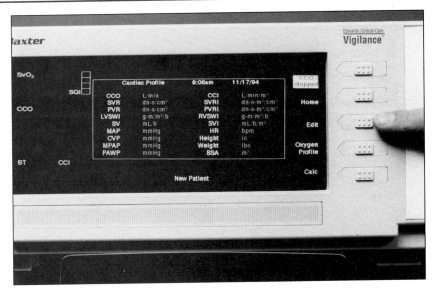

Next, press the CURSOR key until the cursor rests on the specific patient data that you wish to change—in this case, height.

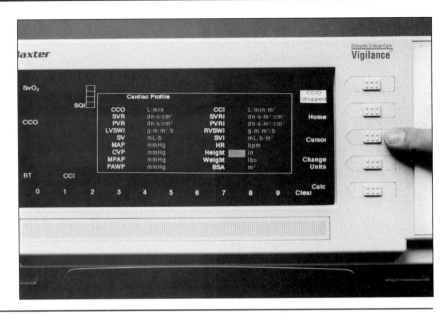

Enter the value by pressing the touch bar below the displayed value that you wish to enter on the screen. Then press the CURSOR key until it highlights the next patient value that you wish to enter.

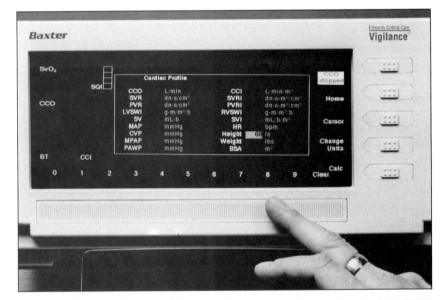

This kind of monitor can accommodate different units of measure, so if the monitor shows a U.S. measurement such as pounds (lb), and you're entering a metric measurement such as kilograms (kg), simply press the CHANGE UNITS key to select the other unit.

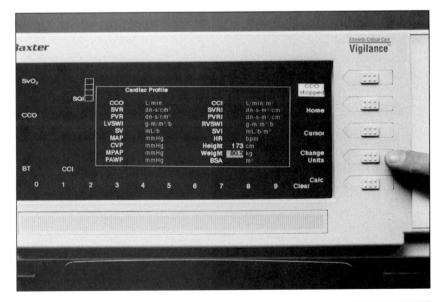

Once you enter the values, press the CALC key to display the calculated values—in this case, BSA for body surface area.

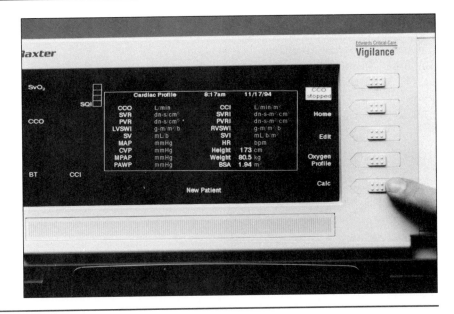

Finish by pressing the HOME key to save the values that you entered and to return to the trend screen.

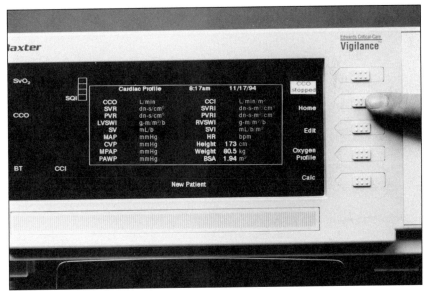

Next, press the SETUP key beside the trend screen, and watch for another screen to appear.

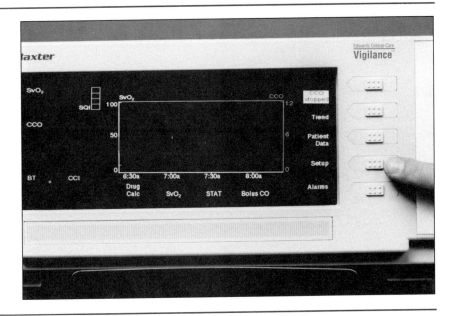

This display screen allows you to choose various systems or units of measure. If you wish to change any index on this screen, press CURSOR until the selection is highlighted.

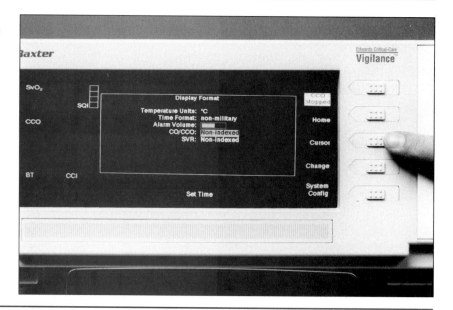

Next, press the CHANGE key to choose Fahrenheit or Celsius temperature, customary (12-hour) or military (24-hour) time, alarm volume, or indexed or nonindexed values for cardiac output and systemic vascular resistance (SVR). Then press the HOME key to store the changes and to return to the trend screen.

▶ *Clinical tip:* Cardiac output must be identified as a parameter for it to be displayed. (When you enter the patient's height and weight, the cardiac index is automatically computed.)

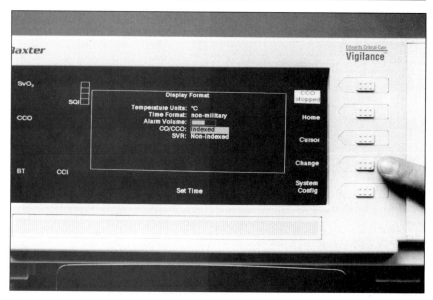

Now press the ALARMS key and watch for the alarm screen to appear.

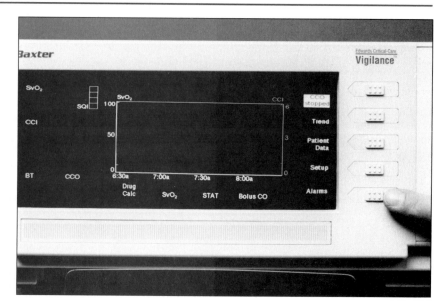

To change the alarm limits for continuous cardiac output, first press the touch bar to select CCO.

▶ *Clinical tip:* You can also change the alarm limits for SvO₂ by subsequently pressing the touch bar to select SvO₂.

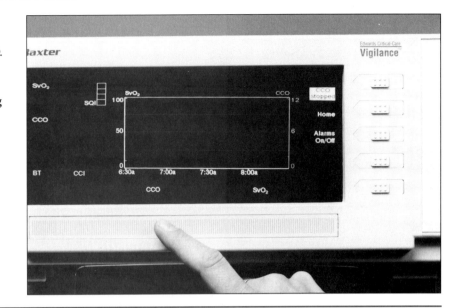

Next, press the HI/LOW key (as shown), and select the desired limits using the touch bar. Then press HOME to store the desired entry and to return to the trend screen.

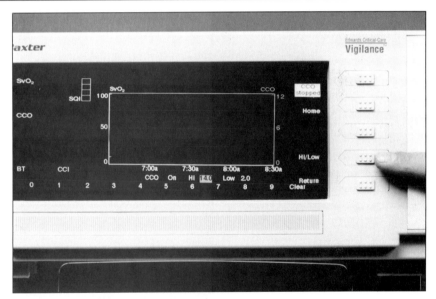

Look at the trend screen to make sure that the alarms aren't disabled. If they are, you'll see a bell covered by an X on the display screen. In such a case, press ALARMS and watch for the alarm screen to appear. Then press the ALARMS ON/OFF key to reactivate the alarm (as shown). When you're done, press the HOME key to return to the trend screen.

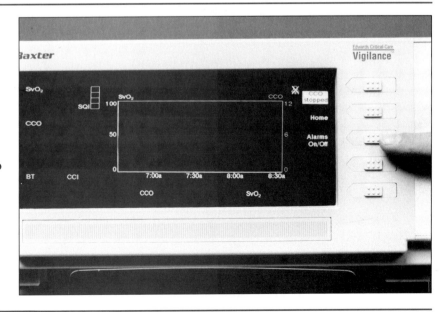

Next, locate the thermistor connection port and the continuous cardiac output port on the patient's PA catheter. Remove the covers from the ports (as shown).

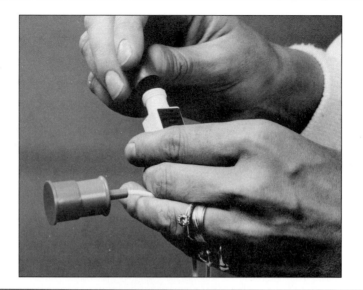

Connect the color-coded (blue) thermal filament connector to the same color port of the patient cable.

Connect the color-coded (white) port of the patient cable from the console to the color-coded (white) thermistor port of the PA catheter. Line up the ridge inside the rim of the thermistor port with the indentation on the patient cable and push them together. Don't twist the connection because this can damage the wire filaments inside the thermistor port.

▶ *Clinical tip:* On color-coded cardiac output monitors, be sure to match the connections, such as the thermal filament and the thermistor connector, according to color.

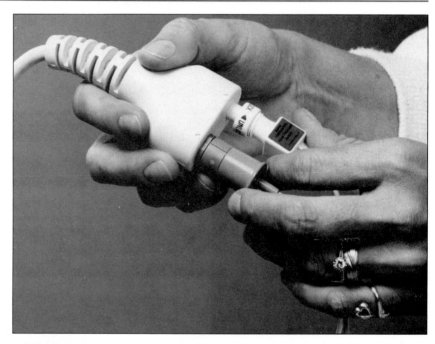

Screw the outer round cover from the patient cable onto the outer area of the thermistor port to secure the connection.

You are now ready to begin continuous cardiac output monitoring.

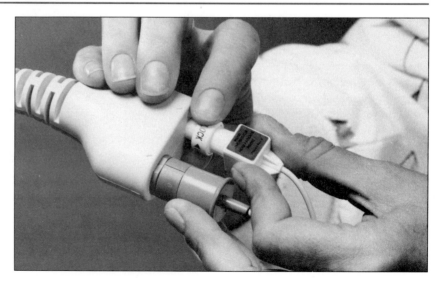

Setting up for S⊽O₂ monitoring

To use this monitor's S⊽O₂ function, first insert the optics module connector (blue) on the PA catheter into the optics module on the S⊽O₂ cable.

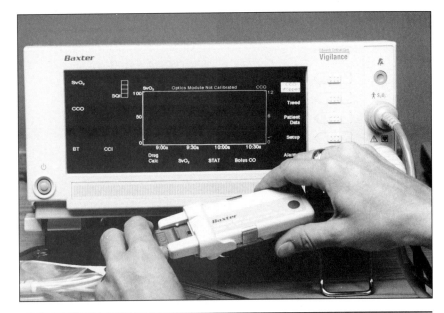

Press the touch bar under "S⊽O₂," which calls up a screen to access S⊽O₂ calibration options.

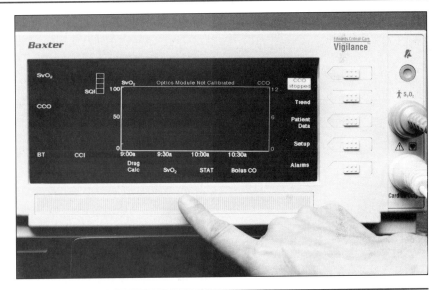

Then press the touch bar below the words "In Vitro Calibration" (as shown). A screen displaying hemoglobin and hematocrit values will appear.

Enter the laboratory values for the patient's hemoglobin or hematocrit by pressing the CURSOR key to select hemoglobin or hematocrit and then pressing the touch bar below the appropriate numbers. If the values are unknown, use the default values already displayed.

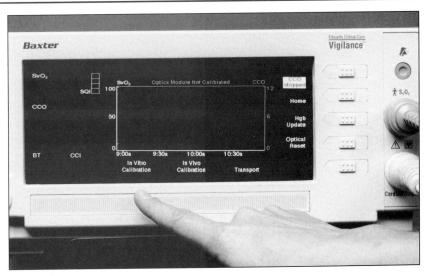

Next, press the CAL key (as shown) to complete the calibration process.

Note: You'll need to perform an in vivo calibration of the SvO_2 system every 24 hours. To do this, consult the manufacturer's directions.

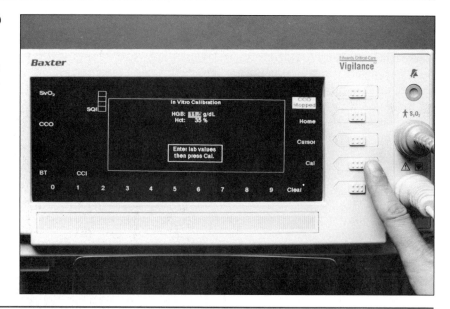

The message "In Vitro Calibration in progress" will appear on the screen along with the amount of time remaining until the calibration is complete.

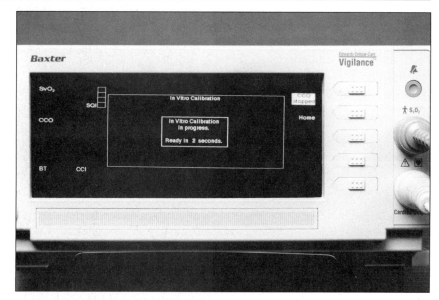

Next, the screen will show "In Vitro Calibration OK." You are now ready to initiate SvO_2 monitoring.

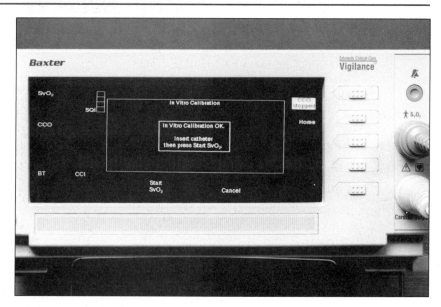

Monitoring the patient

Assist with the insertion of the special PA catheter. (See "Preparing for Catheter Insertion," pages 38 to 42, and "Assisting with Catheter Insertion," pages 43 to 50.)

Once the catheter is properly positioned in the pulmonary artery, remove your gloves (if desired) and press the touch bar below "START SvO₂" to begin monitoring SvO₂, if you'll be measuring this parameter.

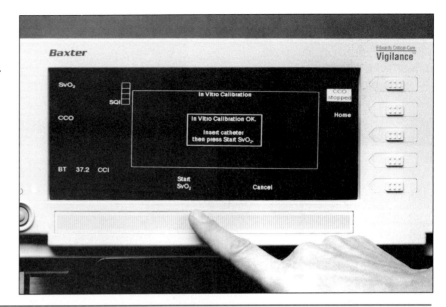

Pressing START SvO₂ will return the trend screen and cause the SvO₂ value to appear in the upper left corner of the screen.

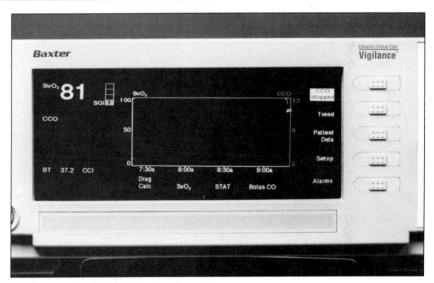

Next, press the CCO STOPPED key beside the upper right corner of the trend screen. It will become the CCO RUNNING key.

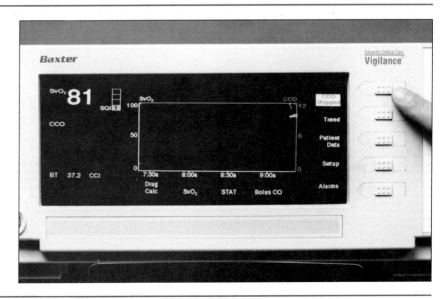

The message "Collecting CCO data" will appear on the trend screen. About 3 minutes later, the cardiac output value will appear (as shown). Thereafter, the cardiac output value will be updated every 30 seconds.

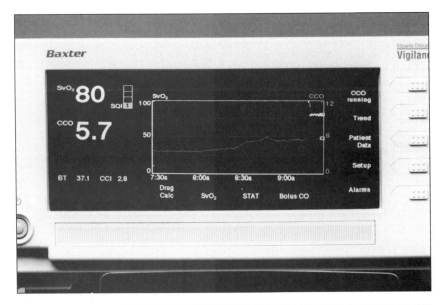

Press the touch bar under "STAT" if you wish to display the history of cardiac output data. Ten boxes will appear, with the most recent data in the top left box and the oldest data in the bottom right box.

Then press the HOME key to return to the trend screen.

Finally, document the procedure, including the time monitoring was initiated, the results, and the patient's tolerance of the procedure, in your progress notes.

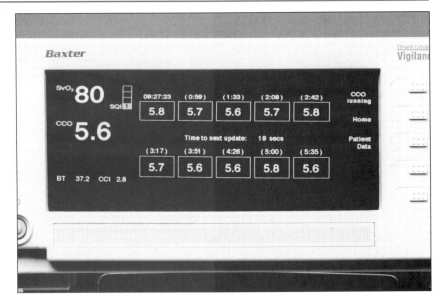

MONITORING LEFT ATRIAL PRESSURE

Left atrial pressure (LAP) monitoring provides information about left ventricular function after open-heart surgery. A catheter inserted in the left atrium allows direct measurement of LAP. After being sutured to the pericardium, the catheter is drawn through a mediastinal incision on the chest wall and sutured to the skin.

LAP is created by blood volume in the left side of the heart and reflects the filling pressures in the left ventricle when the mitral valve is open. Unless the patient has mitral valve disease, LAP and the waveform produced during monitoring are reliable indicators of left ventricular end-diastolic pressure and, therefore, left ventricular function. Normal LAP ranges from 4 to 12 mm Hg. The LAP waveform resembles the pulmonary artery wedge pressure (PAWP) waveform.

LAP monitoring isn't performed routinely because pulmonary artery pressure (PAP) monitoring provides essential hemodynamic data with fewer risks. By monitoring PAP, you can approximate the LAP from the PAWP value. If the patient has a pulmonary artery catheter with a cardiac output port, you can measure cardiac output as well.

INDICATIONS

LAP monitoring is used primarily in heart transplant patients and in patients with left ventricular dysfunction who are undergoing cardiac surgery. It may also be used to evaluate treatment in patients with pulmonary hypertension, tricuspid or pulmonic valve disease, or abnormal cardiac anatomy. (In these patients, PAWP values may be unreliable indicators of left ventricular pressure.) Additionally, LAP monitoring may be initiated for patients with severe right ventricular failure who require infusion of prostaglandins and vasoconstrictors.

COMPLICATIONS

A major complication of LAP monitoring is systemic, cerebral, or coronary embolism, which may result from the introduction of air into the heart. (Using an air filter connected to a pressure transducer system can reduce the risk of this complication.) Another potential complication, bleeding at the insertion site may follow removal of the left atrial catheter and lead to life-threatening cardiac tamponade.

Setting up the system

Before the patient returns from the operating room, prepare a pressure transducer system with a fast flush device. You'll use heparin flush solution in the flush line. (To decrease the chance of flushing drugs and the risk of infection, this I.V. line should flow only to the left atrial catheter.)

Besides an I.V. pole, you'll need clean gloves, a gown, a face shield, an air filter, a 10-ml syringe, a monitor pressure cable, hypoallergenic tape, povidone-iodine ointment, sterile 4″ × 4″ gauze pads, a linen saver pad, a marking pen, and a carpenter's level or a ruler. You'll also need a monitor with LAP monitoring capabilities.

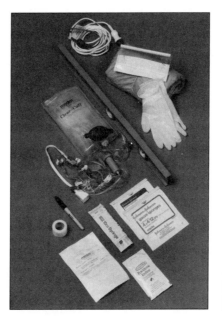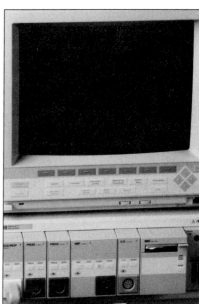

Cindy Tryniszewski, RN, MSN, Susan Galea, RN, MSN, CCRN, and *Cynthia Possanza, RN, MSN, CCRN,* contributed to this section. Ms. Tryniszewski is a clinical manager with Springhouse Corporation. Ms. Galea and Ms. Possanza are independent nurse consultants for Springhouse Corporation. The publisher thanks the following organizations for their help: *Medtronic, Inc.,* Minneapolis; *Medex, Inc.,* Hillard, Ohio; and *Hewlett-Packard Co.,* Andover, Mass.

After you assemble the equipment, unwrap the air filter. Then put on gloves and attach the air filter to the pressure transducer line at the end of the pressure transducer tubing. Secure all connections.

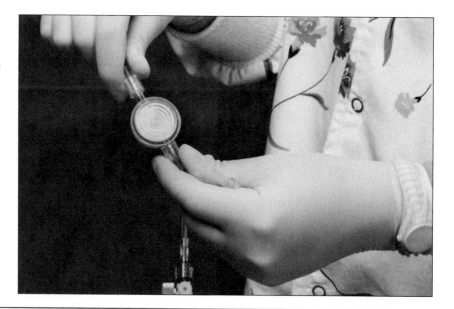

To expel air from the filter, remove the end cap on the filter, and squeeze the fast flush device (as shown). Let the filter fill completely with the heparin flush solution while you hold the filter upright to expel the air.

▶ *Clinical tip:* Completely saturate the filter with the flush solution by letting it rest for several minutes and then flushing it again.

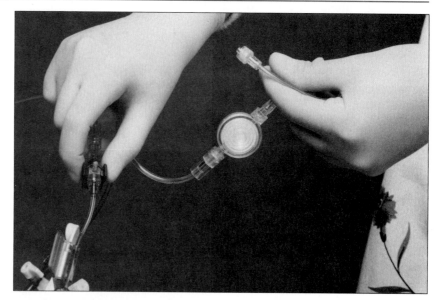

Now rotate the filter from front to back and check for air bubbles. If you see any, gently tap the filter and continue flushing.

▶ *Clinical tip:* Be sure to expel air from every part of the line. Otherwise, an air bubble may be forced into the patient's left atrium, causing an embolism.

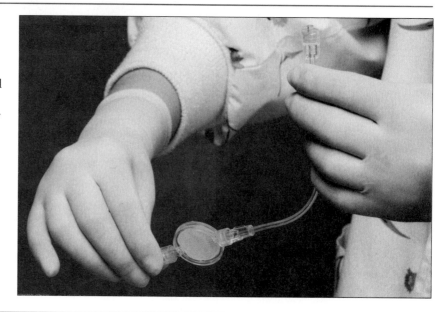

Take the prepared pressure transducer system and air filter to the patient's room and hang them on an I.V. pole. Insert the LAP module into the monitor if it's not already in place, and connect the monitor pressure cable to the LAP module. Then connect the transducer cable to the monitor pressure cable (as shown).

If you're using a manifold mount and it's not already in place, attach the mount to the I.V. pole and put the transducer into the mount.

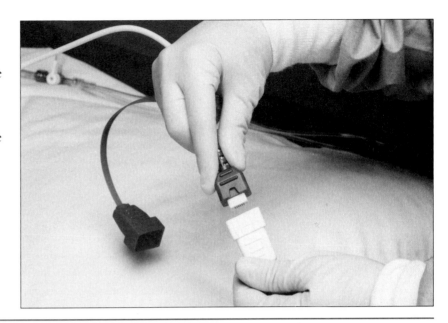

To ensure accurate pressure readings, position the transducer at the phlebostatic axis—the fourth intercostal space midway between the anterior and posterior chest wall. Position the transducer's air-fluid interface (located at the vent, or zero, port of the transducer's stopcock) level with this point (as shown).

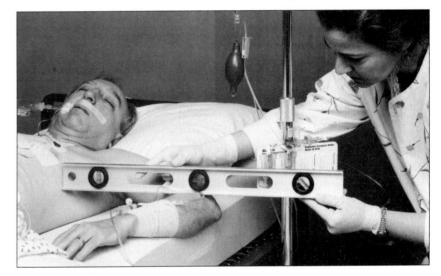

Use a marking pen to pinpoint the phlebostatic axis on the patient's chest or on a piece of tape applied to the patient's chest. This mark allows every nurse to use the same reference point when measuring LAP.

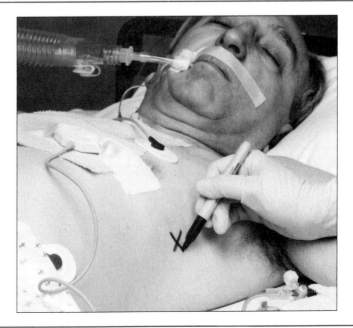

Turn the stopcock off to the patient, thereby opening the transducer to air. Then remove the cap from the vent port of the transducer (as shown).

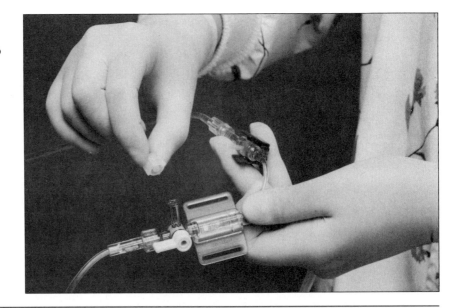

Following the manufacturer's manual, press the ZERO key on the monitor. Then press the CALIBRATE key. Keep in mind that some monitors require manipulation of a calibration key or knob, whereas others calibrate automatically. When you've finished zeroing, turn the stopcock on the transducer so that it's closed to air and open to the patient.

Continuing to follow the manufacturer's directions, select the appropriate mode and scale.

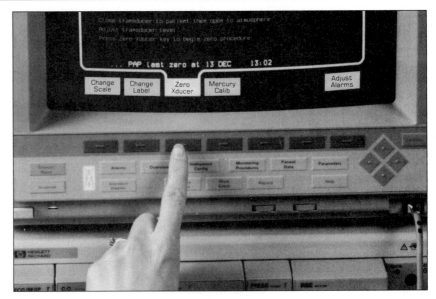

Before attaching the pressure transducer tubing to the left atrial catheter, put on clean gloves, a gown, and a face shield. Then remove the protective cap from the air filter at the end of the pressure transducer tubing. Be sure to turn the stopcock off to the patient before removing the cap from the left atrial catheter (as shown).

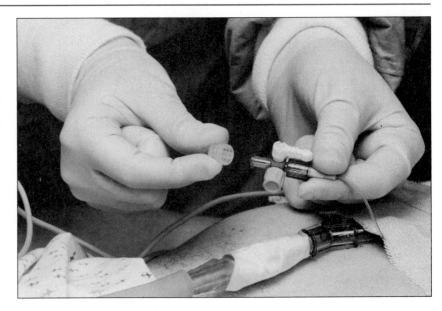

Place a linen-saver pad on the patient's chest. Then attach a 10-ml syringe to the open port of the stopcock. Pull back on the syringe to flush the stopcock and expel any air within the pressure tubing and stopcock.

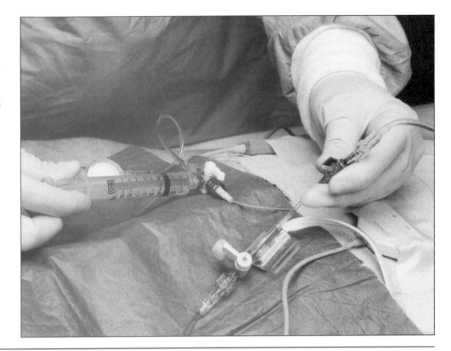

After you connect the tubing to the catheter, turn the stopcock to open the transducer to the patient. The patient's left atrial waveform should appear on the monitor.

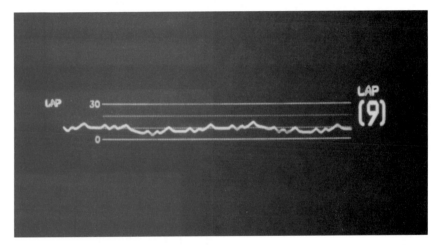

Review the alarm limits. If they need adjustment, set the high and low monitor alarms for the LAP limits determined by the doctor. Usually, you'll set the high alarm at 2 mm Hg above the baseline reading and the low alarm at 2 mm Hg below the baseline.

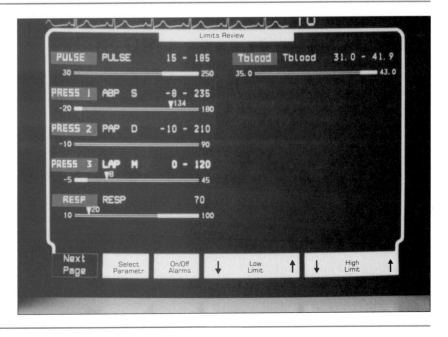

Alternatively, if the pressure transducer system and air filter were connected to the left atrial catheter in the operating room, connect the monitoring cable to the transducer (as shown). And turn the stopcock so that it's open to the patient.

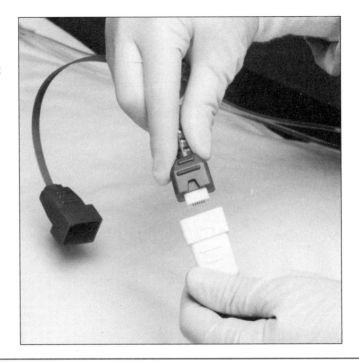

Once you've connected the patient to the pressure transducer system and the monitor, assess and care for the catheter site. Although the surgeon sutured the catheter to the skin, you can reinforce security by taping the catheter (as shown).

▶ *Clinical tip:* Alternatively, tape the air filter to a tongue blade and then to the patient's chest.

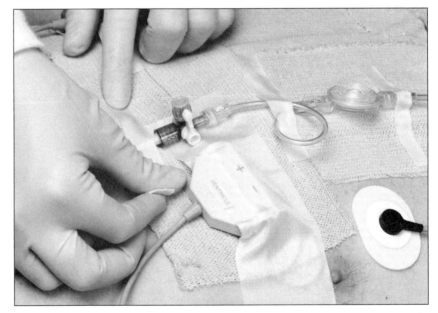

Taking the reading

Rezero the pressure transducer as described previously. Obtain the mean LAP measurement from the digital readout on the monitor screen (as shown). Note the LAP value at the end-expiration stage of respiration.

Then document the procedure and the first reading, noting the concentration of the heparin flush solution.

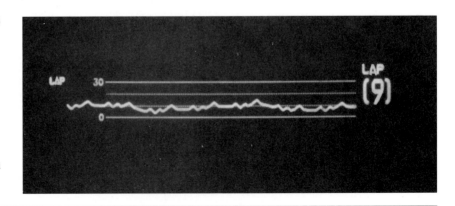

Continuously monitor the LAP waveform and pressure readings and compare them to other hemodynamic indices, such as cardiac output. Notify the doctor of any abnormal waveforms, including those revealing the catheter's migration to the left ventricle (as shown), damping, or a rise or fall of 2 mm Hg or more in the height of the A and V waves.

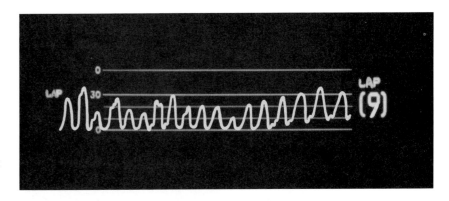

Document each reading as ordered or according to hospital protocol—usually hourly.

▶ ***Clinical tip:*** Remember that evaluating trends and changes in trends provides a more accurate picture of your patient's hemodynamic status and response to therapy than measuring isolated values alone.

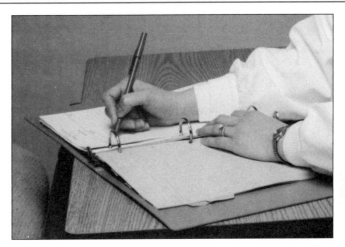

Discontinuing LAP monitoring

To assist with catheter removal, assemble the following equipment: sterile gloves, clean gloves, hypoallergenic tape, povidone-iodine ointment, a suture removal set, and sterile 4″ × 4″ gauze pads.

You'll also need equipment for observing universal precautions, including a face shield (or goggles and a mask), a gown, and gloves.

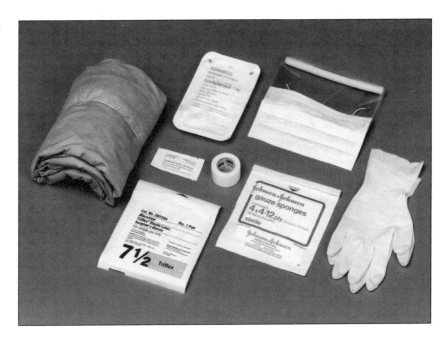

Explain the procedure to the patient. Then place him comfortably in the supine position with the head of the bed elevated 30 to 45 degrees. This decreases the risk of air embolism formation.

Turn off the monitor's LAP alarm while taking care not to turn off other alarms. Then put on the clean gloves, gown, and face shield.

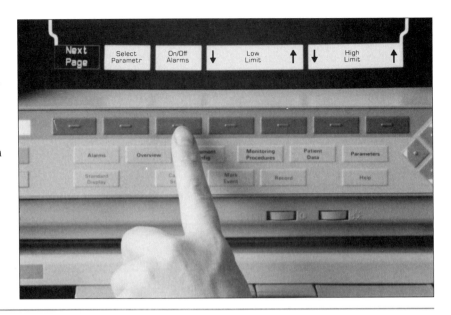

Close the flow clamp on the tubing of the pressurized heparin flush solution.

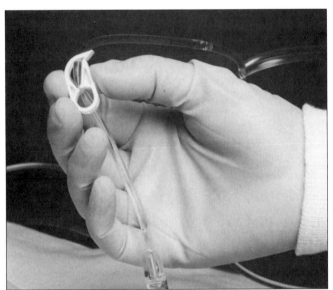

Turn the stopcock closest to the patient off to the patient.

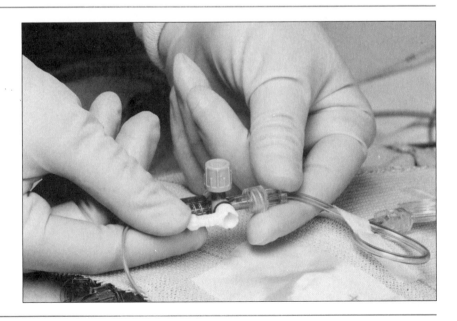

Remove the dressing. Then remove and discard your gloves and put on a pair of sterile gloves.

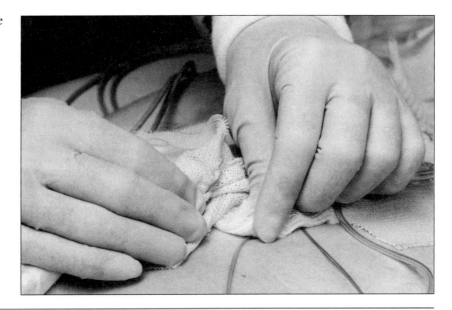

Immediately after the doctor cuts the sutures that hold the catheter to the patient's skin and removes the catheter, apply direct pressure to the exit site with sterile 4″ × 4″ gauze pads. Continue applying manual pressure for 10 minutes to prevent hemorrhage.

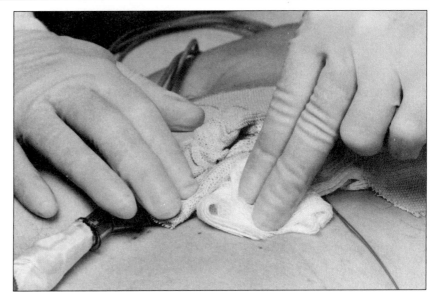

Once you're sure that the bleeding has stopped, apply povidone-iodine ointment to the site and cover it with dry, sterile 4″ × 4″ gauze pads. Tape the dressing in place.

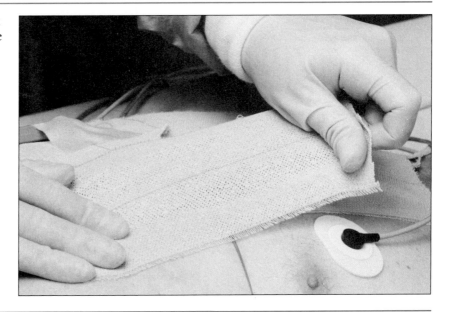

Check the catheter to make sure that it's intact. If you see evidence of breakage or other damage, notify the doctor immediately and save the catheter for the doctor to examine. Otherwise, dispose of the equipment according to hospital policy.

Auscultate the patient's breath and heart sounds and check vital signs and chest tube drainage every 15 minutes for the first hour, every 30 minutes for the next hour, and every hour thereafter or according to hospital protocol. Notify the doctor if you detect a significant increase or decrease in chest tube drainage or abnormal vital signs.

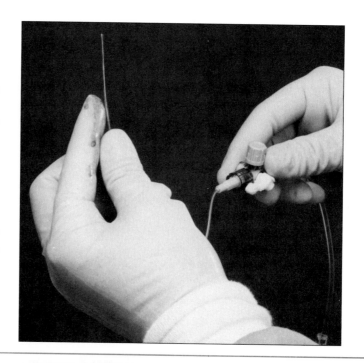

About 1 hour after catheter removal, check the dressing for signs of bleeding and the exit site for signs of a hematoma. If you observe such signs, apply pressure to the site and notify the doctor. If you don't observe any bleeding or a hematoma, redress the site as you dressed it initially.

As ordered, arrange for a chest X-ray about 1 hour after catheter removal to assess for cardiac tamponade. Then document the procedure.

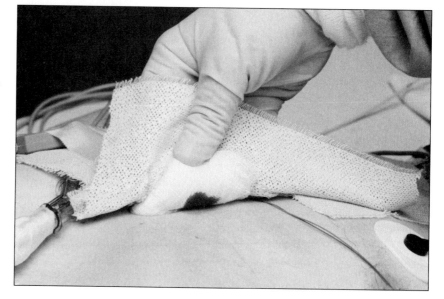

Understanding LAP waveforms

The normal left atrial pressure (LAP) waveform reflects low pressure. Similar to the pulmonary artery wedge pressure waveform, it has two positive deflections and consists of four distinct components: the A wave, the X descent, the V wave, and the Y descent.

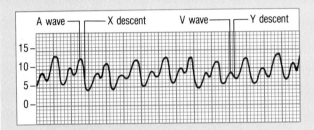

The first positive deflection, the *A wave,* represents left atrial contraction (also referred to as left atrial kick), which forces blood from the left atrium through the mitral valve and into the left ventricle.

After the left atrium contracts and before the mitral valve closes, the pressure in the left atrium falls and the waveform begins a downward slope, identified as the *X descent.*

During ventricular systole, the left atrium fills with blood and the mitral valve closes. At this point, the second positive deflection—the *V wave*—appears as the closed mitral valve bulges into the left atrium.

At the end of ventricular systole, the pressure in the left atrium decreases. This is represented as a downward slope of the V wave called the *Y descent.*

Abnormal LAP waveforms

Various conditions can produce abnormal LAP waveforms with the following features:

• *Absent A wave.* In atrial fibrillation, no A wave will appear in the LAP waveform because the atria only quiver and the left atrium doesn't contract. The mean LAP will increase in atrial fibrillation.

• *Prominent A wave.* Any condition that increases pressure or volume in the left atrium during atrial contraction will produce a prominent A wave. In patients with complete heart block or atrioventricular dissociation, the left atrium may contract against a closed mitral valve at times. The result: increasing LAP, which causes a prominent A wave.

In patients with mitral stenosis, the narrowing of the mitral valve obstructs blood flow from the left atrium to the left ventricle. To pump blood effectively to the left ventricle, the LAP must be high enough to force the blood through the stenotic valve. If the patient is in normal sinus rhythm, the LAP waveform will reveal a prominent A wave.

• *Prominent V wave.* This waveform abnormality may result from any condition that causes an increase in left atrial volume or pressure during left ventricular systole. In mitral insufficiency, for example, the incompetent mitral valve allows blood from the left ventricle to flow back into the left atrium during systole. This results in a prominent V wave unless the left atrium has enlarged enough to accommodate the regurgitated volume.

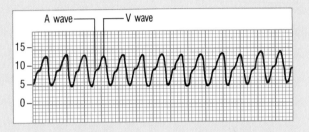

Evaluating the data

Before interpreting the data from the LAP waveforms, always remember to take pressure readings on the monitor's mean mode. Also, be sure to take readings at the end-expiration stage of respiration. Normally, a patient's LAP will fall during inspiration because of the drop in intrathoracic pressure and will rise to baseline during expiration.

Mean LAP ranges between 4 and 12 mm Hg. If your monitoring system doesn't automatically display the mean LAP value, use this equation:

$$\text{Mean LAP} = \frac{(\text{LAP diastolic} \times 2) + (\text{LAP systolic})}{3}$$

Decreased LAP

Expect LAP to decline as a result of hypovolemia from reduced fluid intake, postoperative hemorrhage, and postoperative rewarming that causes vasodilation.

Increased LAP

Expect LAP to rise from such conditions as mitral stenosis, tachyarrhythmias, a noncompliant left ventricle, and hypervolemia. In *mitral stenosis,* obstructed blood flow from the left atrium to the left ventricle increases left atrial volume and pressure. In *tachyarrhythmias,* the left ventricle's inability to eject a normal volume of blood raises LAP. In a *noncompliant left ventricle,* decreased myocardial contractility reduces blood ejection from the left ventricle, resulting in increased left ventricular pressure and LAP. In *hypervolemia,* increased fluid volume returning to the heart augments pressure within the heart.

COMPLICATIONS

Managing hazards of LAP monitoring

PROBLEM AND SIGNS	POSSIBLE CAUSES	NURSING INTERVENTIONS
Clotted catheter tip • Damped or straight waveform on the monitor	• Localized coagulation • Blood clot or air bubble • Sluggish flush solution flow • Insufficient heparin in flush solution	• Notify the doctor. He may attempt to aspirate the clot to prevent its release into the general circulation. Once he removes the clot, he may flush the catheter; if the clot resists removal, he'll usually remove the catheter.
Blood loss • Bloody dressing • Blood flowing from disconnected line	• Disconnected line • Dislodged catheter	• If the line disconnects, turn the stopcock closest to the patient off to the patient, and replace the equipment. • If the catheter pulls out, apply direct pressure to the site and notify the doctor. Also notify him if blood loss is great and vital signs change.
Hemorrhage • Increased sanguineous drainage from mediastinal chest tubes • Any or all of the following: hypotension, tachycardia, irritability, oliguria, pallor, and cool, clammy skin • Decreased pulmonary artery wedge pressure, decreased left atrial pressure (LAP)	• Bleeding from insertion site into mediastinum	• Notify the doctor immediately. • Check the patient's vital signs. • Administer fluids, blood products, and oxygen as prescribed. • In cases of inadequate gas exchange, prepare the patient for intubation. • If bleeding continues, prepare the patient for surgical intervention.
Embolism (air embolism or cerebral, coronary, or systemic thromboembolism) • Fall in blood pressure • Rise in central venous pressure (CVP) • Weak, rapid pulse • Cyanosis • Loss of consciousness or change in level of consciousness	• Air in tubing • Loose connections	• Notify the doctor and monitor vital signs. • Place the patient in Trendelenburg's position on his left side. If air has entered the heart chambers, this position may keep the air in the heart and out of circulation. • Check the line for a leak or a disconnection. • If the line disconnects, don't rejoin it. Replace the part with sterile equipment. Meanwhile, turn the stopcock off to the patient or clamp the line with a rubber-shod hemostat. • Administer oxygen if ordered. • Alert the doctor if you detect any systemic abnormalities.
Systemic infection • Sudden rise in patient's body temperature and pulse rate • Chills and shaking • Blood pressure changes	• Poor aseptic technique or contamination of equipment during manufacture, storage, or use	• Look for other sources of infection first. Obtain specimens of urine, sputum, and blood for culture as ordered. • Notify the doctor, who will probably discontinue the line and send the catheter tip for culture and sensitivity tests. • Administer antibiotics as prescribed.
Endocarditis • Intermittent fever, night sweats • Loud, regurgitant heart murmur • Weakness, fatigue • Weight loss, anorexia • Arthralgia	• Poor aseptic technique or contamination of equipment during manufacture, storage, or use	• Notify the doctor, who may discontinue the line. • Administer antibiotics as prescribed.
Catheter displacement • Ventricular arrhythmias • Heightened V waves • Absent valve click in a patient with a prosthetic mitral valve	• Catheter improperly sutured or taped to skin	• Notify the doctor if you think that the catheter moved; prepare to assist with catheter repositioning or removal. • Administer antiarrhythmic agents as prescribed.
Cardiac tamponade • Reduced cardiac output • Muffled heart sounds • Pulsus paradoxus • Neck vein distention • Reduced arterial blood pressure • Markedly elevated CVP or an equalization of CVP and pulmonary artery pressure • Decreased voltage reflected in the QRS complex • Sudden increase or decrease in chest tube drainage	• An accumulation of blood or fluid in pericardial sac	• Notify the doctor, who may order surgery. • Assess and document electrocardiogram rhythm patterns, vital signs, mental status, heart and breath sounds, and urine output. • Initiate I.V. volume therapy, as prescribed, with fluids and volume expanders. • Administer oxygen if ordered. • Administer inotropic agents as prescribed. • Begin resuscitative measures if necessary.

Caring for the patient with a left atrial catheter

During the insertion of a left atrial catheter and during the critical postoperative period after its insertion, you'll need to monitor your patient's hemodynamic status, ensure that the monitoring equipment is working effectively and safely, and prevent complications. Here are some guidelines.

Monitor hemodynamic status

• Measure and record left atrial pressure (LAP) at least hourly. Obtain the mean LAP at end expiration.
• Take your patient's vital signs at least hourly. To ensure accurate interpretation of values, take LAP readings at the same time that you measure the patient's blood pressure, heart rate, central venous pressure, pulmonary artery pressure, and urine output.
• Monitor the patient's LAP waveform. Watch for any increase in the height of the baseline V waves and a rise of 2 mm Hg or more in pressure. If you detect such an increase, notify the doctor.

Ensure effective operation

• To keep the left atrial catheter line and connecting tubing patent, make sure that a pressurized heparin flush solution continuously flows through the line. Check the flow rate hourly and maintain it at 3 to 4 ml/hour. Add more heparin to the solution if ordered.
• Balance and calibrate the pressure transducer at least once every 8 hours.
• Continuously monitor the LAP waveform, the electrocardiogram, and other pressure tracings. If you notice waveform damping, notify the doctor. Consult the manufacturer's manual as needed.
• If the patient has a prosthetic mitral valve, auscultate for the valve click sound. Notify the doctor immediately if you don't hear this sound; it may indicate that the left atrial catheter has slipped through the prosthetic valve.

Prevent complications

• Review and maintain sterile technique.
• Change the dressing at the insertion site every 24 hours or as recommended by hospital protocol. Check for redness, drainage, or broken sutures. If you detect any of these problems, notify the doctor immediately.
• Watch for bleeding from the insertion site (and, possibly, hemorrhage or cardiac tamponade if bleed-

ing affects the pericardial sac). This may occur if the catheter's size and position were inappropriate for the patient. To minimize complications that may accompany bleeding, check the patient's prothrombin and partial thromboplastin times. Also check the platelet count, which should be higher than 60,000/mm^3. If any results are abnormal, notify the doctor.
• Avoid contaminating the catheter site when bathing the patient.
• Don't rejoin any portion of a disconnected line. Instead, replace the portion with sterile equipment.
• Never infuse any I.V. fluids or medications other than the prescribed flush solution through the left atrial catheter line. If the catheter clogs, don't flush it or attempt to aspirate the occlusion. Notify the doctor immediately.
• Change the components of the system as recommended by hospital policy. For example, change a flush solution bag before it empties or every 24 hours. Change the pressure bag holding the flush solution at least once every 24 hours and the pressure tubing and the filter once every 48 hours.
• Frequently check the catheter connections and the insertion site. Check the taped connections for security, and make sure that the tape holding the catheter in place remains secure.
• Be alert for air bubbles in the system. If you detect any, attempt to expel the air. If you're unsuccessful, notify the doctor immediately. Always expel all air from the line before attaching it to the left atrial catheter.
• Measure and record chest tube drainage hourly. Notify the doctor of a significant increase or decrease in sanguineous drainage, which may indicate hemorrhage or developing cardiac tamponade.
• Monitor the patient and his waveform for signs of ventricular arrhythmias, and notify the doctor at once should any occur.
• Auscultate the patient's heart at least once every 4 hours or whenever you see a significant change in the LAP value or waveform. Notify the doctor of significant changes.
• Keep the patient on bed rest at all times.
• Be sure to arrange for a daily X-ray of the patient's chest to verify correct placement of the left atrial catheter.

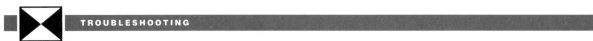

Solving LAP monitoring problems

PROBLEM	POSSIBLE CAUSES	NURSING INTERVENTIONS
Damped waveform Interference with transmission of the physiologic signal to the transducer	• Air in the system	• Check the entire system for air, including the tubing and transducer diaphragm. If air is present, flush it from the system through a stopcock port. Do not flush fluid into the patient.
	• Loose connections	• Check and tighten all connections.
	• Occluded catheter tip	• Notify the doctor, who may try to aspirate the occlusion. If successful, he'll flush the line to restore patency; if unsuccessful, he'll remove the line.
	• Catheter tip resting against the left atrium wall	• Reposition the patient.
	• Kinked tubing	• Unkink the tubing.
	• Inadequately inflated pressure bag	• Inflate the pressure bag to 300 mm Hg.
False-high pressure reading Values are higher than the patient's normal values with no significant change in baseline clinical findings. Before responding to the high reading, recheck the system for accuracy.	• Improper calibration	• Recalibrate the system.
	• Transducer placed below the level of the phlebostatic axis	• Reposition the transducer so that it's level with the phlebostatic axis.
	• Kinked catheter	• Unkink the catheter.
	• Occluded catheter tip	• Notify the doctor, who may try to aspirate the occlusion. If he's successful, he'll flush the line to restore patency; if he's unsuccessful, he'll remove the catheter.
	• Catheter tip resting against the left atrium wall	• Reposition the patient.
	• Small air bubbles in the tubing closest to the patient	• Flush air bubbles from the system through a stopcock port. Do not flush fluid into the patient.
False-low pressure reading Values are lower than the patient's normal values with no significant changes in baseline clinical findings. Before responding to the low reading, recheck the system for accuracy.	• Improper calibration	• Recalibrate the system.
	• Transducer placed above the level of the phlebostatic axis	• Reposition the transducer so that it's level with the phlebostatic axis.
	• Loose connections	• Check and tighten all connections.
	• Kinked catheter	• Unkink the catheter.
	• Catheter tip resting against the left atrium wall	• Reposition the patient.
	• Large air bubble close to the transducer	• Reprime the transducer.
Artifact Waveforms are erratic or form unrecognizable patterns.	• Electrical interference	• Check electrical equipment in the area.
	• Patient movement	• Instruct the patient to lie quietly while you read the monitor.
Drifting waveform Waveform floats above and below the baseline.	• Temperature change in the flush solution	• Allow temperature of the flush solution to stabilize.
	• Kinked or compressed monitor cable	• Check the cable and fix the kink or compression.
Absent waveform	• No power supply	• Turn on the power.
	• Loose connections	• Check and tighten all connections.
	• Stopcock turned off to the patient	• Properly position the stopcock. Be sure that the pressure transducer line is open to the catheter.
	• Transducer disconnected from the monitor module	• Reconnect the transducer to the monitor module.
	• Occluded catheter tip	• Notify the doctor, who may try to aspirate the occlusion. If he's successful, he'll flush the line to restore patency; if he's unsuccessful, he'll remove the line.
	• Catheter tip resting against the left atrium wall	• Reposition the patient.

USING THORACIC ELECTRICAL BIOIMPEDANCE MONITORING

Available for general use since the early 1990s, thoracic electrical bioimpedance monitoring provides a noninvasive alternative for tracking hemodynamic status. This technique provides information about a patient's cardiac index, preload, afterload, contractility, cardiac output, and blood flow by measuring low-level electricity that flows harmlessly through the body from electrodes placed on the patient's thorax. These electrodes detect signals elicited from the changing volume and velocity of blood flow through the aorta. The signals are interpreted by the bioimpedance monitor as a waveform. Cardiac output is computed from this waveform and the electrocardiogram (ECG).

BENEFITS

Thoracic electrical bioimpedance monitoring eliminates the risk of infection, bleeding, pneumothorax, emboli, and arrhythmias associated with traditional invasive monitoring. And the accuracy of results ob-

tained by this method proves comparable to that obtained by thermodilution. What's more, the bioimpedance monitor automatically updates information every second to tenth heartbeat (see *Understanding hemodynamic indices*).

INDICATIONS

Thoracic electrical bioimpedance helps to monitor patients who would have a high risk of complications from thermodilution monitoring. Because of its portability, the thoracic electrical bioimpedance unit may be used in the operating room, postanesthesia care unit, and intensive care unit.

However, baseline bioimpedance values may be reduced in patients who have conditions that are characterized by increased fluid in the chest, such as pulmonary edema and pleural effusion. Also, bioimpedance values may be lower than thermodilution values in patients with tachycardia and other arrhythmias.

Understanding hemodynamic indices

Once you connect your patient to a thoracic electrical bioimpedance monitor, you can easily obtain the hemodynamic data needed to determine his stability and to plan treatment and care. With a thoracic electrical bioimpedance monitoring unit, you can measure the following values:
- **cardiac index:** cardiac output (CO) divided by body surface area, which puts CO in perspective for the patient's size
- **cardiac output:** the volume of blood pumped through the heart (measured in liters/minute)
- **dZ/dt:** indicator of peak flow
- **ejection fraction (EF):** the volume of blood ejected from the left ventricle in a single myocardial contraction (expressed as a percentage)
- **end-diastolic volume (EDV):** the volume of blood in the left ventricle at the end of diastole, also known

as the preload volume (measured in milliliters)
- **heart rate (HR):** the number of heartbeats in 1 minute
- **left cardiac work index (LCWI):** myocardial oxygen consumption is reflected
- **preejection period (PEP):** the time between the onset of ventricular activity and the opening of the aortic valve (measured in seconds)
- **stroke volume (SV):** the amount of blood pumped from the ventricle with each myocardial contraction (measured in milliliters)
- **systemic vascular resistance (SVR):** resistance against which the left ventricle pumps
- **ventricular ejection time (VET):** the amount of time that blood is flowing out of the ventricles
- **Zo:** base impedance, or the amount of resistance met by the electrical current passing through the thorax.

Karen E. Michael, RN, MSN, a case manager for Greater Atlantic Health Service, Philadelphia, contributed to this section. The publisher thanks *Renaissance Technologies, Inc.,* Newtown, Pa., for its help.

To begin thoracic electrical bioimpedance monitoring, assemble the equipment at the patient's bedside. You'll need a thoracic electrical bioimpedance unit, such as the IQ System (manufactured by Renaissance Technologies) shown here.

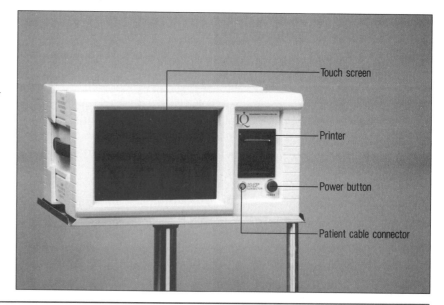

You'll also need a patient harness with color-coded leadwires, a connecting cable, four sets of thoracic electrical bioimpedance electrodes, three ECG electrodes, 3″ × 3″ or 4″ × 4″ gauze pads, a tape measure, and gloves.

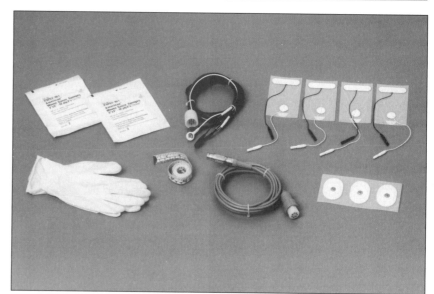

Explain the procedure to the patient, wash your hands, and put on gloves. Plug the thoracic electrical bioimpedance unit into a power supply, and press the POWER button. The initial display screen will appear.

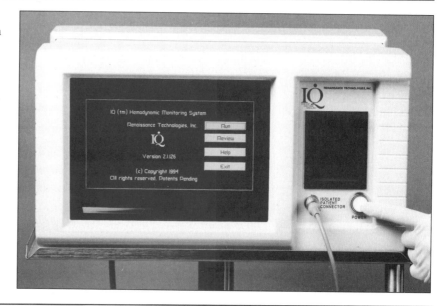

Now press the RUN key on the initial display screen. The patient data screen will appear.

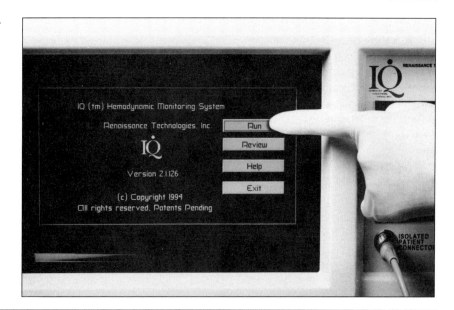

Enter the basic patient data by pressing each patient data block on the screen. Choose METRIC or ENGLISH for numbers, MALE or FEMALE, and ADULT or PED-NEO. When you press the appropriate block on the screen, a dot will appear beside your choice.

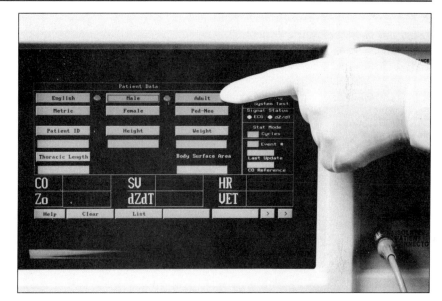

To enter data for the patient's ID number, thoracic length, height, and weight, press the block that identifies the index you wish to include (as shown). Afterward, the numeric keypad screen will appear.

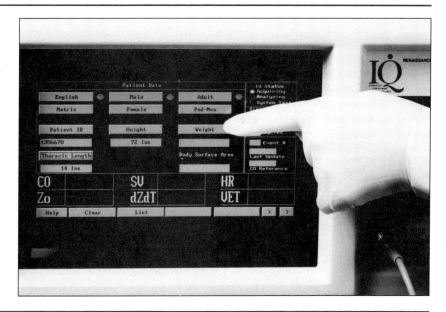

Enter the actual value for the chosen index by pressing the smaller blocks on the keypad (as shown). When you've entered all the data for the chosen index, press ENTER. This returns you to the patient data screen. Now repeat the process for each index you wish to include.

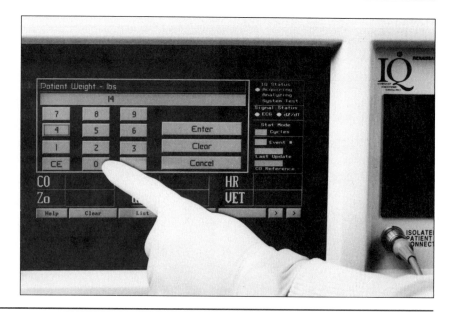

When you've entered your data, press the > block on the patient data screen to call up the waveform screen.

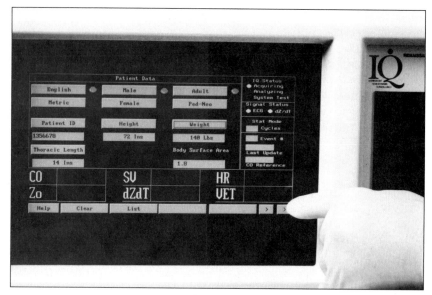

You'll routinely use this screen to monitor the patient's status. It displays the ECG and pulmonary artery pressure waveforms as well as six parameters that you choose. To select a parameter, press the block labeled PARAMETERS.

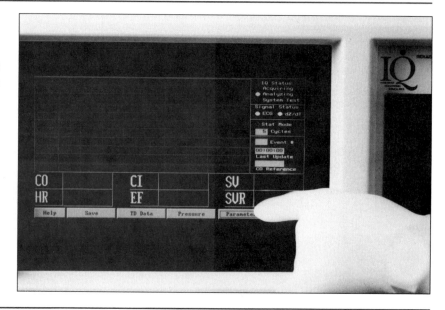

The parameter screen will appear (as shown). Press the blocks labeled with the parameters you wish to display on the waveform screen. Then press > at the bottom of the parameter screen to return to the waveform screen. All of the selected parameters will now appear on the waveform screen.

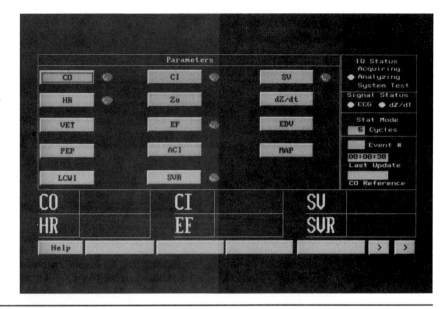

Assist the patient onto his back. Provide privacy and expose his chest. Then wet some 4″ × 4″ or 3″ × 3″ gauze pads with warm water, and clean the skin on each side of his neck from the base of the neck to 2″ (5 cm) above the base (as shown). Also clean the skin on both sides of the chest at the midaxillary line directly across from the xiphoid process.

▶ **Clinical tip:** To ensure that you've cleaned a large enough area for electrode placement, clean at least two fingerbreadths above and below the site.

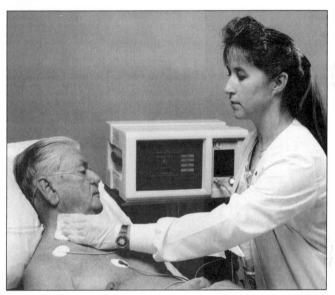

Place one electrode set vertically at the neck base below the ear with the arrow end (containing the round electrode) pointing down. Place the bar electrode at least 2″ above the round electrode. If the two electrodes are an attached set, place the bar electrode directly above the round one (as shown).

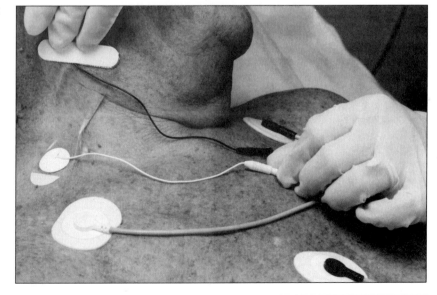

Place the second set of electrodes on the opposite side of the neck in line with the ear and about 180 degrees from the first set.

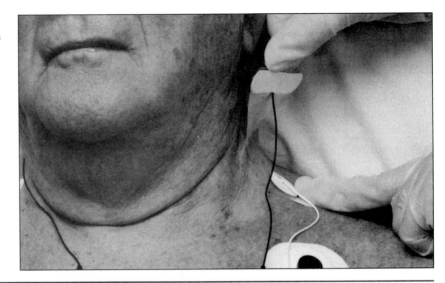

Alternatively, place the bar electrode on each side of the patient's forehead. If you fail to get a clear waveform, this placement, which increases the distance between the electrodes, often improves the waveform quality. It's also convenient if the patient has a beard.

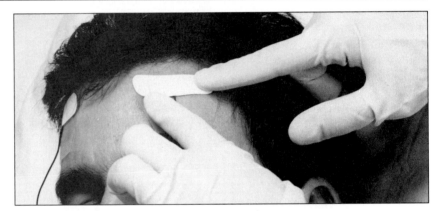

Place the remaining two sets of electrodes on either side of the patient's chest. To determine the correct location, draw a line with your finger from the xiphoid process to the midaxillary line on one side of the chest. This is the site for the first chest electrode. Place the round electrode here with the arrow pointing up.

Place the second (bar) electrode at least 2″ below the first. Or, if you're using an attached set of electrodes, place the bar electrode directly below the round one (as shown).

Next, place the final set of electrodes on the midaxillary line directly opposite the first set of electrodes.

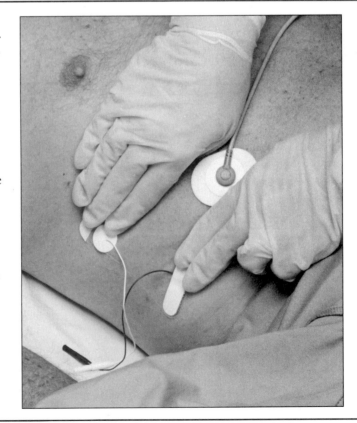

Attach ECG electrodes (as shown) and try different lead selections until you obtain a consistent QRS signal.

▶ *Clinical tip:* Don't remove the patient from the primary monitor. The regular system must still be maintained to ensure monitoring at the central station and to keep the alarms intact.

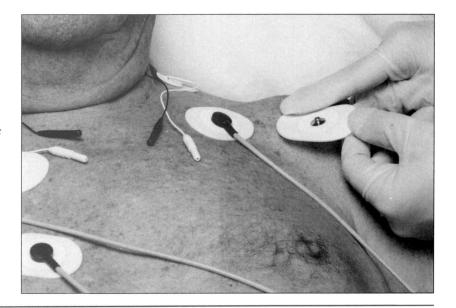

Now attach the leadwires of the bioimpedance harness to the thoracic electrical bioimpedance electrodes and the ECG electrodes.

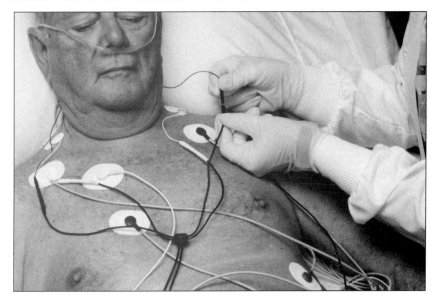

Attach the harness cable to the cable from the bioimpedance monitor.

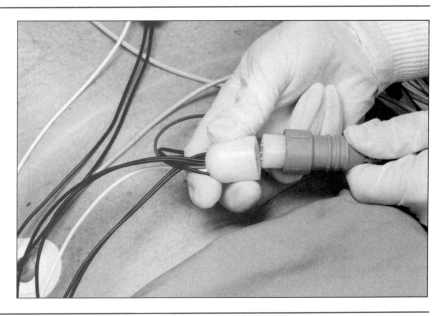

Next, measure the distance between the round electrode on one side of the patient's neck and the round electrode on the same side of his chest. This distance, the thorax length, is the numeric value required by the monitor's computer to calculate accurate stroke volume.

Enter this value by calling up the patient data screen, entering the value, and returning to the waveform screen.

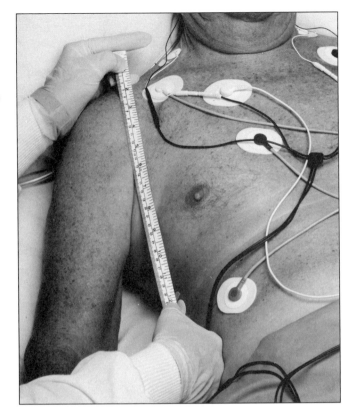

Finally, note the waveforms and values on the monitor, and document the values by pressing PRINT on the waveform screen to print a strip containing all the values monitored. Place the strip on the patient's chart.

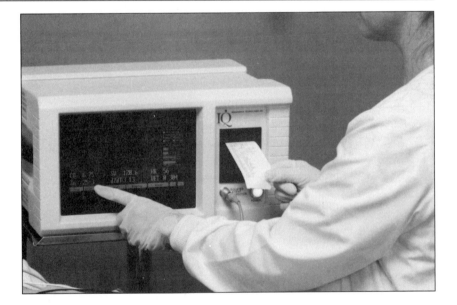

Respiratory Monitoring

LEARNING ABOUT CONTINUOUS Sv̄O₂ MONITORING

Mixed venous oxygen saturation ($S\bar{v}O_2$) monitoring measures the balance between oxygen supply and tissue oxygen demand. Considered one of the most useful and sensitive procedures currently available, $S\bar{v}O_2$ monitoring also shows trends in oxygen supply and tissue consumption.

Continuous $S\bar{v}O_2$ monitoring aids assessment and intervention in hemodynamically unstable patients and allows early detection of impaired oxygen delivery before significant hypoxia can occur. $S\bar{v}O_2$ monitoring may be useful for patients with diminished cardiac output and low SaO_2 or hemoglobin (Hb) levels. It also helps evaluate a patient's response to drugs, suctioning, or ventilator setting changes.

Knowing the patient's $S\bar{v}O_2$ level, however, isn't useful alone. The balance between available oxygen and tissue consumption depends on other factors, such as cardiac output, arterial oxygen saturation (SaO_2), and Hb levels on the supply side and tissue oxygen needs on the demand side. Any change in the patient's $S\bar{v}O_2$ level typically reflects a change in one or more of these factors.

OXYGEN SUPPLY AND TISSUE DEMAND

Cardiac output refers to the volume of blood pumped from the heart each minute. A normal cardiac output of 4 to 8 liters/minute is maintained by a normal heart rate and stroke volume.

SaO_2, expressed as a percentage, represents the actual amount of oxygen bound to Hb divided by the maximum amount of oxygen that could possibly bind to Hb. Because Hb carries most of the blood's oxygen, a normal SaO_2 level is 95% to 100%. Of course, if the patient doesn't have a normal Hb level—14 to 18 g/dl for men and 11.5 to 15.5 g/dl for women—tissue oxygenation will be poor despite a normal SaO_2 level. What's more, the oxygen supply may be adequate or inadequate, depending on tissue demand for oxygen.

Normally, tissues use about 250 cc of oxygen/minute. $S\bar{v}O_2$ is the amount of oxygen that returns to the heart from the tissues. Normal $S\bar{v}O_2$ levels range from 60% to 80%.

Some conditions that raise $S\bar{v}O_2$ levels and lower the demand for oxygen include increased cardiac output, elevated SaO_2 levels, vasoconstriction, septic shock, hypothermia, anesthesia, sedation, and chemical paralysis.

Conditions that lower $S\bar{v}O_2$ levels and raise the demand for oxygen include decreased cardiac output, reduced SaO_2 levels, vasodilation, cardiogenic shock, hyperthermia or fever, shivering, seizures, positive end-expiratory pressure, and high airway pressure.

HOW THE MONITOR WORKS

The $S\bar{v}O_2$ monitoring system consists of a flow-directed, thermodilution pulmonary artery catheter with fiber-optic filaments, an optical module, and an oximeter.

The device works this way: Oxygen-saturated hemoglobin (oxyhemoglobin) in the bloodstream reflects light emitted by a fiber-optic filament under the catheter's balloon tip. Then another light-receiving fiber-optic filament detects the reflected light and transmits it to a photodetector in the optical module. The optical module converts the light into an electrical signal and averages the value.

The display screen on the computerized oximeter then projects a continuous graphic trend of the oxyhemoglobin levels along with a digital reading. The oximeter displays a new reading every second.

NURSING CONSIDERATIONS DURING CONTINUOUS MONITORING

Because $S\bar{v}O_2$ monitoring is an invasive procedure that requires the patient to have a pulmonary artery catheter, be alert for complications. For example, the insertion procedure increases the risk of infection, especially if the patient is already immunocompromised because of illness or tracheal intubation.

To prevent potential infections, you'll need to implement specific measures. For example, maintain sterility at the insertion site by changing the sterile dressing every 24 hours or more often if it becomes wet or soiled. Also, inspect the insertion site each time you change the dressing, change the tubing every 24 hours, and use a continuous heparin flush to prevent clot formation.

Other nursing measures include monitoring the patient for related complications, such as pneumothorax, air emboli, and cardiac arrhythmias.

Michelle Conlon, RN, BSN, CCRN, who contributed to this section, is manager of clinical education services at Abbott Critical Care Systems, Mountainview, Calif. The publisher also thanks *Abbott Critical Care,* Chesterfield, Mo., for its help.

MONITORING S$\bar{v}$O$_2$ LEVELS

To monitor S$\bar{v}$O$_2$ levels, you'll need to follow several procedures to set up the equipment correctly and calibrate the monitor. The following pages will show you how to perform these tasks. Keep in mind, of course, that you'll always consult the manufacturer's directions for your specific monitoring system.

Setting up the equipment

To perform continuous S$\bar{v}$O$_2$ monitoring, you'll need to obtain a kit that contains a flow-directed, thermodilution pulmonary artery catheter with fiber-optic filaments (to be inserted by the doctor). You'll need an optical module and a computerized oximeter. You may also need a strip recorder for documenting the S$\bar{v}$O$_2$ measurements. A printer, an optional piece of equipment, lets you record the graphic display.

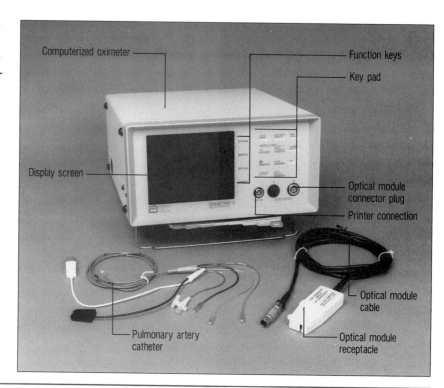

To begin, connect the optical module cable to the oximeter by aligning the red dot on the connector plug at the end of the cable with the red mark on the oximeter. Then push in the plug until it locks in place.

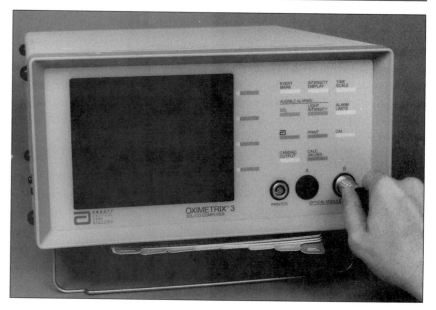

Turn on the oximeter by flipping the power switch to a forward position. On the display screen, you should see a version number in the upper left corner, the correct date and time under the version number, and the mode SṽO₂.

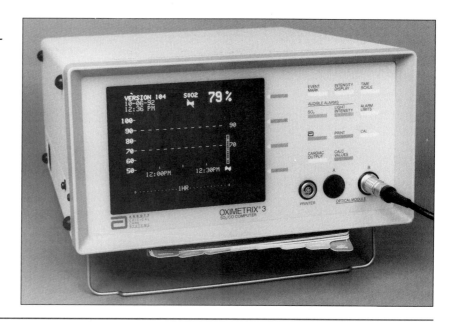

Inspect the pulmonary artery catheter package for any rips or tears. Then remove the outer wrapping from the package while leaving the inner wrapping over the catheter intact.

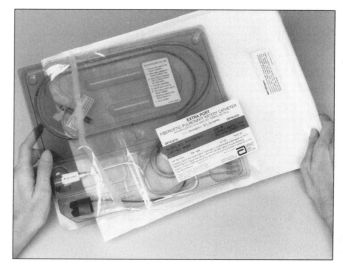

Peel back the lift tab on the inner wrapping to uncover the optical connector (as shown near right). Place the optical module in the specially designed recess in the tray.

With the optical module still in the tray, open the optical module lid by pulling the lid straight out in the direction of the arrow and then lifting. A LOW LIGHT message will appear on the display screen when you open the lid. Next, slide the optical connector, located at the distal end of the pulmonary artery catheter, into the optical module (as shown far right). Make sure that the word TOP on the connector faces up. Then close the lid.

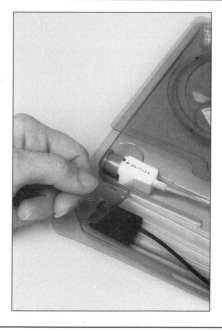
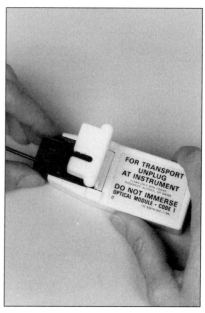

Next, check that the black optical reference is in position by verifying that the catheter tip is in the reference.

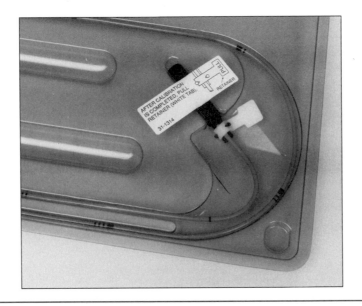

Calibrating the monitor before catheter insertion

Before the doctor inserts the pulmonary artery catheter, calibrate the equipment so that it's ready to function. First, press the oximeter key labeled CAL. The display screen should list the calibration options shown here. Then, with the catheter still in the package, select the preinsertion function by pressing the key next to the block labeled P.

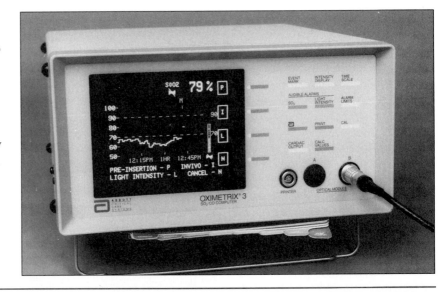

The message shown here should then appear on the display screen. To initiate calibration, press the function key next to the block labeled Y. Expect the screen to display only the letters CAL and the monitoring mode ($S\bar{v}O_2$) for up to 1 minute. When the system completes the calibration, the screen will display the message CAL OK in the upper right corner. If the message CAL FAIL appears, repeat the calibration steps.

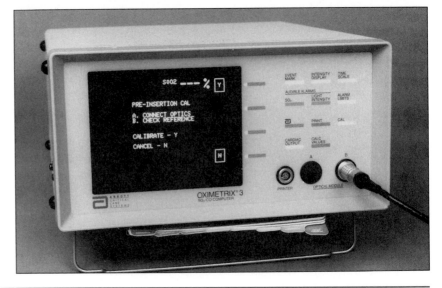

Calibrating the monitor after catheter insertion

You may need to calibrate the monitor once the catheter is in place—for example, if calibration wasn't done before insertion, if the catheter disconnects from the optical module, if the fiber-optic filaments sustain damage, if you suspect an incorrect reading, or if a catheter has simply been in place for an extended period.

Before doing so, make sure that the patient's SaO_2 level is relatively stable. Also, set the intensity of the signal display so that it's within normal limits. Then press the computer key labeled CAL (as shown).

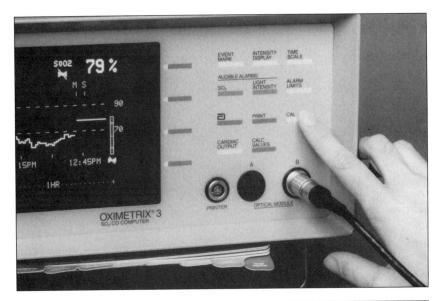

Press the function key next to the block labeled I. This selects in vivo calibration.

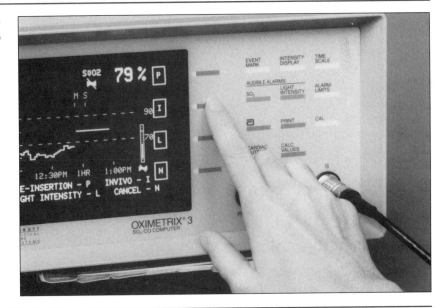

Press the function key next to the block labeled Y to continue with in vivo calibration. In response, the oximeter will store the preceding 5 seconds of oxygen saturation data, and the display screen will signal DRAW BLOOD for 12 seconds.

When this message appears, clear the distal lumen of the pulmonary artery line, draw a blood sample, and send it to the laboratory for $S\bar{v}O_2$ analysis. The screen will display the in vivo calibration process and exhibit the stored oxygen saturation values in the upper left corner.

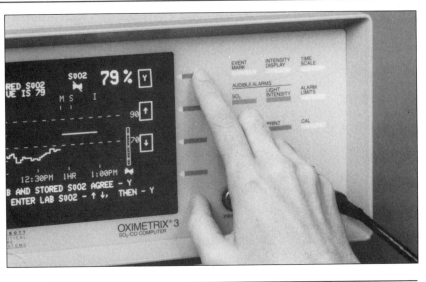

After you receive the laboratory's SvO₂ results, compare them with the stored value that appears in the upper left corner of the display screen. Is the new value within 4 saturation units of the stored value? If not, enter the laboratory value by manipulating the function keys next to the blocks showing the up and down arrows (as shown here).

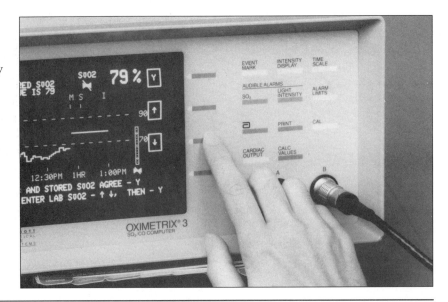

Once you've entered the correct saturation number—or if the laboratory value was within 4 saturation units of the value displayed by the computer—press the key next to the block labeled Y.

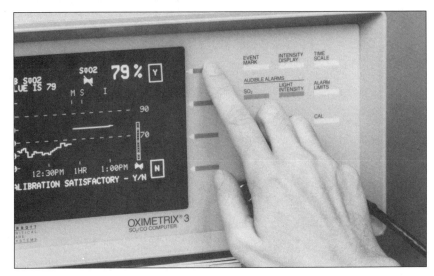

Adjusting the equipment

After calibration, adjust the rest of the equipment. Begin by calibrating the light intensity. First, press the key labeled CAL. Next, press the function key beside the block labeled L for "light intensity" (shown here).

When the next screen display appears, press the function key next to the block labeled Y to confirm that you want to proceed. The computer will then begin calibration, after which the screen will display the letter L and the light intensity signal should center in the vertical intensity bar on the screen's right.

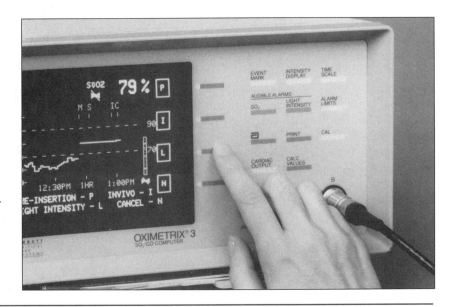

Next, set the alarm limits. To do so, first press the ALARM LIMITS key.

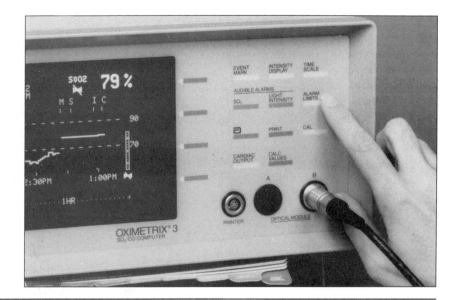

Adjust the alarm limits as necessary by manipulating the function keys next to the blocks labeled with an up or down arrow (as shown here).

After you've set the appropriate limits, again press the ALARM LIMITS key. The on-screen display should return to the monitoring mode.

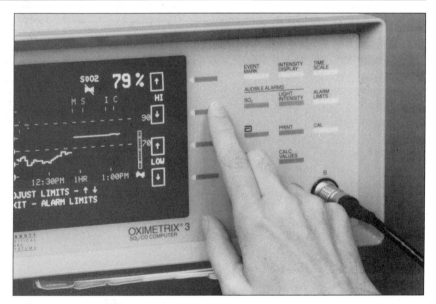

At this point, you may wish to change the time scale on the trend graph. The scale determines the duration covered by the trend graph. For example, the graph may display Sv̄O₂ measurements for 1, 2, 4, 8, or 16 hours. To change the scale, simply press the TIME SCALE key. Each time you depress the key, the time scale will change to the next lowest value.

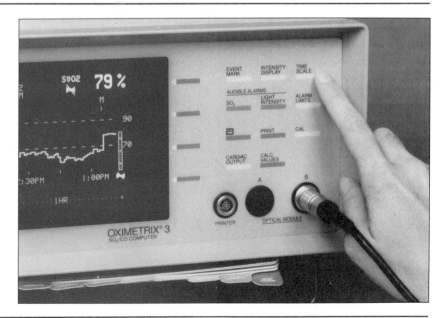

Marking individual events

During monitoring, the computer automatically marks certain functions (called events) on the trend graph. Events may include arterial mode monitoring, calibration, light intensity, and time adjustment. If you want to mark individual events—for example, initial drug administration, ventilator adjustments, or suctioning—press the EVENT MARK key. The event mark looks like a vertical arrow.

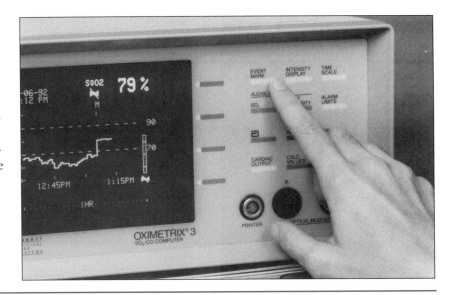

The event mark selection list should appear on the screen. Review the list. Then, after identifying the pertinent event, highlight the letter next to the event by manipulating the function keys next to the up or down arrows (as shown here). Once highlighted, press the function key next to the block containing the number 2.

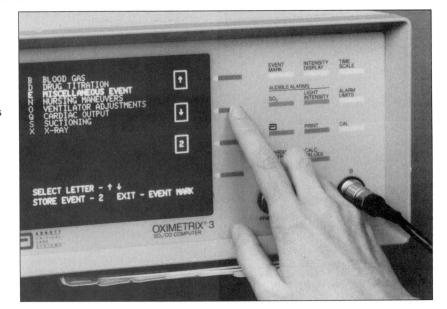

The routine monitoring display should return to the screen. Check the trend graph for the new event mark. Both the vertical event mark and the selected letter code should appear above the trend graph.

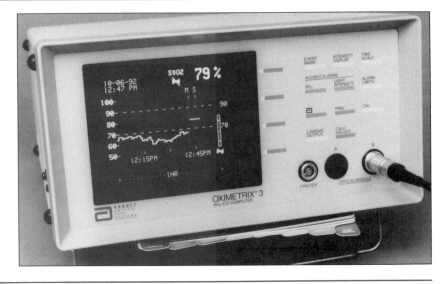

INSIGHTS AND INTERPRETATIONS

Interpreting Sv̄O₂ tracings

Continuous mixed venous oxygen saturation (Sv̄O₂) monitoring allows you to monitor individual readings and trends in venous oxygen saturation. The patient's Sv̄O₂ levels continuously appear in the upper right corner of the display screen. In addition, the computer displays these readings as a graph, portraying the patient's Sv̄O₂ levels for a limited time.

Normal Sv̄O₂ values range from 60% to 80%. If the value drops below 60%, or if it changes by more than 10% for 5 minutes or more, assess the patient's condition and intervene appropriately. If the Sv̄O₂ value doesn't return to the baseline, notify the doctor.

Changing Sv̄O₂ levels

A low continuous Sv̄O₂ level (under 60%) or a level that declines over time signals impaired oxygen delivery. This may result from hemorrhage, hypoxia, shock, arrhythmias, suctioning, an increased demand for tissue oxygen (which may signal hyperthermia), shivering, or seizures.

Changes in the Sv̄O₂ level are a sensitive, early indicator of deteriorating cardiopulmonary function—appearing well before other signs and symptoms. A sudden increase in Sv̄O₂ levels could be one of the first indicators of an intracardiac shunting defect. Increased Sv̄O₂ levels can also signal the early stages of septic shock as oxygen demands increase because of fever and hypermetabolism. In later stages, as cardiac output falls, oxygen delivery decreases, resulting in decreased Sv̄O₂ levels.

Cyanide toxicity caused by nitroprusside administration is also identifiable through Sv̄O₂ levels. As this condition impairs the processing of oxygen, the Sv̄O₂ levels increase.

Use the following examples to help you interpret Sv̄O₂ monitoring results.

Normal readings

This tracing represents a stable, normal Sv̄O₂ level: over 60% and below 80%. Note the relatively constant line.

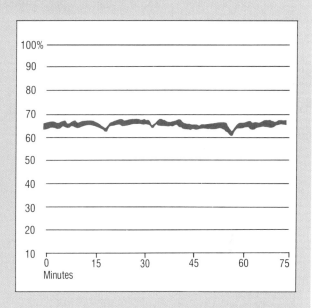

Abnormal readings

The tracings below and on page 19 display abnormal trends. The first tracing shows a falling Sv̄O₂ level in a patient returning from the operating room after coronary artery bypass surgery. Notice the event marks (arrows) that indicate atrial pacing and the cardiac index (CI) at about 1 hour, 15 minutes; administration of a vasoactive drug; the patient's plotted response; and his subsequent return to the operating room.

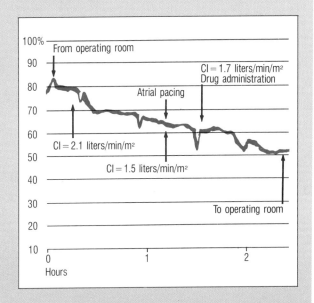

Interpreting SvO₂ tracings (continued)

Because a patient's SvO₂ level may change almost immediately after intervention, the subsequent levels can help you determine the intervention's effectiveness. The tracing below shows a rise in SvO₂ levels and cardiac output (CO) after the patient has received I.V. nitroprusside.

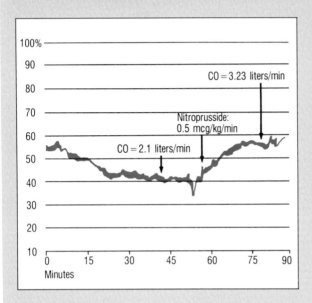

This graph shows the patient's response to changes in ventilator settings. Note that the elevated positive end-expiratory pressure (PEEP) causes an increase in SvO₂ and partial pressure of oxygen in arterial blood (PaO₂); therefore, the fraction of inspired oxygen (FIO₂) can be decreased.

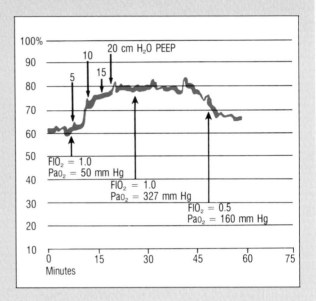

The tracing below represents the patient's response to a muscle relaxant.

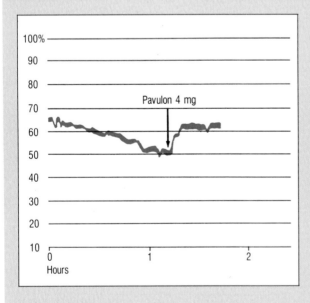

This tracing shows typical changes in the SvO₂ level as a result of various activities.

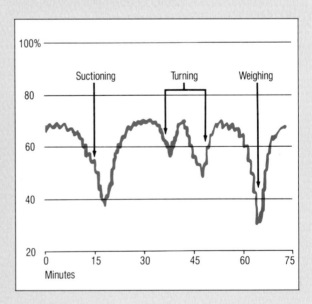

LEARNING ABOUT PULSE OXIMETRY

Pulse oximetry allows continuous, noninvasive electronic monitoring of a patient's arterial oxygen saturation levels painlessly—without needles or other invasive instruments. However, pulse oximetry doesn't provide all the data you need to evaluate your patient's ventilatory status. In some situations, you may still need to withdraw blood for a routine arterial blood gas analysis.

The pulse oximeter measures the absorption (amplitude) of light waves as they pass through areas of the body that are perfused by arterial blood. It can detect changes in the patient's oxygen status within seconds, compute an accurate pulse rate, and monitor pulse amplitude (see *How pulse oximetry works,* page 22).

Note: The pulse oximeter monitor shown on the following pages usually denotes arterial oxygen saturation values with the symbol SpO_2. This symbol differentiates arterial oxygen saturation measured electronically from arterial oxygen saturation [SaO_2] measured by invasive means.

APPLICATIONS

First used to detect hypoxemia in patients under general anesthesia, pulse oximetry currently is used in various inpatient and outpatient settings. By safely calculating SpO_2 trends, pulse oximetry helps evaluate the progression of such underlying disorders as cardiac or respiratory failure, interstitial lung disease, or pulmonary emboli as well as treatment effectiveness. Pulse oximetry also helps assess the effects of suctioning or postural drainage and helps monitor SpO_2 levels during normal activities of daily living in patients with chronic lung disease or sleep apnea and during diagnostic tests or surgery.

NORMAL LEVELS

Normal SpO_2 values vary with a patient's age, medical history, and current condition. For most patients, though, the normal SpO_2 level ranges between 95% and 100%. Lower levels suggest hypoxemia, which may warrant intervention.

Although SpO_2 measurements are usually accurate, certain factors may skew results. For example, the dyes used in cardiac output studies and high levels of carboxyhemoglobin in patients who smoke will produce false-high readings.

SYSTEM COMPONENTS

A pulse oximetry system consists of a pulse oximeter, a sensor, and an extension cable. A key component, the sensor contains light-emitting diodes (LEDs) and a photodetector, which pick up the arterial pulse signal. Depending on the manufacturer and the patient's needs, the system will use one of two kinds of sensors: a transmission sensor (the most common) or a reflectance sensor.

Positioned opposite the LEDs (over a vascular bed perfused by arterial blood, such as a finger or a toe), the *transmission sensor* measures light transmitted by the LEDs through vascular tissue.

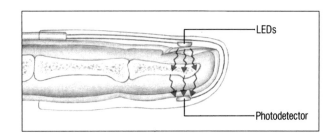

In contrast, a *reflectance sensor* measures light reflected by the vascular bed. The photodetector is positioned side by side with the LEDs on a flat surface such as the forehead.

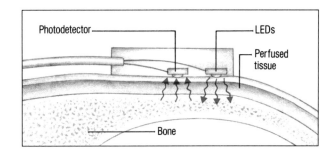

The sensor relays data to the monitor by way of the extension cable, which amplifies and clarifies the pulse signal. The monitor then displays the patient's pulse rate, SpO_2 level, and pulse strength. It also displays alarm settings and status messages.

Patricia A. McGaffigan, RN,C, MS, clinical education manager at Nellcor, Inc., Hayward, Calif., contributed to this section. The publisher thanks the following organizations for their help: *Dynatech Nevada, Inc.,* Carson City, Nev.; *Hewlett-Packard Co.,* Waltham, Mass.; *Hill-Rom,* Batesville, Ind.; and *Nellcor, Inc.,* Hayward, Calif.

Equipment variations

Some pulse oximeters can transmit a patient's SpO_2 values to a central monitoring station at the nurses' station. And some synchronize the pulse signal with the patient's electrocardiogram (ECG), which helps decrease interference with the pulse signal. This is an important feature because patient movement at the sensor site can mimic an arterial pulse signal and interfere with accurate SpO_2 measurement.

If your system has synchronization capability, implement it by connecting a special patch cable from the oximeter to the patient's ECG monitor. This al-lows the pulse oximeter to use only the light absorption changes occurring after a QRS complex to compute the SpO_2 measurement. Light absorption changes occurring at other times are assumed to result from movement or artifacts and are discarded. The result: a more reliable SpO_2 measurement.

Although most pulse oximeters function similarly, the setup and operating procedures may vary. Consult the manufacturer's instructions before beginning. Also, ensure patient comfort at all times during monitoring.

How pulse oximetry works

Pulse oximetry monitors arterial oxygen saturation levels by using two light-emitting diodes (LEDs) to send red and infrared light through pulsating vascular tissue, such as the fingertip, toe, nose, or forehead. A photodetector placed near the LEDs measures the absorption of transmitted light as it passes through the vascular bed.

Surrounding bone, tissue, veins, and pigmentation absorb some of the red and infrared light at a constant rate. However, because the volume of blood in the arterial bed changes with each heartbeat (re-flecting systole and diastole), the amount of light absorbed also changes. It is this changing condition that determines the arterial blood supply.

Oxygenated and deoxygenated hemoglobin absorb red and infrared light at different rates. From these rates, the pulse oximeter calculates the exact amount of oxygen-carrying hemoglobin in the arterial blood. The monitor displays this value as SpO_2 along with the pulse rate. The monitor may also display a pulse amplitude bar or a pulse waveform.

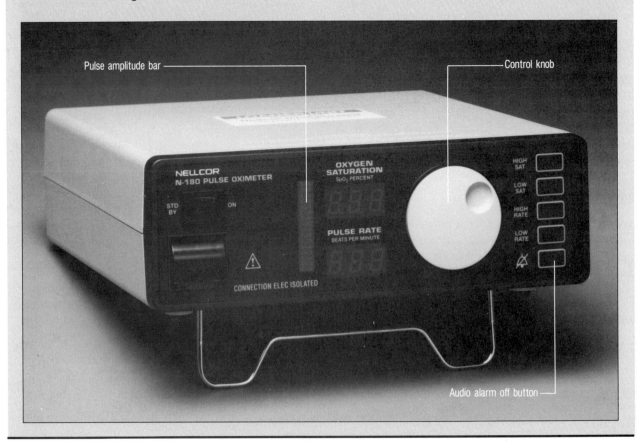

Pulse amplitude bar — Control knob — Audio alarm off button

PERFORMING PULSE OXIMETRY

Your main concerns when performing pulse oximetry include placing the sensor correctly and securely, and setting up the monitor according to the manufacturer's directions.

You'll need a pulse oximeter, a monitor (and grounded power cord, if required), a compatible sensor, and an extension cable. Depending on the situation, you may also need alcohol wipes, nail polish remover, or a special patch cable compatible with the patient's ECG monitor. To transmit data to a central monitoring station, you'll need a special bedside transmitter and fiber-optic connector.

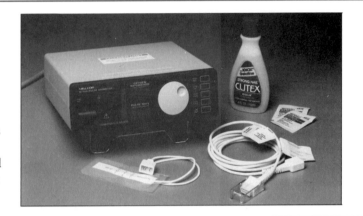

Take the equipment to the patient's room, and explain the procedure. Then plug the pulse oximeter into a grounded outlet.

If you'll be transmitting the pulse oximetry data to a central monitoring station, place the pulse oximeter on top of the special bedside transmitter. Insert the fiber-optic connector into the rear of the pulse oximeter and then into the bedside transmitter. Plug the bedside transmitter into a grounded outlet.

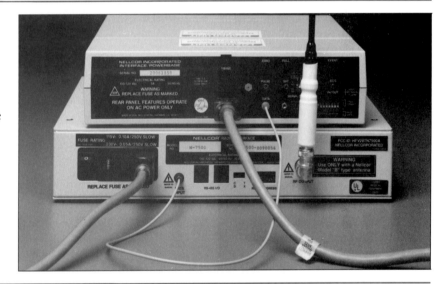

Like a radio, the bedside transmitter transmits data across radio frequencies to the central monitor (shown).

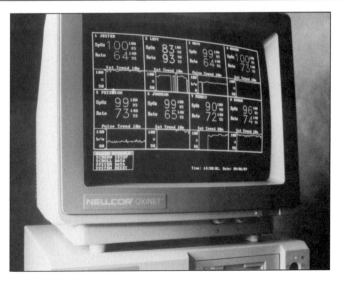

Select a sensor site that the manufacturer recommends. Check the strength of the patient's pulse and the adequacy of capillary refill at the proposed site. If the patient has poor peripheral perfusion, consider applying the sensor to her nose or using a reflectance sensor (these primarily monitor central rather than peripheral blood flow). Also, avoid placing a sensor on an extremity with a blood pressure cuff, an arterial or intravenous line, or a pressure dressing.

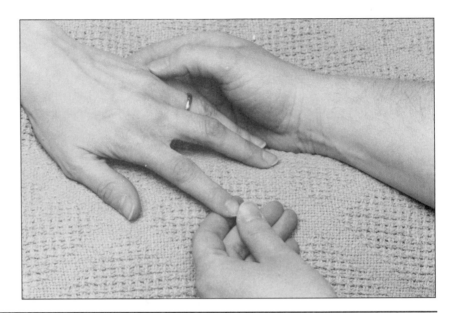

If you're placing the sensor on the patient's finger, remove any nail polish, which could block light transmission and lead to unreliable readings. Although skin preparation isn't necessary, you may want to remove oil from the patient's skin with an alcohol wipe before applying a reflectance sensor. If you're applying a sensor on the nose, use the supplies in the sensor package to prepare the skin site.

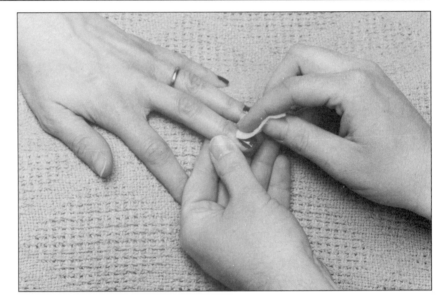

Apply the sensor according to the manufacturer's instructions. Properly align the LEDs and photodetector as indicated by the markings on the sensor.

▶ *Clinical tip:* If you're placing a sensor on the patient's finger, position the patient's hand at heart level to eliminate venous pulsations and to promote accurate readings.

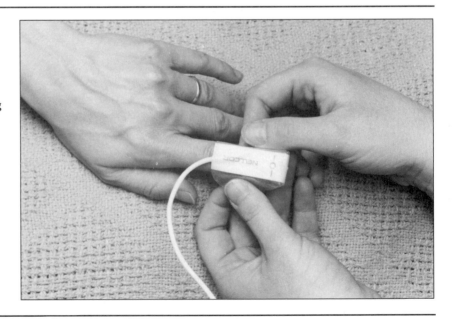

If necessary, protect the sensor from bright light by covering it with an opaque cloth such as the blanket.

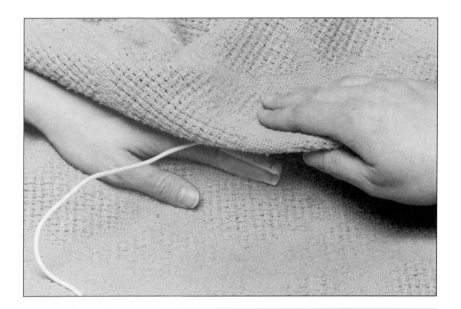

Connect the sensor to the extension cable.

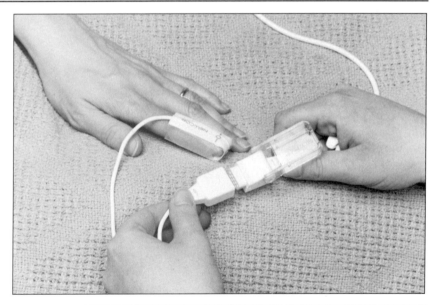

Switch on the power. A self-test display should flash on the monitor. After a few seconds, an SpO₂ value and pulse rate will appear on the screen. Note the initial information provided, including the SpO₂ measurement, pulse rate, pulse amplitude, and any status messages.

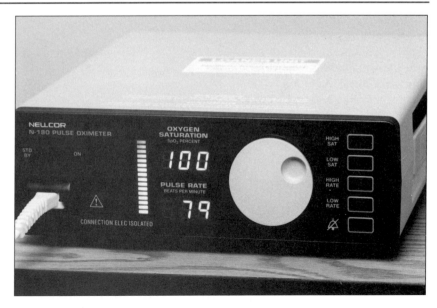

Depending on the type of oximeter you're using, you may hear a beep with each heartbeat. Typically, the beep rises in pitch as SpO$_2$ increases and falls as SpO$_2$ decreases. You can adjust the beep's volume by turning the control knob clockwise to increase the volume and counterclockwise to decrease it.

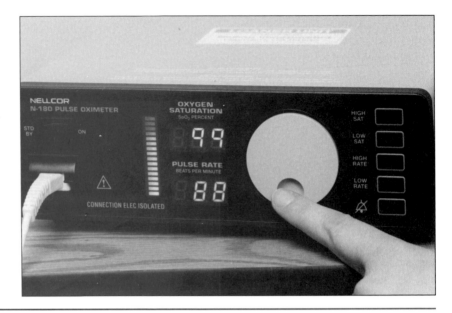

Even if your system has preset alarm limits, you'll need to check the high- and low-limit alarms. The high limit for SpO$_2$ is 100% for adults and 95% for neonates; the low limit is 85% for adults and 80% for neonates. The high pulse limit is 140 beats/minute for adults and 200 beats/minute for neonates; the low limit is 50 beats/minute for adults and 100 beats/minute for neonates.

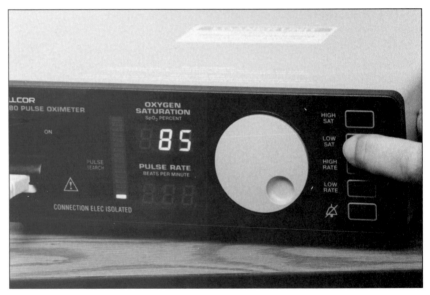

If necessary, adjust the alarm limits according to hospital policy, the patient's condition, or the doctor's order. On the model shown here, you would press the appropriate alarm limit button as you turn the control knob.

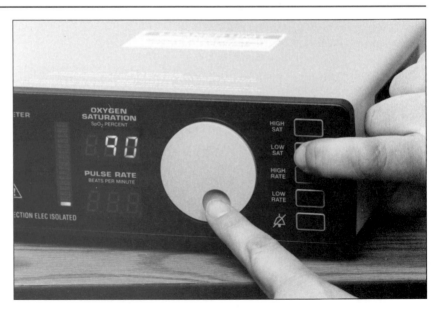

Set the averaging mode according to the patient's activity level. Press the HIGH RATE and LOW RATE buttons simultaneously as you turn the control knob. Continue turning the control knob until the desired mode number appears in the oxygen saturation display.

▶ ***Clinical tip:*** Usually, for inactive patients you'll select mode 1, which takes a reading over 5 to 7 seconds and averages the data to produce the SpO_2 value. For sleep studies, choose mode 2, which averages data over 2 to 3 seconds. For active patients, select mode 3, which averages readings over 10 to 15 seconds. In any mode, document SpO_2 values as often as required by the patient's condition or unit policy.

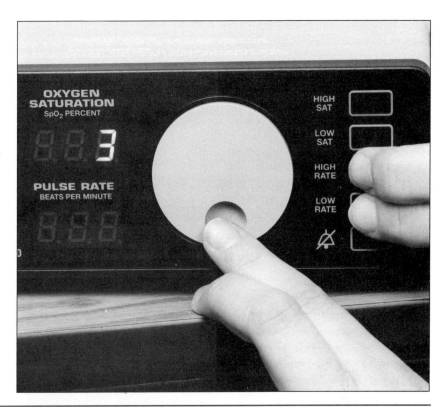

If you need to silence the alarm at any point, press the appropriate button (as shown). Doing so will silence the audible alarm for 60 seconds; however, the visual alarm will continue to flash as long as the triggering situation exists. Although the audible alarm will reset after 60 seconds, make sure that you've turned the alarms back on before leaving the patient's bedside.

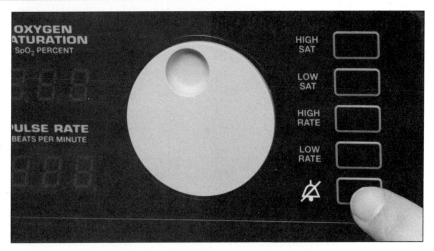

Most pulse oximeters contain a battery that operates the unit in case of a power failure. Refer to the manufacturer's directions for information about battery life and recharging requirements. The unit shown here contains a battery that charges whenever the monitor is plugged in; when fully charged, the battery will operate the unit for at least 6 hours. When 5 or fewer minutes remain on the battery's life, the LOW BATT indicator will flash.

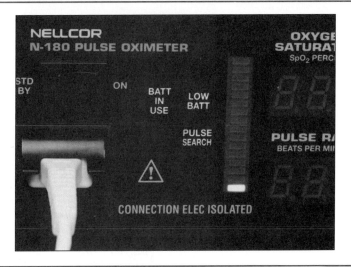

If the patient's activity frequently triggers oximeter alarms, you may need to synchronize the oximeter and the ECG. To do so, connect the pulse oximeter to the ECG monitor with a special patch cable, and watch for the message ECG IN USE to appear on the pulse oximeter monitor.

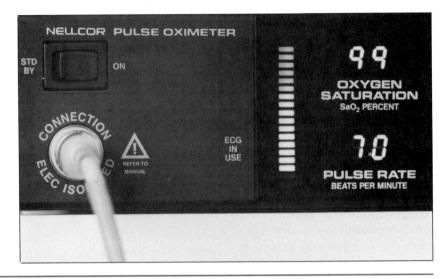

Once the equipment is operating, frequently inspect the sensor site, and rotate it according to the manufacturer's recommendations and your hospital's policy. If the patient is at risk for skin breakdown, inspect and change the site more frequently.

When removing a sensor, take care not to injure the patient or damage the sensor. Document the date and time of each sensor site change, the location of the sensor, and the condition of the skin.

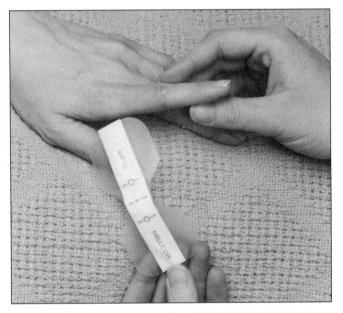

When monitoring is no longer required, remove the sensor and turn off the power on the pulse oximeter. Clean the sensor as recommended by the manufacturer. If you've been using an adhesive sensor, recycle it if that's an option or discard it.

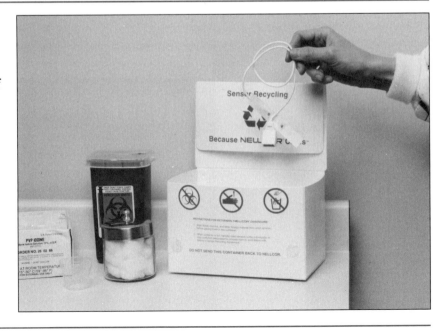

PERFORMING CAPNOGRAPHY

In this procedure, a capnometer measures changes in exhaled carbon dioxide (CO_2) concentrations and records these changes as waveforms on a display screen or a paper strip.

More and more, capnography is used for noninvasively evaluating a patient's respiratory status—especially during anesthesia, mechanical ventilation, cardiopulmonary resuscitation, and endotracheal intubation. Used continuously at the bedside, capnography warns caregivers of developing complications, permits early therapeutic intervention, and reduces the need for multiple arterial punctures for blood gas analyses.

A capnometer monitors ventilation and perfusion by measuring the partial pressure of end-tidal CO_2 ($ETCO_2$) in expired air. A by-product of cellular metabolism, CO_2 is carried by mixed venous blood to the right side of the heart and then to the lungs. There, CO_2 diffuses across the pulmonary capillaries and exits from the alveoli during expiration.

Typically, capnometers use infrared light to measure CO_2 in the airway at the end of expiration. Here's how: The capnometer has a sensor that contains an infrared light source and a photodetector. Depending on the equipment, the sensor may be positioned directly at the patient's airway, or it may be used with an adapter. Once in place, the sensor passes an infrared light beam through expired air. Of the normally exhaled gases, only CO_2 and water vapor absorb infrared light. The capnometer dehumidifies the expired air, leaving only CO_2 to be measured as it absorbs the light. Now the sensor's photodetector can compute the amount of infrared light absorbed. The collected data are transmitted to a microprocessing unit, which converts the data to a numerical value and a corresponding $ETCO_2$ waveform called a capnogram.

UNDERSTANDING CAPNOMETRIC VALUES

Depending on the equipment, CO_2 values may be measured in various ways—for example, as a percentage (%), in millimeters of mercury (mm Hg), or in kilopascals (kPa). Higher CO_2 concentrations absorb more light and, therefore, appear as higher values. If pulmonary perfusion and alveolar ventilation are adequate, the $ETCO_2$ value will approximately equal the partial pressure of CO_2 in arterial blood ($PaCO_2$). If pulmonary perfusion and alveolar ventilation are significantly compromised—as occurs in cardiac arrest—$ETCO_2$ will be lower than $PaCO_2$ or may be absent altogether.

Gather the necessary equipment, including the monitor, the CO_2 module for the monitor, and the sensor cable with the attached calstick and the attached sensor (which houses the transducer). You'll also need a Velcro strap, gloves, and an airway adapter.

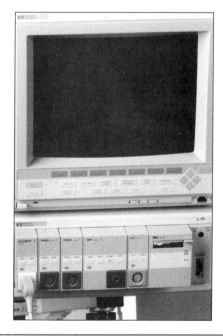
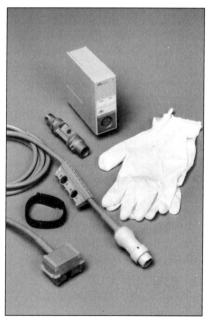

Contributors to this section include *Linda Murphy, RN, MSN,* applications district manager, Hewlett-Packard Co., Valley Forge, Pa.; *Mary E. Kruitwagen, RN,* clinical application specialist, Hewlett-Packard Co., Valley Forge, Pa.; and *Loraine Hopkins Pepe, RN, MSN, CCRN, CS,* staff nurse, medical-surgical intensive care unit, Chestnut Hill Hospital, Philadelphia. The publisher thanks *Doylestown (Pa.) Hospital;* Hewlett-Packard Co., Waltham, Mass.; and *Hill-Rom,* Batesville, Ind., for their help.

Insert the CO_2 module into the rack, and plug the sensor cable into the module.

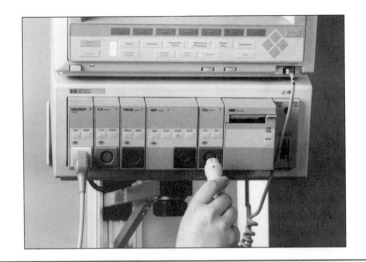

Watch for the message CO_2 SENSOR WARMUP to appear on the screen. When it disappears, you'll check the instrument's accuracy.

▶ **Clinical tip:** When plugging in a cold sensor, wait about 20 minutes before checking the instrument's accuracy (and, if needed, calibration).

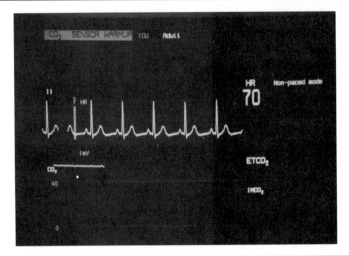

To check accuracy, slide the sensor over the calstick cell labeled 0.0 mm Hg. If the instrument is accurate, the value displayed on the screen should be within 1 mm Hg of the cell value within 1 minute. Next, slide the sensor over the remaining calstick cell. The numbers displayed on the monitor screen should be within 1 mm Hg of the value labeled on this cell.

Do an accuracy check if you move the sensor cable from one module to another and if you're using the module for another patient. If the transducer is used many times each day, check its accuracy at least once a day. If the values on the screen don't match the values on the calstick cells, you'll need to recalibrate.

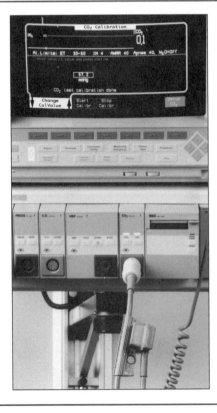
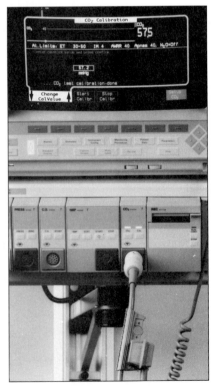

Calibrating the system

You can proceed with monitoring once you verify accuracy. But if you can't verify accuracy, you'll need to calibrate the transducer. To do so, press the CAL key on the front of the module (as shown). Note the value displayed in the center of the screen. This value should match the value indicated on the calstick cell. (Each sensor cable has its own calstick cell value printed on the calstick.)

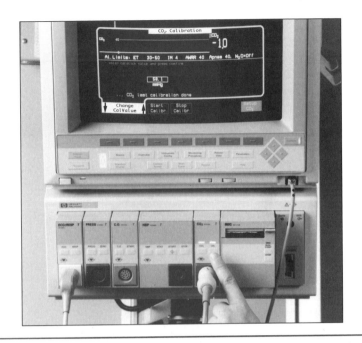

If the values match, press the CON-FIRM key. If they don't match, adjust the values by pressing the appropriate up and down arrow keys until they do. Then press the CONFIRM key (as shown) to store the value. (Keep in mind that each time you adjust the values, you'll need to recalibrate.)

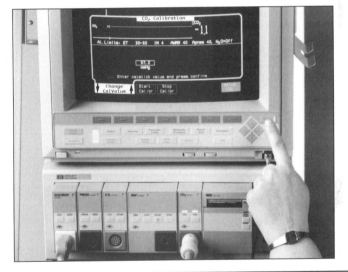

Next, press the START CAL key. Note that the screen provides instructions, such as PLACE SENSOR ON CALSTICK or PRESS START CAL-IBR. After placing the sensor on the calstick cell, watch for the message CO_2 CAL RUNNING on the monitor screen. This is the first part of calibration, which may take up to 4 minutes, after which a single tone will sound, and the message CO_2 CAL 1 DONE will appear.

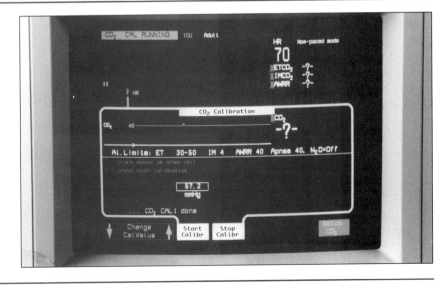

Repeat the previous step with the second calstick cell. Again wait for a single tone and the message CO_2 CAL DONE to appear on the monitor screen. This confirms a successful calibration. Should the calibration falter, expect a prompt to appear on the screen with directions on how to proceed.

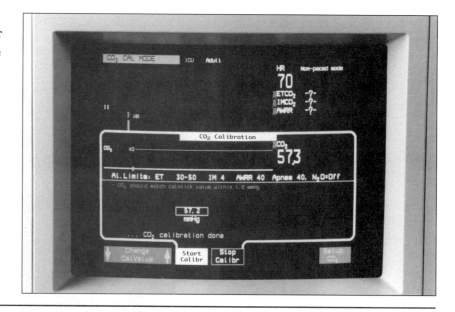

Once calibration has been completed, exit the calibration mode by pressing the STANDARD DISPLAY key.

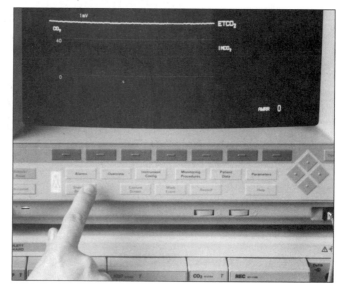

Monitoring CO₂

To continue setting up, snap the sensor onto the airway adapter. Wrap the Velcro strap around the juncture to secure the connection.

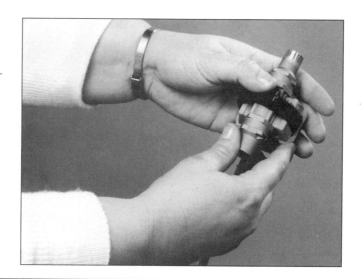

Next, put on gloves and connect the airway adapter to the patient's breathing circuit. Wear gloves whenever you handle the airway adapter to prevent cross-contamination.

▷ *Clinical tip:* To ensure accuracy, the airway adapter should be as close to the patient's airway as possible (to minimize the effect of increased dead space on the CO_2 value), and any in-line suction device should be proximal to the airway adapter.

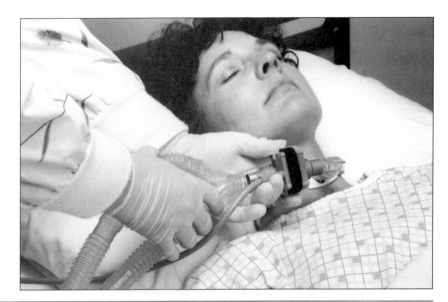

After making the proper connections, observe the $ETCO_2$ waveform and value (which appear below the electrocardiogram) on the monitor. Both will appear continuously on the screen. Assess the $ETCO_2$ waveform for height, frequency, rhythm, baseline, and shape.

▷ *Clinical tip:* Normal $ETCO_2$ values (which approximate $PaCO_2$ values) range from 35 to 45 mm Hg. They're usually 2 to 5 mm Hg less than the values obtained by arterial blood gas analysis. This variation assumes that the patient has normal ventilation, perfusion, and physiology and that you're correctly sampling his exhaled CO_2.

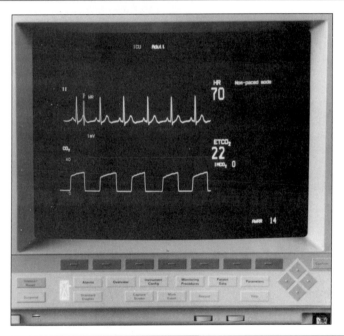

Adjusting alarm limits

Most systems have preset alarm limits, which may need adjustment depending on the patient's condition. To change these limits, press the CO_2 key on the module. The CO_2 task window should appear on the screen (as shown) and display the adjustments that can be made to the alarms. Begin setting the $ETCO_2$ alarms by pressing the $ETCO_2$ ALARMS key.

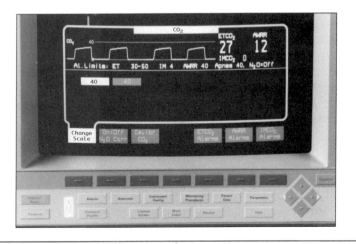

To adjust the alarm limits, press the up and down arrow keys (as shown) and then press the SETUP ETCO$_2$ key. To exit this alarm mode, press the SETUP CO$_2$ key.

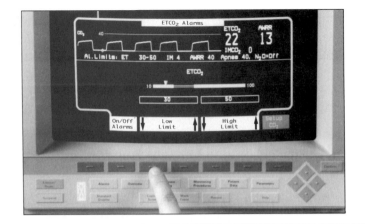

Set additional alarms similarly. For example, to set the airway respiratory rate (AWRR) alarm, press the AWRR ALARMS key. To change or adjust this alarm, press the up and down arrows as you did when adjusting the ETCO$_2$ alarms.

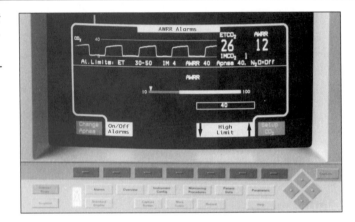

To adjust the apnea alarm time (measured in seconds) in the AWRR mode, press the CHANGE APNEA key (as shown). Then choose the desired time by continuing to press the CHANGE APNEA key until the value you want is highlighted. This value is the number of seconds between breaths. When the equipment fails to detect a breath in the number of seconds chosen, the alarm will sound.

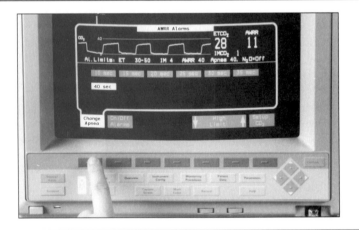

To return to the standard display mode, press the SETUP CO$_2$ key. When the CO$_2$ task window appears, press the STANDARD DISPLAY key.

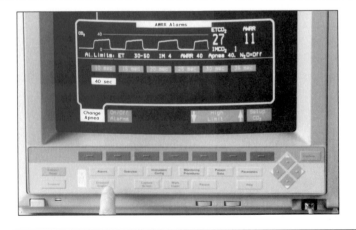

INSIGHTS AND INTERPRETATIONS

Understanding the normal capnogram

A capnogram (the waveform produced by capnography) shows changes in the blood's carbon dioxide (CO_2) levels during the respiratory cycle. The waveform has four phases.

Phase 1
This phase represents inspiration and alveolar gas exchange. The baseline pressure of zero (0 mm Hg) indicates the absence of carbon dioxide (CO_2) during inspiration.

Phase 2
Occurring during expiration, this phase is characterized by a sharp, nearly vertical upstroke that reflects CO_2 moving past the capnometer's sensor. In this phase, alveolar gases replace inspired gases in the patient's anatomic dead space.

Phase 3
In this phase (also called the plateau), the waveform reflects expired alveolar gas and the period during which no gas moves before the next breath. Normally, the plateau appears flat but slightly inclined to the right. Its width varies with changes in the patient's respiratory rate. The peak value of the plateau determines the end-tidal CO_2 ($ETCO_2$) value.

Phase 4
A sharp downstroke to the baseline represents phase 4, which marks the beginning of inspiration when CO_2-free gas moves past the sensor. This phase ends when the downstroke levels out at the baseline and the cycle continues.

Normal capnogram

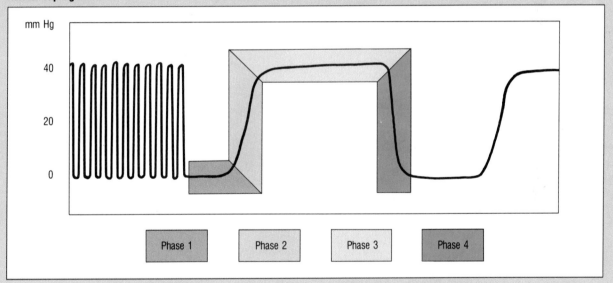

Recognizing abnormal capnograms

Once you're familiar with a normal capnogram, recognizing abnormal ones isn't difficult. Naturally, you'll interpret abnormal waveforms in light of the patient's clinical condition and other physical and mechanical factors. Keep in mind that waveform changes during phases 2 and 3 of the respiratory cycle reflect expiratory problems, whereas changes during phases 1 and 4 represent inspiratory problems.

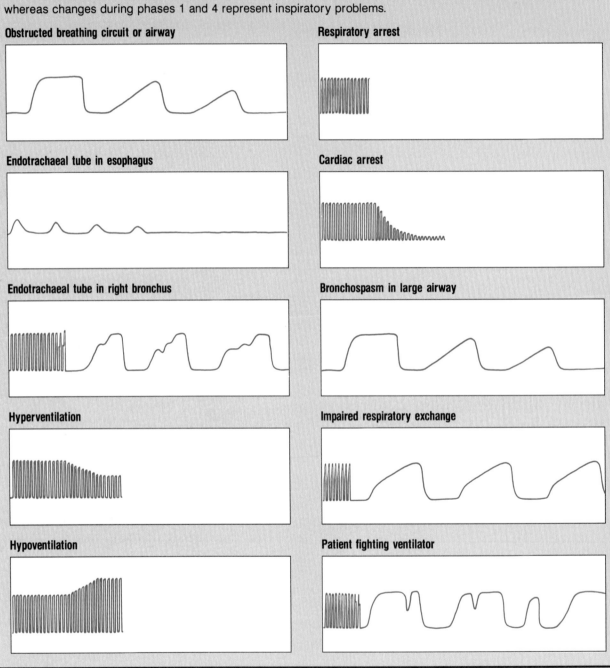

Obstructed breathing circuit or airway

Respiratory arrest

Endotrachaeal tube in esophagus

Cardiac arrest

Endotrachaeal tube in right bronchus

Bronchospasm in large airway

Hyperventilation

Impaired respiratory exchange

Hypoventilation

Patient fighting ventilator

MONITORING END-TIDAL CARBON DIOXIDE

Every nurse knows the importance of correct endotracheal (ET) tube placement. Even a brief displacement may deprive a patient of oxygen and expose him to additional complications such as GI distention. Now, a new and effective device—an end-tidal carbon dioxide (CO_2) detector—is available to help you confirm tube placement.

This device works simply by changing colors within a transparent dome. The color reflects CO_2 expired from the lungs through the ET tube during ventilation.

In a patient receiving adequate ventilation, the device will detect CO_2. If it doesn't, you should suspect a problem—assuming that ventilation is being performed properly. For example, the ET tube could be misplaced in the esophagus or the stomach, where CO_2 isn't normally present. In such a case, you'd withdraw the ET tube immediately, ventilate the patient with a hand-held resuscitation bag, and intubate him again.

The end-tidal CO_2 detector doesn't replace traditional methods of confirming ET tube placement. You'll still need to assess bilateral breath sounds, watch for the symmetrical rise and fall of the chest wall, listen over the epigastric area for gurgling sounds (indicating that the tube is in the esophagus), and obtain a chest X-ray to verify proper placement.

In some circumstances, the end-tidal CO_2 detector's findings may mislead you. For example, a patient who was recently resuscitated with a hand-held device or who recently drank an alcoholic or carbonated beverage may have detectable CO_2 in his stomach.

Like the Easy Cap device described on these pages, most end-tidal CO_2 detectors are inexpensive and disposable after one use. The Easy Cap detector uses a range of colors to evaluate the volume of CO_2 present.

Store end-tidal CO_2 detectors in the crash cart or in any other place in which ET intubation supplies are kept. When needed, take the detector package to the patient's bedside along with a pair of gloves and a hand-held resuscitation bag. You'll also need a stethoscope.

Use the following directions to operate the Easy Cap end-tidal CO_2 detector.

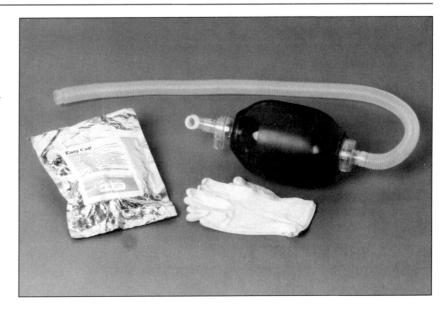

Karen E. Michael, RN, MSN, a case manager for Greater Atlantic Health Service, Philadelphia, contributed to this section. The publisher thanks *Nellcor Inc.*, Hayward, Calif., for its help.

Put on your gloves and check the expiration date on the package. Then open the package and remove the end-tidal CO_2 detector. Look at the color inside the dome. In natural or fluorescent light, it should either match the color of the indicator card or appear darker than the purple segment labeled CHECK on the dome's rim. Discard the device if the dome is a lighter color than it should be.

▶ **Clinical tip:** Under incandescent lighting, the dome looks pink. Always check its color under fluorescent or natural light.

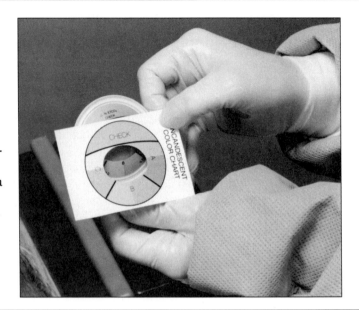

Once you've intubated the patient and inflated the ET tube's cuff, firmly attach the CO_2 detector to the ET tube (as shown). The dome should be parallel to the patient's face. Then attach the hand-held resuscitation bag to the detector.

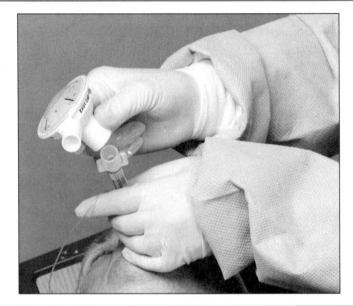

Ventilate the patient with six breaths of moderate tidal volume. Six breaths should wash out any CO_2 retained from a previous manual resuscitation effort or from ventilation, alcohol, or carbonated drinks. Continue ventilating, and observe the color changes in the dome.

▶ **Clinical tip:** Remember that the effects of manual resuscitation and ingestion of alcohol or carbonated beverages can alter the detector's findings. Color changes detected after fewer than six ventilations can be misleading.

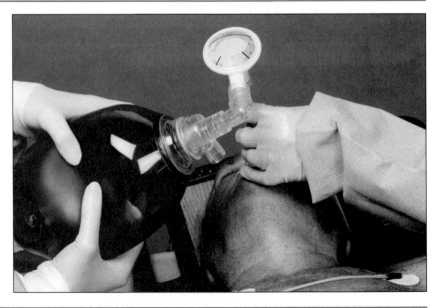

Watch for the color in the dome to fluctuate from purple to yellow. On inspiration, the dome should be purple, which signifies the absence of CO_2.

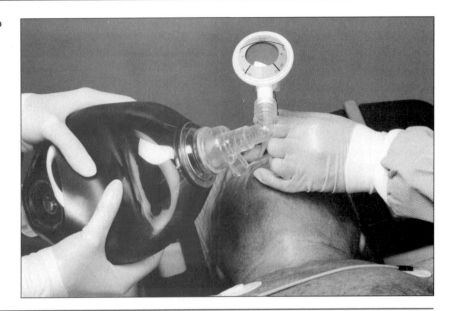

On expiration, watch for the dome color to change to yellow, indicating the presence of CO_2. Compare the color in the dome with the colors on the rim. Use the indicator card supplied by the manufacturer to interpret the changes associated with tube placement.

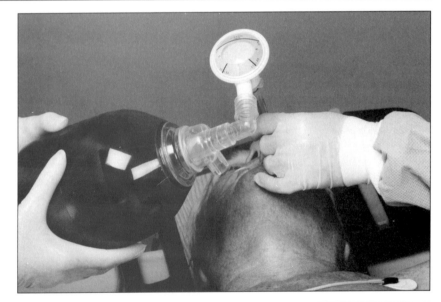

Auscultate the patient's breath sounds and observe his chest movements. Also arrange for a chest X-ray. Tape the ET tube securely and connect the patient to a ventilator. You can leave the end-tidal CO_2 detector in place, but it's accurate for only 15 minutes with high-humidity ventilation.

Once auscultation and X-rays confirm the ET tube's placement, remove the device and discard it. Document the procedure, the results obtained, your auscultation findings, and the X-ray findings in the progress notes.

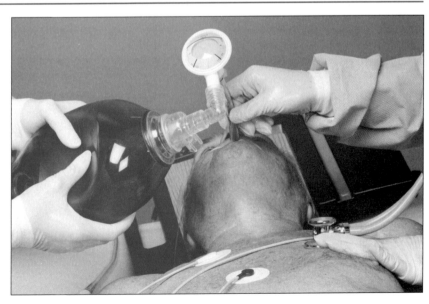

Analyzing CO_2 levels

Depending on which end-tidal carbon dioxide (CO_2) detector you use, the meaning of color changes within the detector dome may differ from the analysis for the Easy Cap detector described below.

• The rim of the Easy Cap is divided into four segments. Clockwise from the top are these sections: CHECK, A, B, and C. The CHECK segment is solid purple—signifying the absence of CO_2.

• The numbers in the other sections range from 0.03 to 5 and indicate the percentage of exhaled CO_2. The color should fluctuate during ventilation from purple (in section A) during inspiration to yellow (in section C) at the end of expiration. This indicates that the end-tidal CO_2 levels are adequate: above 2%.

• An end-expiratory color change from the C to the B range may be the first sign of hemodynamic instability.

• During cardiopulmonary resuscitation (CPR), an end-expiratory color change from the A or B range to the C range may mean the return of spontaneous ventilation.

• During prolonged cardiac arrest, inadequate pulmonary perfusion leads to inadequate gas exchange. The patient exhales little or no CO_2, so the color stays in the purple range even with proper intubation. Ineffective CPR also leads to inadequate pulmonary perfusion.

Color indications on end expiration

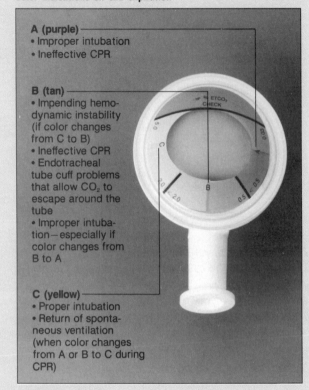

A (purple)
• Improper intubation
• Ineffective CPR

B (tan)
• Impending hemo-dynamic instability (if color changes from C to B)
• Ineffective CPR
• Endotracheal tube cuff problems that allow CO_2 to escape around the tube
• Improper intuba-tion—especially if color changes from B to A

C (yellow)
• Proper intubation
• Return of sponta-neous ventilation (when color changes from A or B to C during CPR)

Using an end-tidal CO_2 detector: Some do's and don'ts

When using an end-tidal CO_2 detector, check the instructions and ensure ideal working conditions for the device. Here are some additional guidelines.

Avoiding high humidity, moisture, and heat
• Watch for changes that indicate the CO_2 detector's decreasing life span. A detector may be used for about 2 hours. However, using it with a ventilator that delivers high-humidity ventilation may shorten its usefulness to no more than 15 minutes. Watch for sluggish color changes from breath to breath.

• Don't use the detector with a heated humidifier or nebulizer.

• Keep the detector protected from secretions, which will render the device useless. If secretions enter the dome, remove and discard the detector.

• Use a heat and moisture exchanger to protect the detector. In some detectors, this filter fits between the endotracheal (ET) tube and the detector.

• If you're using a heat and moisture exchanger, remember that it will increase your patient's breathing effort. Be alert for increased resistance and breathing difficulties, and remove the exchanger if necessary.

Taking additional precautions
• Instilling epinephrine through the ET tube can damage the detector's indicator (the color may stay yellow). If this happens, discard the device.

• Take care when using a CO_2 detector in a child who weighs less than 30 lb (14 kg). A small patient who rebreathes air from the dead space air (about 38 cc) will inhale too much of his own CO_2.

• Spot-check the CO_2 detector you're using often for effectiveness. If you must transport the patient to another area for testing or treatment, use another method to verify the tube's placement.

• Never reuse a disposable end-tidal CO_2 detector. It is intended for one-time, one-patient use only.

Artificial Airways

ESTABLISHING AN OROPHARYNGEAL AIRWAY

Artificial airways help alleviate upper airway obstructions that result when soft tissue occludes the posterior pharynx. The occlusion may occur when the patient is lying on his back and his pharyngeal and laryngeal muscles relax, allowing his tongue to fall backward and obstruct his airway.

How will you know that your patient's airway is blocked? Watch for stridor, accessory muscle use in breathing, sternal retractions, tracheal tug (a downward jerking of the trachea), rocking chest motion (chest falling and abdomen rising on inspiration), limited chest excursion, diminished or absent breath sounds, and cyanosis.

If your patient exhibits these signs, immediately attempt to open the airway mechanically. First, try repositioning his head to realign airway structures. You have three ways to do this: You may place the patient's head in the sniffing position, extend the patient's neck, or perform a jaw-thrust maneuver. If these measures fail, your next step will be to insert an oropharyngeal airway.

Caution: Don't perform any maneuver if you suspect that the patient has a cervical spine injury. Instead, insert an artificial airway.

Made of firm plastic, an oropharyngeal airway curves in such a way that it separates the base of the tongue from the posterior pharynx and allows air to pass. The airway also facilitates oropharyngeal suctioning.

Available in several sizes and two styles (known as the Berman and the Guedel), oropharyngeal airways are intended only for short-term use—for example, in postictal, anesthetized, or unconscious patients. Occasionally, they may be used for longer periods—for example, in orally intubated patients to prevent them from biting their endotracheal tubes. Oropharyngeal airways are easy to use and relieve most types of obstructions, but they do have the following disadvantages:

• Once inserted, the airway may dislodge easily.

• Conscious or semiconscious patients tolerate the airway poorly. Its insertion may stimulate vomiting and laryngospasm, thereby increasing the risk of aspiration.

• Airway insertion may damage teeth, oropharyngeal tissue, or both. For this reason, the airway shouldn't be used in a patient who has recently had oral surgery or who has loose or avulsed teeth.

Opening the airway: Initial measures

With the patient supine, place a folded sheet or firm head ring under her head to elevate it about 4" (10 cm) above her mattress. This straightens the cervical spine and aligns the pharynx and larynx. The patient is now in the sniffing position.

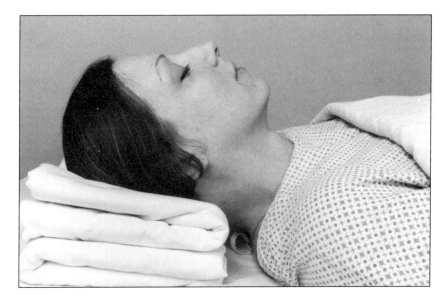

By extending the patient's neck, you may also be able to reestablish the airway. Straighten the patient's neck but be careful not to hyper-extend it.

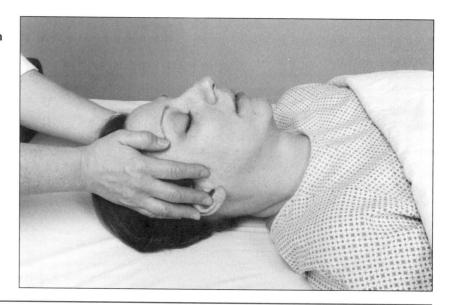

To perform the jaw-thrust maneu-ver, position your body behind the patient's head. Rest your thumbs on her cheeks, curve your index fingers under her jaw, and lift.

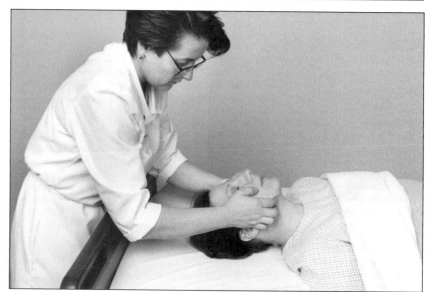

Inserting the airway

To insert an oropharyngeal airway, first obtain several airways of both types in several different sizes. You'll need a gown, a tongue blade, gloves, a face shield (or safety goggles and a mask), and a stethoscope. You may also need suction equipment.

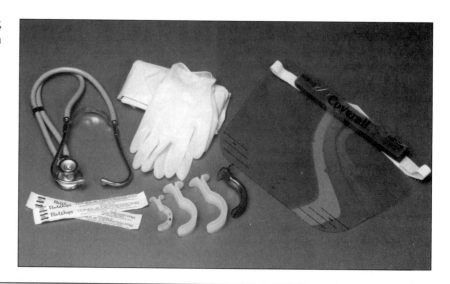

Explain the procedure to the patient even though she may not appear to be alert. Provide privacy. Use universal precautions as appropriate.

Place the patient in the supine position and, if necessary, remove the pillow and suction her mouth. If she's wearing dentures, remove them. Doing so prevents damage to them and ensures that they don't dislodge during the procedure and further obstruct the airway.

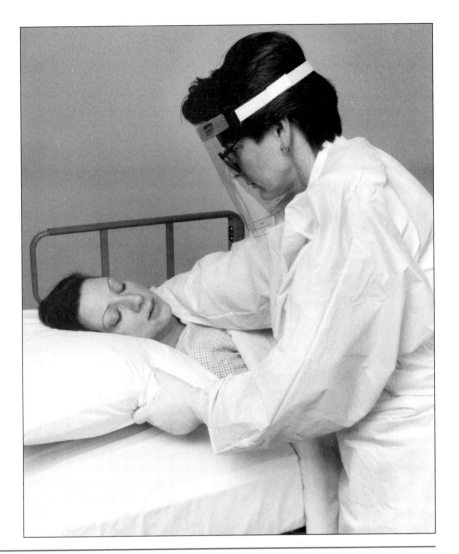

Select the appropriate size of airway. To estimate the correct size, hold the airway alongside the patient's upper jaw, with the front of the airway even with the patient's teeth (as shown). The airway's curve should reach the angle of the jaws. Usually, a child requires a small airway; an average-sized adult, a medium one; and a large adult, a large.

▶ *Clinical tip:* The airway's size is important. An oversized airway can exacerbate the obstruction and induce gagging, vomiting, and aspiration. An undersized airway may also exacerbate the obstruction—especially if the tip rests on the middle of the patient's tongue and pushes the rear of the tongue into the back of the mouth.

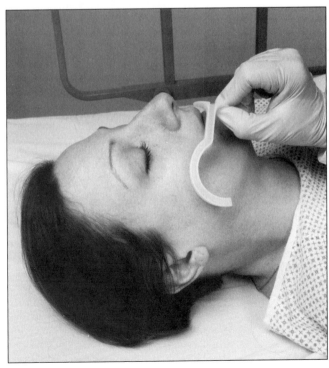

Hyperextend the patient's neck, unless contraindicated.

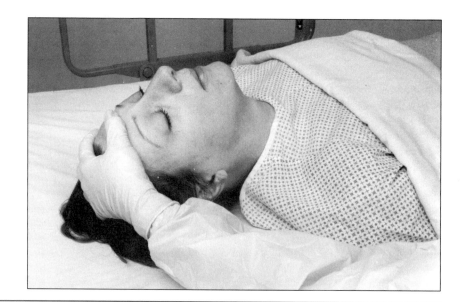

Open the patient's mouth using the scissors technique: Place the index or middle finger of your nondominant hand on the patient's upper teeth and your thumb on her lower teeth (as shown). Push your fingers apart to open the patient's mouth.

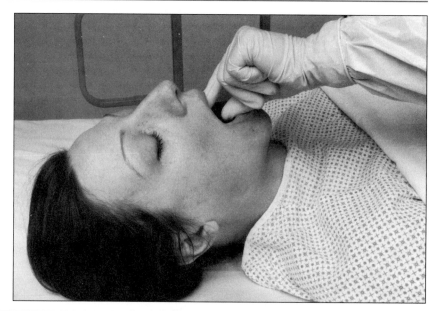

If you use a tongue blade when inserting the airway, hold it in your nondominant hand and place it on the back of the patient's tongue. Depress the tongue by pulling the tongue blade forward slightly. Then, with your dominant hand, slide the oropharyngeal airway over the depressed tongue until the flange of the airway sits just in front of the upper incisors.

▷ *Clinical tip:* If your patient has a dry tongue, wet the airway with water to ease insertion.

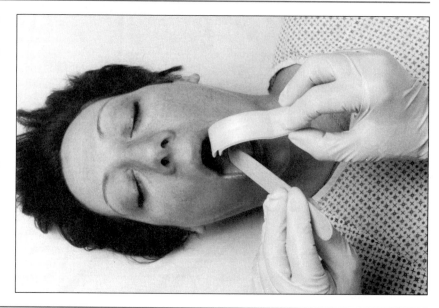

If you insert the airway without using a tongue blade, first open the patient's mouth using the scissors technique. Then insert the airway upside down, with the tip pointing toward the roof of the patient's mouth. Gently advance the airway over the patient's tongue, being careful not to scrape the hard palate or place pressure on the upper teeth.

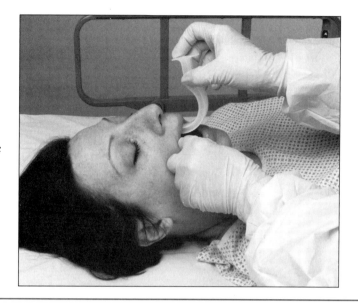

As the airway approaches the posterior wall of the pharynx, rotate it so that it points downward.

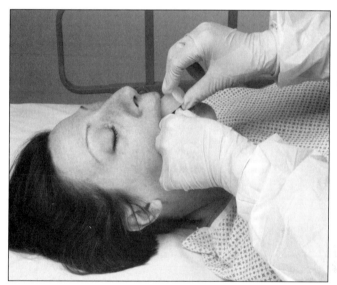

Once inserted, the oropharyngeal airway should bend, following the natural curvature of the oropharynx. Don't tape the airway in place after insertion.

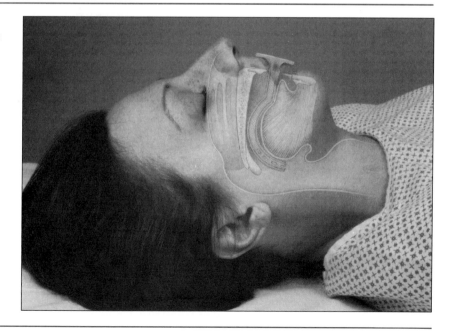

Auscultate the patient's lungs to confirm adequate ventilation and correct airway size and position. Position the patient on her side to decrease her risk of aspiration. Then document the procedure.

▶ *Clinical tip:* Clear breath sounds on auscultation indicate that the airway is the proper size and in the correct position.

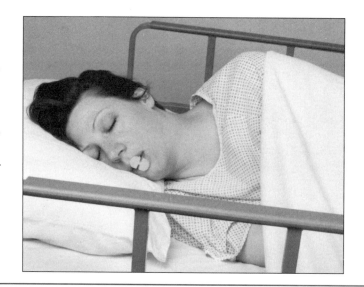

Caring for the patient with an airway

To maintain an inserted airway, you'll need a gown, a premoistened oral cleaning swab (or a lemon-glycerin swab), hydrogen peroxide, water, an emesis basin, gloves, a face shield (or safety goggles and a mask), pipe cleaners, and a clean oropharyngeal airway of the same type and size as the one that's in place. You may also need suction equipment.

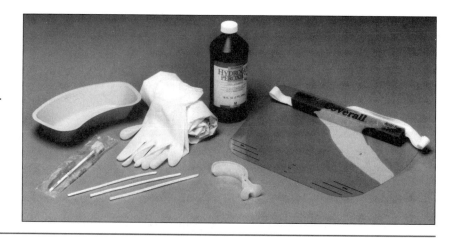

Frequently observe the position of the airway in the patient's mouth. Also, auscultate the patient's lungs to ensure that the airway is correctly positioned.

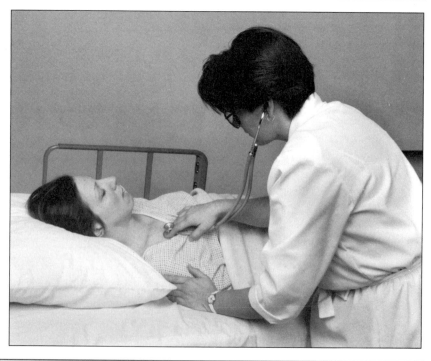

Suction the patient's oral cavity as necessary. Perform mouth care every 2 to 4 hours, as needed, using a premoistened oral cleaning swab (shown here) or a lemon-glycerin swab. Be sure to wear gloves and a face shield whenever you might come in contact with the patient's secretions.

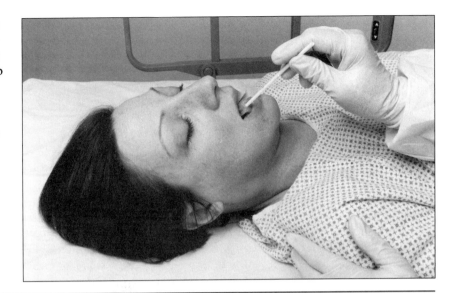

If you see the airway heavily coated with secretions, gently remove it. To do so, pull the airway outward and downward, following the mouth's natural curvature. Place the used airway in the emesis basin and immediately reinsert a clean airway, using the technique described above.

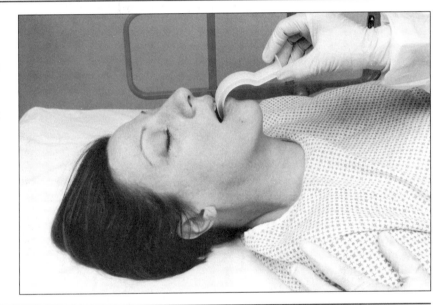

Once you insert the new airway, clean the used airway with hydrogen peroxide and water. If necessary, use a pipe cleaner to remove secretions. Store the clean airway for future use on the same patient.

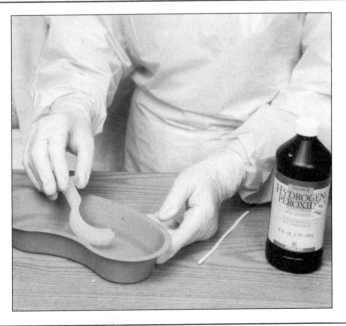

ESTABLISHING A NASOPHARYNGEAL AIRWAY

If your patient's airway is blocked and repositioning his head fails to open it, you'll need to insert an artificial airway. However, if an oropharyngeal airway is contraindicated, a nasopharyngeal airway is the ideal choice. You'll use this airway for a patient who is conscious or semiconscious; who has had recent oral surgery; who has loose, cracked, or avulsed teeth; or who can't or won't open his mouth. A nasopharyngeal airway may also be used to protect the nasal mucosa from injury when the patient needs frequent nasotracheal suctioning.

A nasopharyngeal airway is contraindicated for a patient taking anticoagulants or a patient with a hemorrhagic disorder, sepsis, or a nasopharyngeal deformity caused by disease. It's also contraindi-cated if the patient's condition involves cerebrospinal fluid leaking from the nose.

Made of pliable latex, a nasopharyngeal airway is inserted through the nostrils. The airway follows the curvature of the nasopharynx and extends into the posterior pharynx, where it separates the base of the tongue from the posterior pharyngeal wall. The bevel-shaped pharyngeal end of the airway facilitates insertion; the funnel-shaped nasal end helps prevent slippage. This type of airway can't damage the teeth.

Disadvantages of a nasopharyngeal airway include its potential to cause severe epistaxis and to damage the nasal mucosa. Additionally, it may make suctioning difficult, especially if the procedure kinks or clogs the airway.

Inserting the airway

To insert a nasopharyngeal airway, you'll need several sizes of naso-pharyngeal airways, ranging from #28 to #34 French. Also gather water-soluble lubricant, tongue blades, a gown, gloves, a face shield (or safety goggles and a mask), and a penlight. You may also need suction equipment.

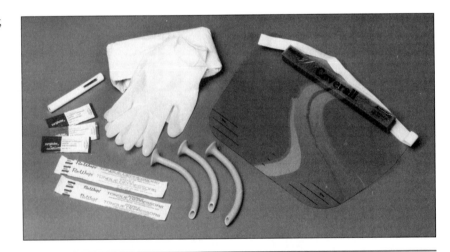

Provide privacy, and explain the procedure to the patient. Use universal precautions, if appropriate. Place the patient in a supine position and, if necessary, suction her. Check the patient's chart to make sure that she isn't allergic to latex.

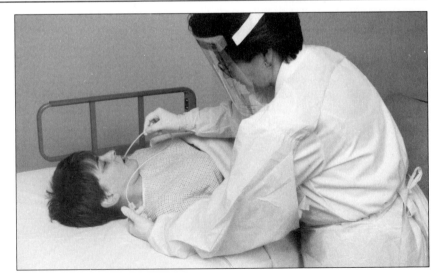

Select the appropriate size of airway. To do so, hold the airway next to the patient's cheek (as shown). Compare the diameter of the airway to the diameter of the patient's nostril. The airway diameter should be slightly smaller. Then note the length of the airway. It should be slightly longer than the distance from the tip of the patient's nose to the edge of her jaw.

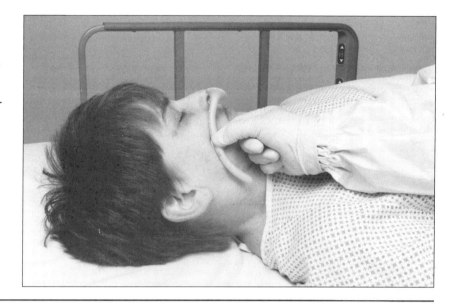

Liberally coat the nasal airway with the water-soluble lubricant.

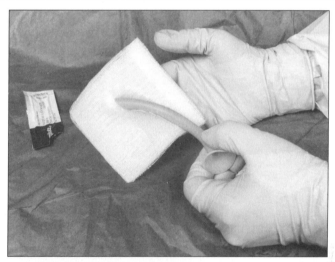

With your dominant hand, slide the airway into the selected nostril. Gently advance the airway along the floor of the nose. Meanwhile, use your other hand to push up the tip of the patient's nose. Once inserted, the airway should follow the nasopharynx's normal curvature.

▶ *Clinical tip:* Avoid threading the airway toward the frontal sinus. Not only will it fail to pass, but its force may also start a nosebleed. If you meet resistance during insertion, carefully twist the airway as you slowly advance it, but *don't force it.* If you still meet resistance, remove the airway, and insert it in the other nostril or switch to a smaller airway.

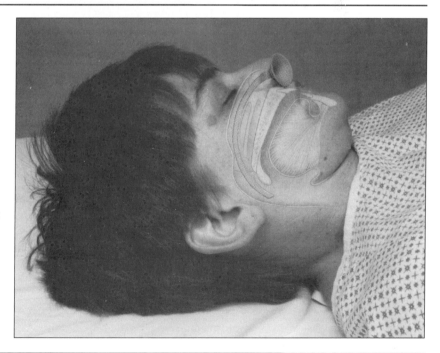

Once you've inserted the airway, confirm its placement. To do so, have the patient close her mouth. Then place your hand over the airway opening. If you feel air, the airway is properly placed. You can also auscultate the lungs to confirm adequate ventilation.

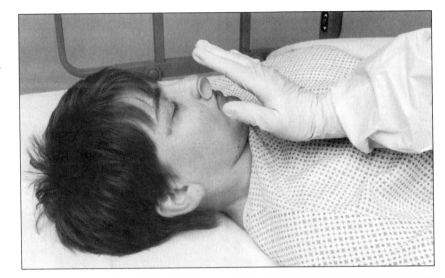

Or, if you can open the patient's mouth, you can confirm placement by depressing the patient's tongue with a tongue blade. Then, using a penlight, look into the patient's mouth. You should see the airway's tip behind the uvula.

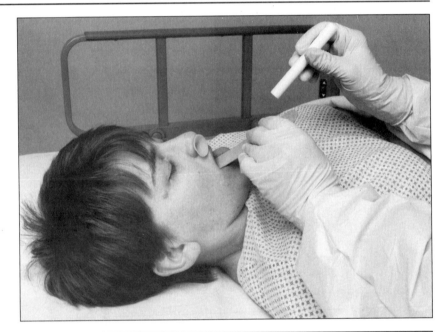

Caring for the patient with an airway

To maintain an inserted nasopharyngeal airway, you'll need a clean airway of the same type and size as the one that's in place. You'll also need hydrogen peroxide, water in an emesis basin, a gown, gloves, water-soluble lubricant, a face shield (or safety goggles and a mask), pipe cleaners, and a penlight.

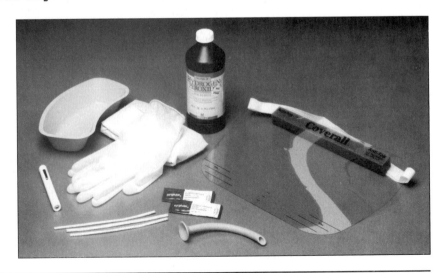

Perform airway maintenance at least once every 8 hours. Begin by putting on gloves and a face shield (or safety goggles and a mask). Then, using one smooth motion, remove the airway.

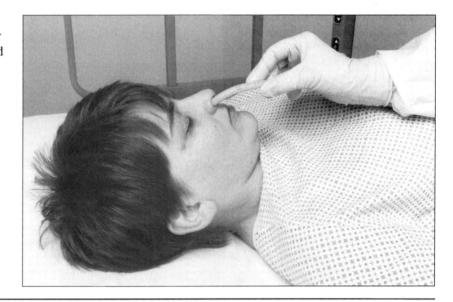

If the airway resists removal, apply water-soluble lubricant around the patient's nostril and the nasal end of the tube. Then gently rotate the tube until it's free. Once removed, check the patient's nasal mucous membranes for irritation and ulceration.

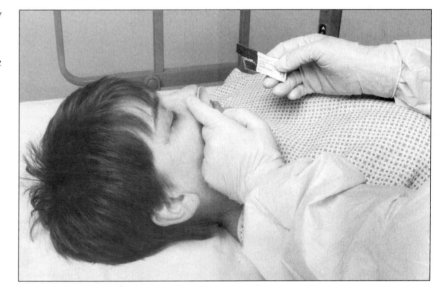

Immediately insert a clean airway into the other nostril, unless contraindicated. Using hydrogen peroxide and water, rinse the airway that you just removed. If necessary, use a pipe cleaner to help remove the secretions. Once the airway is clean, store it for future use on the same patient.

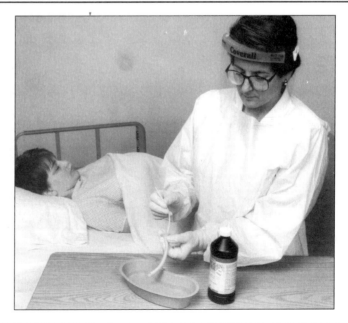

ASSISTING WITH ENDOTRACHEAL TUBE INSERTION

An endotracheal (ET) tube is used to control the patient's airway, to deliver short-term mechanical ventilation, to allow tracheobronchial suctioning, and to administer emergency medications. This flexible, cuffed tube advances through a patient's nose or mouth to the larynx and into the trachea. Performed by a doctor, an anesthetist, a respiratory therapist, or a nurse educated in the procedure, endotracheal intubation usually occurs in an emergency, such as respiratory distress or cardiopulmonary arrest. Emergency medical technicians and paramedics are certified to intubate patients in emergencies in nonhospital settings. Intubation may also occur in the operating room.

Intubation protects the patient from aspiration by sealing off the trachea from the digestive tract with an inflated tracheal cuff. However, it bypasses normal respiratory tract defenses against infection, reduces cough effectiveness, prevents oral communication, risks tracheal injury, and causes discomfort.

TYPES OF TUBES

Used when a patient has facial, oral, or cervical neck trauma or a jaw movement problem, a *nasal ET tube* provides a controlled airway for mechanical ventilation that's more comfortable than an oral ET tube. Contraindications include nasal obstruction, a fractured nose, sinusitis, and bleeding disorders. A nasal ET tube should be used cautiously in basal skull fractures.

An *oral ET tube* provides a controlled airway for mechanical ventilation when the patient has a nasal obstruction or a predisposition to nosebleeds. Most commonly used to ensure an open airway during cardiopulmonary resuscitation, an oral ET tube should not be used in a traumatic injury to the lower face or mouth or after recent oral surgery.

Both kinds of ET tubes are contraindicated in epiglottitis; acute, unstable cervical spine injury; or laryngeal obstruction caused by a tumor, an infection, or vocal cord paralysis.

Preparing for insertion

You'll need two or more ET tubes in appropriate sizes, a 10-cc syringe, a stethoscope, several pairs of gloves, two face shields, two gowns, a sedative, a water-soluble lubricant, a skin preparation, hypoallergenic adhesive tape or a Velcro tube holder, a sterile suction kit, a tonsillar suction device, connecting tubing, a hand-held resuscitation bag with removable mask, an oral airway, and a water-resistant marking pen. You'll also need a lighted laryngoscope with a handle and blades, a local anesthetic spray, a suction source, and a humidified oxygen source.

Obtain a prepared intubation kit (sterile gauze pads, stylet, forceps, sterile water and a sterile basin). If the ET tube will be inserted nasally, you'll need a mucosal vasoconstricting agent.

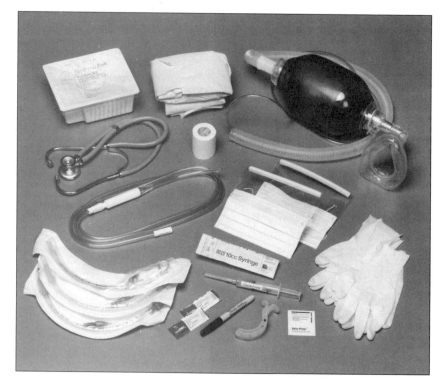

Kate McGovern, RN, BSN, CCRN, and *Marguerite S. Ambrose, RN, MSN, CCRN,* contributed to this section. Ms. McGovern is a clinical leader in the Surgical Trauma Unit at Abington (Pa.) Memorial Hospital. Ms. Ambrose is an assistant professor at LaSalle University, Philadelphia. The publisher thanks *Abington (Pa.) Memorial Hospital* for its help.

Gather the equipment and take it to the patient's bedside. Wash your hands and put on gloves. Then check the battery-operated light in the laryngoscope handle by snapping a blade in place.

If the light fails to flash immediately, replace the bulb or the batteries, whichever is indicated. If necessary, obtain a new laryngoscope and repeat the procedure to check that it functions properly.

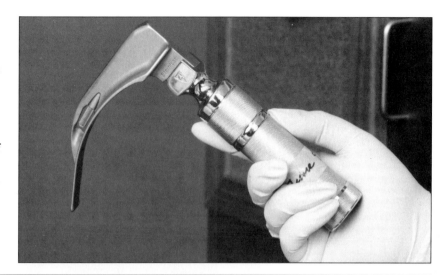

Select the appropriate-sized ET tube. Then pour sterile water into a sterile basin. Attach the 10-cc syringe to the port of the tube's exterior pilot cuff. Slowly inflate the cuff and observe for uniform inflation (as shown). If time permits, submerge the cuff in the sterile water and watch for air bubbles, which indicate a leak and the need for another cuffed tube.

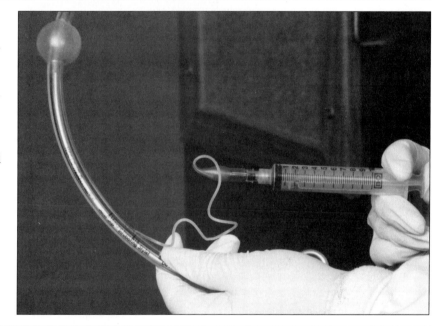

If the patient will be intubated nasally, open the package of water-soluble lubricant and apply some to the tube—either by placing the lubricant on a sterile gauze pad and wiping it on the tube or by squeezing the lubricant directly onto the tube. (You'll rarely use lubricant for oral intubation.)

▶ **Clinical tip:** Use only water-soluble lubricant because lubricant can be absorbed by the mucous membranes.

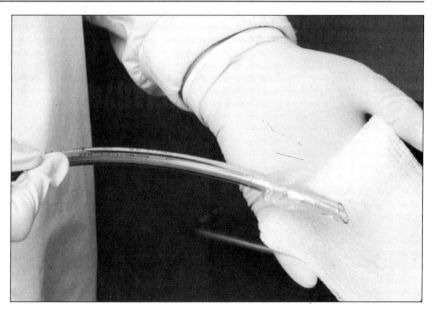

Attach the hand-held resuscitation bag to the oxygen flowmeter. Turn the flowmeter dial to 15 liters. Place the resuscitation bag within easy reach (unless it's already in use for the patient).

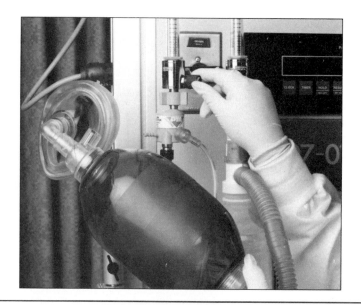

Connect the suction apparatus to the suction source. Next, open the tonsillar suction device, and attach it to the connecting tubing. Turn on the suction briefly to make sure that it's working properly. Note the amount of suction, as indicated by the suction gauge dial (as shown), and listen for the characteristic sound. Place the apparatus near the patient.

Open the suction kit so that it's available for immediate use. If you expect the patient to use mechanical ventilation, have the ventilator ready for use at the bedside. If he will need humidified oxygen and a T-piece, prepare these devices now.

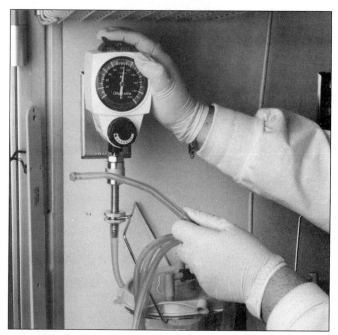

Explain the procedure to the patient and any family members who are present. Put on clean gloves and, if you think that soiling or splattering may occur, a face shield and a gown.

For easy access to the patient, remove the headboard of the bed (as shown). Place the patient in a supine position, and remove any dentures or bridgework, if present.

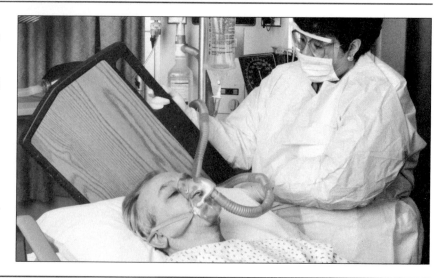

For oral intubation, open the patient's airway (upper right) so that his posterior pharynx can be sprayed with the prescribed anesthetic (lower right). This diminishes the gag reflex and reduces discomfort.

For nasal intubation, spray a local anesthetic and a vasoconstricting agent, as ordered, into the patient's nasal passages. This anesthetizes and shrinks the nasal turbinates and reduces the chance of bleeding.

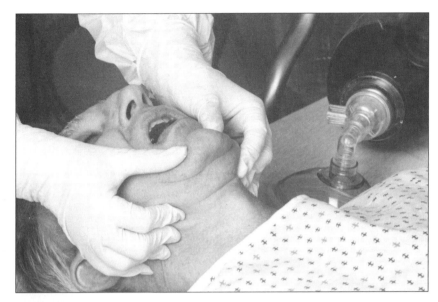

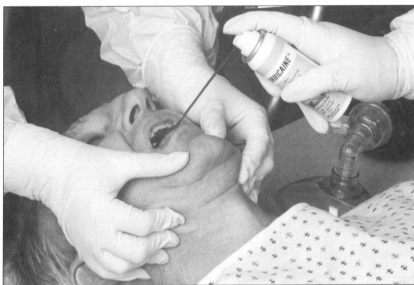

To prevent hypoxia, provide oxygen with a hand-held resuscitation bag until the ET tube is inserted. In some situations (cardiac or respiratory arrest, for example), the patient will already be receiving oxygen this way.

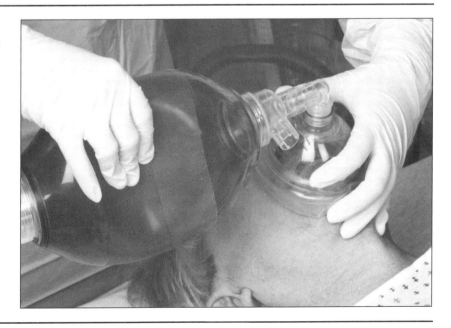

Administer a sedative, as ordered, to decrease respiratory secretions, induce amnesia or analgesia, and help calm and relax the conscious patient.

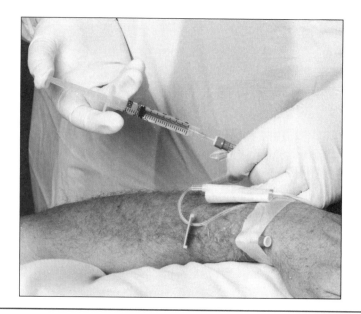

To improve visualization just before tube insertion, suction the patient's pharynx with the tonsillar suction device.

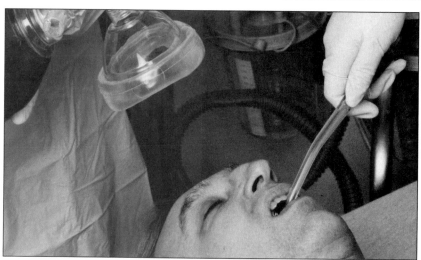

Inserting the ET tube

Stand next to the patient's head at the bedside while the person who will intubate the patient (the doctor or the respiratory therapist, for example) stands at the head of the bed. Hand the ET tube to this person. Then hand him the laryngoscope (as shown). Keep the hand-held resuscitation bag close to the patient's head so that you can ventilate him between intubation attempts.

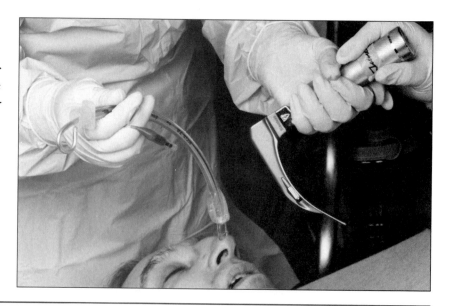

Be prepared to apply pressure to the cricoid cartilage as the person intubating the patient uses the laryngoscope to visualize the vocal cords.

▶ *Clinical tip:* Applying pressure to the cricoid cartilage occludes the esophagus and minimizes gastric regurgitation.

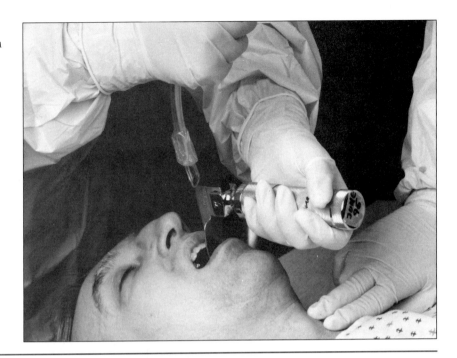

Suction the patient's pharynx with the tonsillar suction device as requested. Once the ET tube advances past the vocal cords, the stylet may be quickly removed (upper right) and the ET tube's cuff inflated (lower right) with 5 to 10 cc of air (until the inflator feels resistance).

▶ *Clinical tip:* Once mechanical ventilation is in effect, use the minimal-leak technique or the minimal-occlusive-volume technique to establish correct cuff inflation.

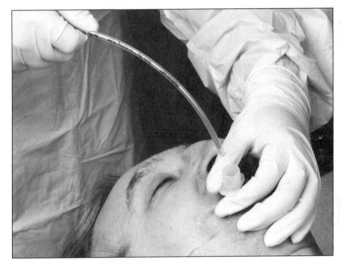

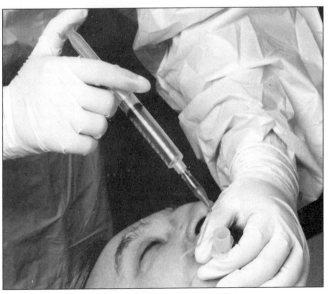

If the patient can breathe spontaneously, listen for air movement and look for condensate inside the tube. Attach the hand-held resuscitation bag to the end of the ET tube, and ventilate the patient while observing his chest for equal lung expansion.

If the patient's lungs don't inflate and you observe stomach distention or hear a gurgling or belching sound (indicating esophageal intubation), expect the person who intubated the patient to deflate the cuff and remove the tube. Again provide oxygen until the next insertion attempt (with a new sterile ET tube to prevent contamination of the trachea).

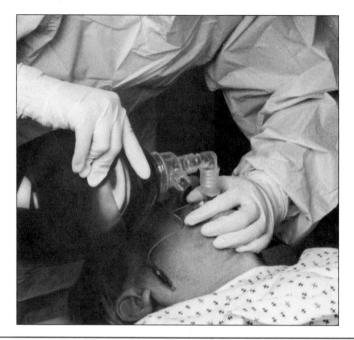

While oxygenation continues, the lungs need to be auscultated bilaterally. If breath sounds aren't heard on both sides of the chest, the ET tube may have entered the right mainstem bronchus (usually the right one because of its wider angle at the bifurcation). Expect the person who intubated the patient to deflate the cuff and withdraw the tube 1 to 2 cm, auscultate for breath sounds, and then reinflate the cuff.

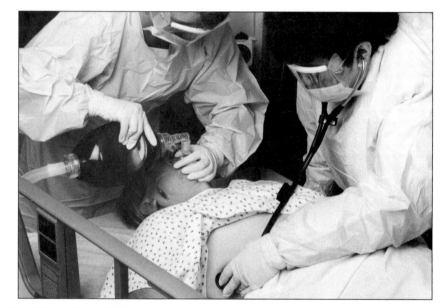

Place an oral airway in the patient's mouth if he tends to obstruct airflow by biting the ET tube.

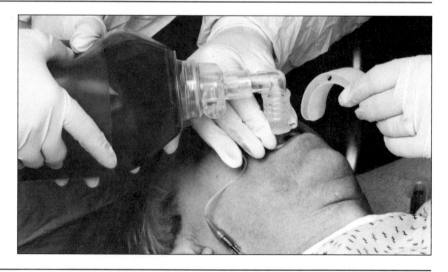

Apply a skin preparation to both cheeks, and let it dry to enhance tape adherence. Then secure the tube firmly with hypoallergenic adhesive tape or a Velcro tube holder, if available.

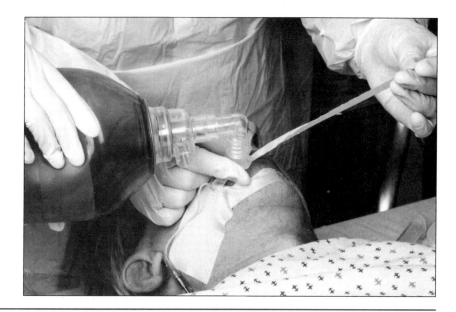

Clearly mark the tube's exit point from the mouth or nose with tape or a marking pen (as shown). Arrange for a chest X-ray to verify tube position. Depending on the X-ray findings, the tube's position may need to be adjusted (by qualified personnel).

Document the date and time of the procedure, noting success or failure, tube type and size, exit point (in centimeters) from the patient's mouth, cuff size, and inflation volume. Also record the administration of medication and supplemental oxygen or ventilation therapy, results of chest auscultation and X-ray studies, complications and nursing interventions, and the patient's tolerance of the procedure.

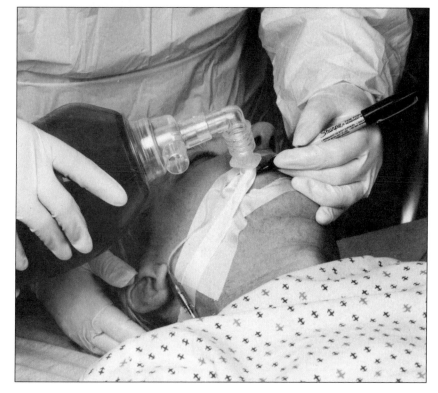

PROVIDING ENDOTRACHEAL TUBE CARE

When caring for a patient with an ET tube, provide meticulous care to ensure airway patency and prevent complications until the patient can maintain independent ventilation. ET tube care includes frequently assessing airway status, maintaining proper cuff pressure to prevent tissue ischemia and necrosis, carefully repositioning the tube to avoid traumatic manipulation, closely monitoring for complications, and offering emotional support to the patient. Possible complications from ET tube use include airway obstruction, injury to the larynx or trachea, and injury to oral or facial skin.

For some patients, you'll need to reposition an oral ET tube to improve comfort, to prevent pressure ulcers, or to correct improper placement. In such cases, make sure that the ET tube remains securely in place to provide continuous airway access and to prevent tube displacement.

Maintaining airway patency

You'll need a stethoscope, suction equipment, a gown, a face shield, and gloves. You may also need an oropharyngeal airway (sized appropriately for the patient).

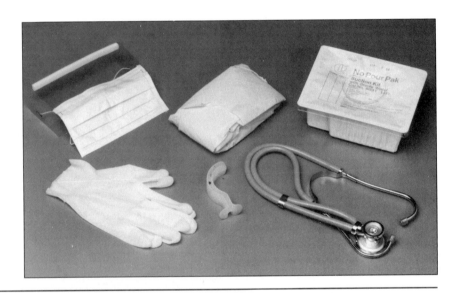

Position the patient's head comfortably so that he's less likely to move around and kink the tubing or obstruct the airway. Auscultate both sides of the anterior chest, and observe chest movement to ensure correct tube placement and full lung ventilation. Do this at least every 2 hours and at any sign of respiratory distress. If you don't hear breath sounds over a lung, notify the doctor, who will order a chest X-ray. Then reposition the ET tube if necessary.

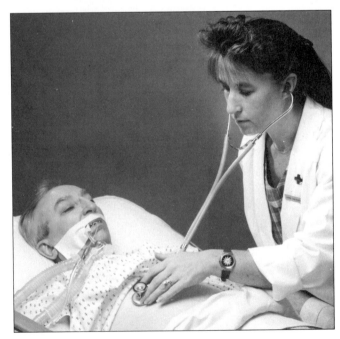

Put on a gown, a face shield, and gloves. Suction secretions from the ET tube whenever necessary.

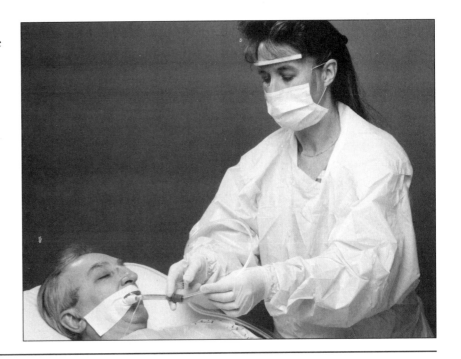

If the patient tends to bite on the ET tube, insert an oral airway beside the tube to prevent obstruction.

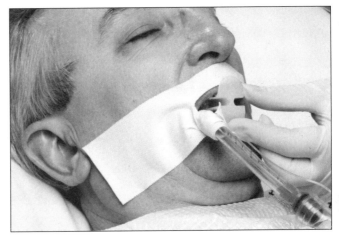

Securing an ET tube

Anchor the ET tube securely after inserting or repositioning it or after replacing the tape that holds it in place. You can use one of many methods. Some of the most common are described on the following pages. If the patient is coughing and you suspect that the tube's position may be unstable, have another colleague assist you.

To begin, explain the procedure to the patient, put on gloves, a gown, and a face shield, and then suction his mouth and tube just before taping the tube.

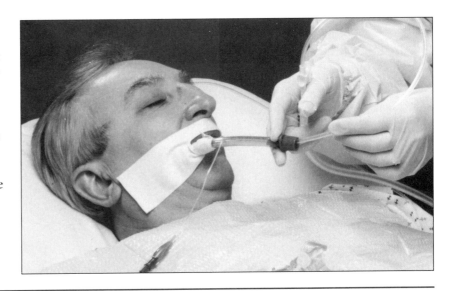

Taping the tube: Method 1

When securing an ET tube using this method, you'll typically need 1″ adhesive tape, 2″ adhesive tape, a skin preparation (such as compound benzoin tincture), gloves, a gown, and a face shield. If your patient's skin is excoriated, you may substitute two transparent semipermeable dressings for the 2″ adhesive tape.

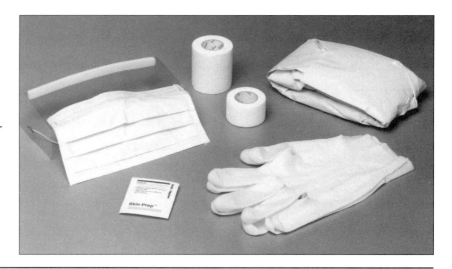

Tear two 2″ (5-cm) strips of the 2″ tape and one 15″ (38-cm) strip of the 1″ adhesive tape.

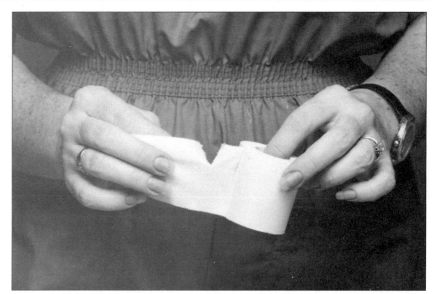

Then make a 13″ (33-cm) slit down the center of the 15″ strip.

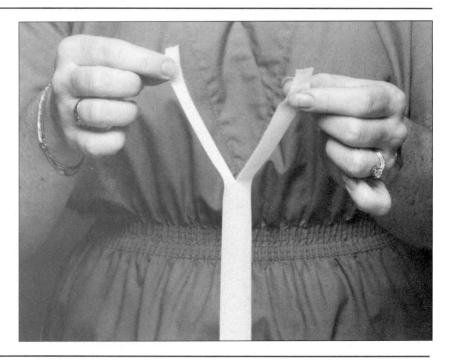

Put on gloves, a gown, and a face shield. Hold the ET tube in place as you remove the soiled tape. Then make sure the patient's face is clean, dry, and free of stubble. If possible, have another nurse hold the tube in place while you remove the soiled tape and apply clean tape.

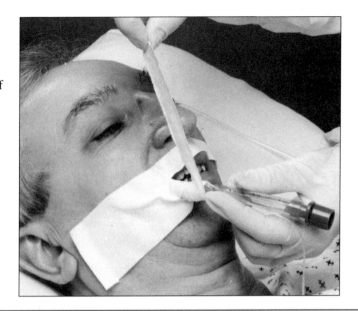

Apply a skin preparation to the patient's cheeks. If you use a spray preparation, be careful to protect the patient's eyes from contact with the preparation.

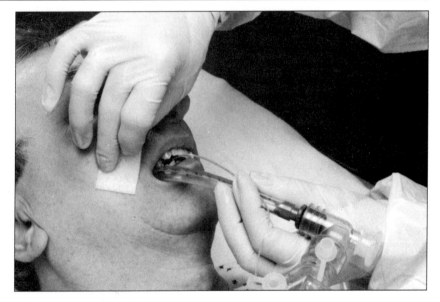

Then place the 2″ tape strips on the patient's cheeks, creating a new surface on which to anchor the tape securing the tube. When the patient's ET tube needs frequent retaping, this preparation helps prevent damage to the patient's skin. If his skin is excoriated or at risk, use a transparent semipermeable dressing to protect the skin.

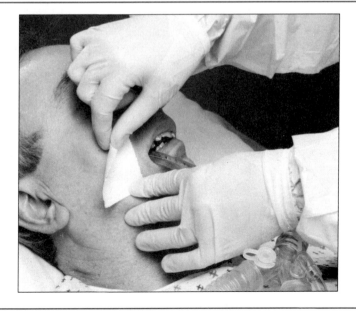

On the side of the mouth where the tube will be anchored, place the unslit end of the 15″ piece of tape on top of the tape on the patient's cheek.

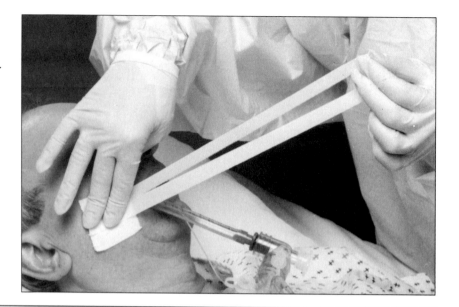

Wrap the top half of the split tape twice around the ET tube, pulling the tape as tightly as possible around the tube. Then, directing the tape over the patient's upper lip, place the end of the tape on the 2″ piece of tape on the patient's other cheek. Cut off any excess tape.

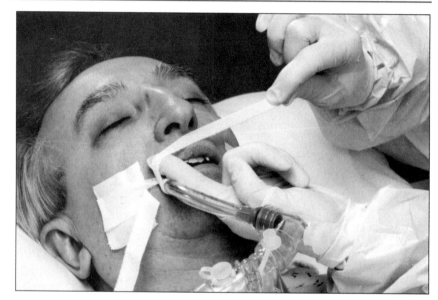

Wrap the lower half of the tape twice around the tube.

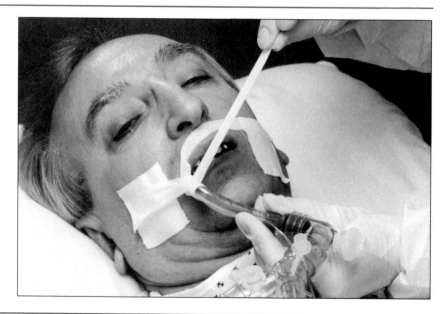

Then attach this lower half of the tape to the 2″ piece of tape on the patient's other cheek.

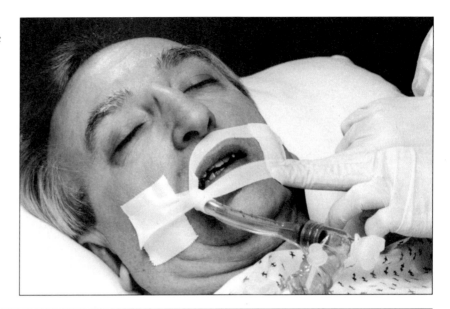

If the patient has an oral airway, bring the lower end of the tape across the lower lip and over the oral airway to secure the airway.

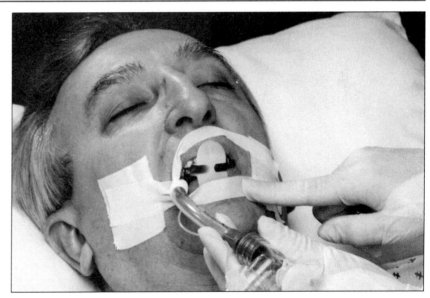

If you've taped an oral airway or are concerned about the tube's stability, apply another 15″ strip of tape in the same manner as the first, starting on the other side of the patient's face.

▶ **Clinical tip:** If the tape around the tube is too bulky, use only the upper part of the tape; cut off the lower part. If the patient has copious oral secretions, seal the tape by cutting a 1″ piece of paper tape, coating it with compound benzoin tincture, and placing the paper tape over the adhesive tape on the tube.

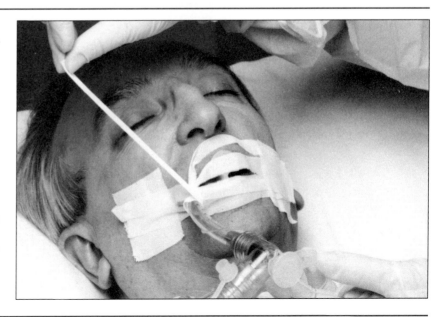

Taping the tube: Method 2

To secure an ET tube in another way, you'll need 1″ adhesive tape, gloves, a face shield, a gown, and skin preparation pads.

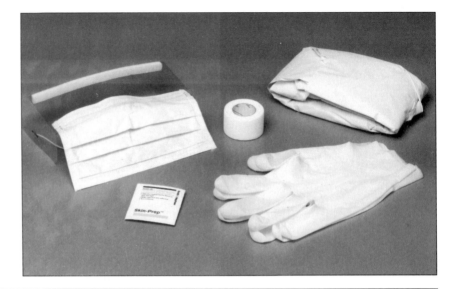

Tear one piece of 1″ adhesive tape long enough to wrap around the patient's head and overlap in front (at least 18″ [46-cm] long). Then tear an 8″ (20-cm) piece of 1″ tape and center it on the longer piece, sticky sides together.

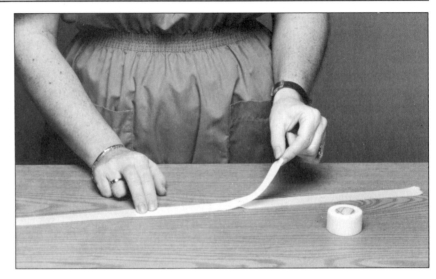

Next, make a 5″ (13-cm) slit down the center of each end of the longer tape.

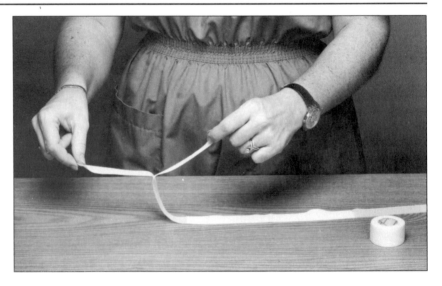

Put on a gown, a face shield, and gloves. Hold the ET tube in place as you remove the tape. Then make sure that the patient's face is clean, dry, and free of stubble. If possible, have another nurse hold the tube in place while you remove the soiled tape and apply clean tape. Apply a skin preparation to the patient's cheeks and under his nose (as shown). Place the middle portion of the tape (the part with the sticky sides together) behind the patient's head.

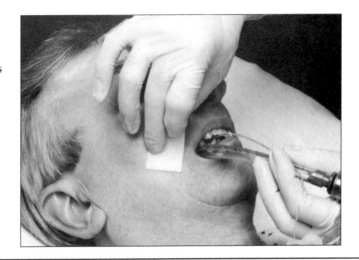

Place the top half of one end of the tape under the patient's nose and secure it to his cheek. Then wrap the lower half of the tape around the ET tube (as shown), bring the tape up over the top lip, and secure it to the area above the upper lip.

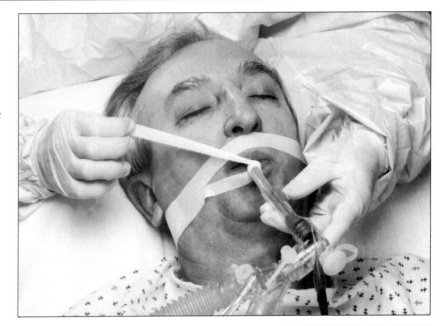

Wrap the lower half of the other end of the tape around the tube in the opposite direction of the first piece of tape. Bring this tape up over the top lip and secure it to the area above the upper lip on the opposite side.

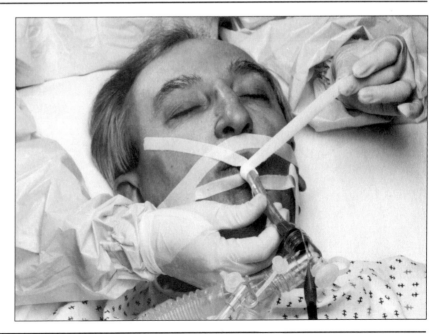

Bring the remaining upper half of tape across the upper lip and over both pieces of tape already there (as shown). Secure the tape to the patient's cheek.

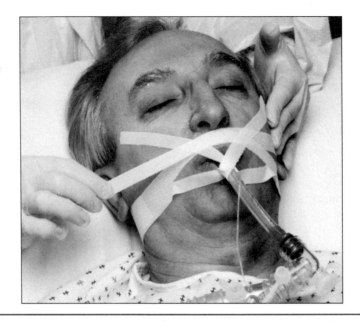

Taping the tube: Method 3

A third way to secure an ET tube requires 3″ adhesive tape, skin preparation pads, gloves, a gown, and a face shield.

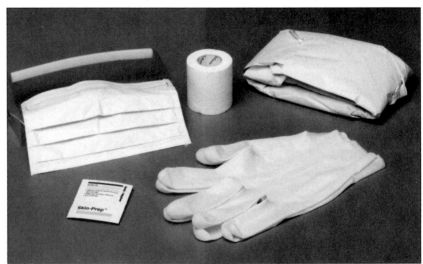

Tear a piece of 3″ tape about 12″ (30.5 cm) long, or long enough to go across the patient's face from one cheek to the other. Then tear a slit three-quarters of the way down one side of the tape (as shown).

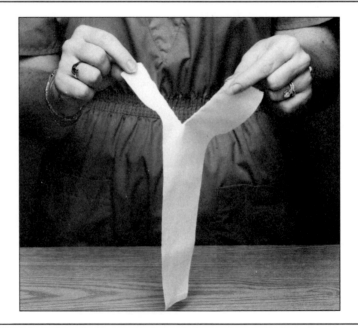

Next, tear a second lengthwise slit three-quarters of the way down other side of the tape (dividing tape into three 1″ wide strips).

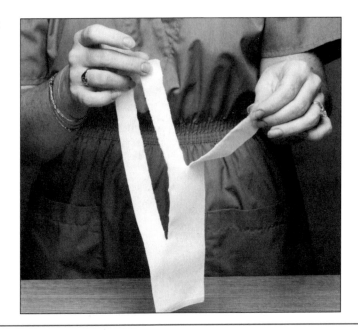

Put on a gown, a face shield, and gloves. Apply a skin preparation to the patient's cheeks. Then stick the unslit end of the tape on the patient's cheek closest to the ET tube.

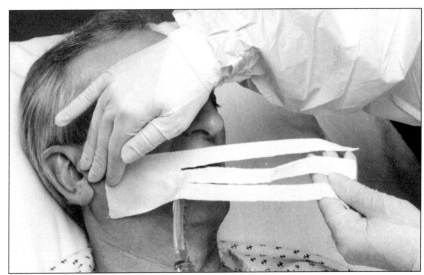

Place the top 1″ tape strip above the patient's upper lip.

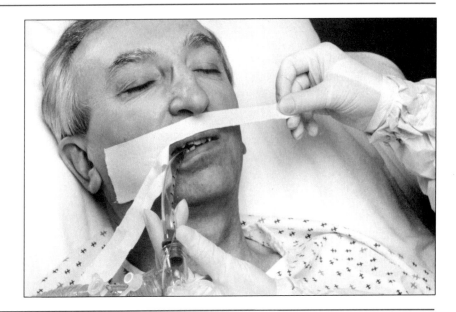

Take the middle 1″ strip and wrap it around the ET tube.

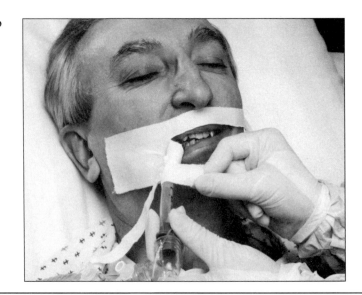

Then wrap the bottom 1″ strip around the ET tube, and place the remaining part of this strip under the patient's lower lip.

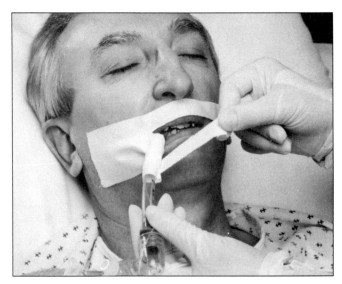

Adjusting an oral ET tube

You'll need a washcloth and towel, skin preparation pads, a suction kit and tonsillar suction device, hypoallergenic adhesive tape or a Velcro tube holder, gloves, and a hand-held resuscitation bag (with mask in case of accidental extubation). You may also need a water-resistant marker.

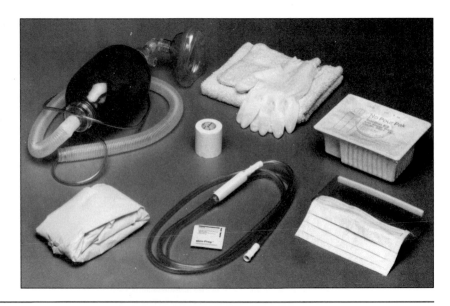

Explain the procedure to the patient, and position him so that he's comfortable and the inserted ET tube is easy for you to reach. Connect the hand-held resuscitation bag to an oxygen source and place it nearby. Then wash your hands and put on gloves, a gown, and a face shield. Using the hand-held resuscitation bag, deliver extra oxygen before performing tracheal suction to remove any secretions.

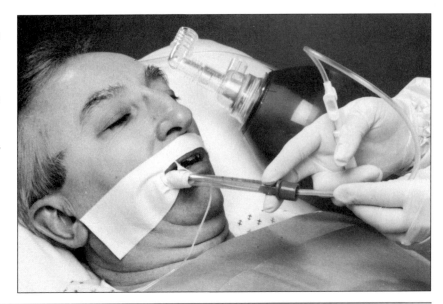

Then, using the tonsillar apparatus, suction the patient's pharynx to remove secretions above the cuff anchoring the ET tube.

▶ *Clinical tip:* Removing secretions reduces the patient's chance of coughing, which can injure the vocal cords, and helps to prevent aspiration during cuff deflation.

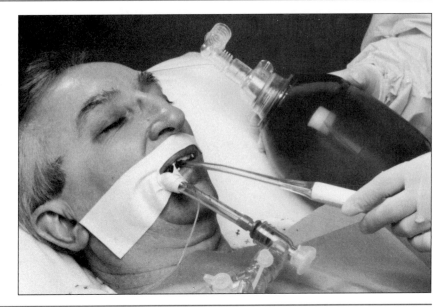

Untape the ET tube or unfasten the Velcro tube holder. If the patient is coughing a lot and the tube seems unstable, have an assistant hold the ET tube to prevent traumatic manipulation or accidental extubation.

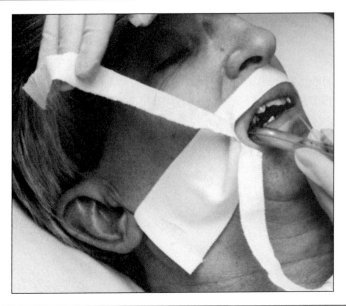

Locate the number (in centimeters) on the tube at the exit point from the mouth. If the tube doesn't have centimeter marks, clearly mark the exit point with a water-resistant marker or a piece of tape. Use this as a reference point when removing the tube.

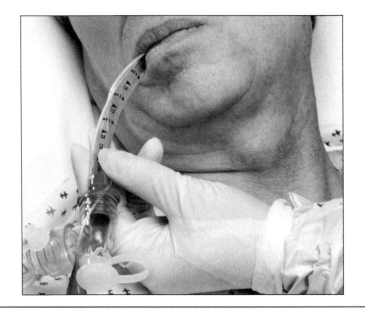

Reposition the tube as necessary. If you're moving it from one side of the mouth to the other, make sure that it exits the mouth at the reference mark you made before the move.

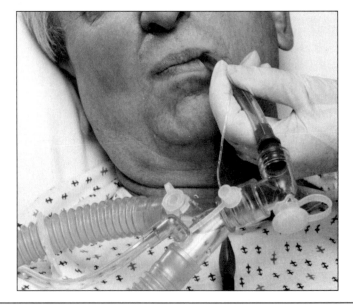

Clean the patient's face and dry it thoroughly (near right). Note any areas of skin breakdown and treat them appropriately. Apply the skin preparation (far right) to create better adhesion when retaping the ET tube.

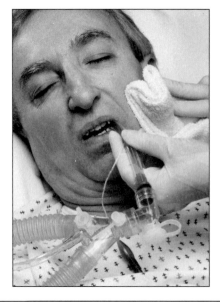
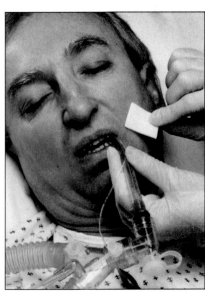

Secure the tube by using adhesive tape or a Velcro tube holder. Finally, document the procedure and the patient's tolerance of it.

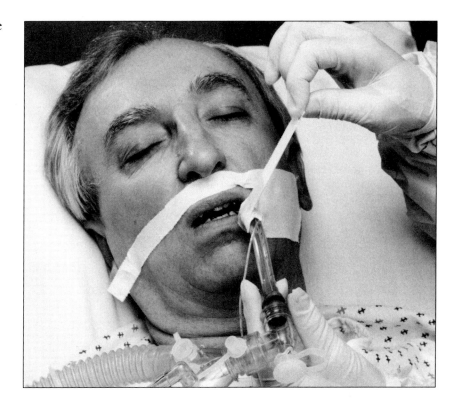

REMOVING THE ENDOTRACHEAL TUBE

An ET tube or any breathing tube is removed when you're certain that the patient has a patent upper airway; that he can clear secretions by coughing; that he has adequate spontaneous tidal volume, vital capacity, minute volume (also called minute ventilation), and negative inspiratory pressure; and that he can breathe without the mechanical ventilator's support. His regular respiratory rate should be 24 breaths/minute or less, and he should have deep, symmetrical chest expansion, a partial pressure of arterial oxygen ranging between 70 and 90 mm Hg on 5 cm H_2O of continuous positive airway pressure (CPAP), and a fraction of inspired oxygen (FIO_2) of 0.4 or less. His pH should be at least 7.35 after 30 minutes on CPAP, and he should be able to grip your hand appropriately on command. Make sure that his vital signs are stable and that he has no serious cardiac arrhythmias.

To remove the ET tube, take the following equipment to the patient's' bedside: a suction kit, tonsillar suction equipment, a 10-ml luer-lock syringe, a hand-held resuscitation bag with an appropriately sized mask, gloves, a gown, a face shield, an oxygen delivery system (usually a face mask), and a linen-saver pad. You'll also need an oxygen flowmeter attached to an oxygen source.

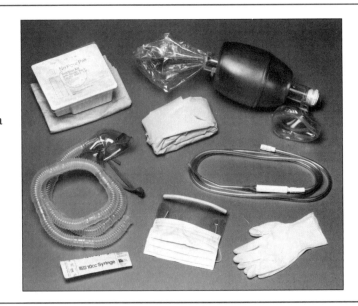

Wash your hands, explain the procedure to the patient, and put on the gown, gloves, and face shield. Place the patient in semi-Fowler's position, and lay the linen-saver pad across his upper chest (as shown). Then set up the oxygen delivery system that the patient will use after extubation.

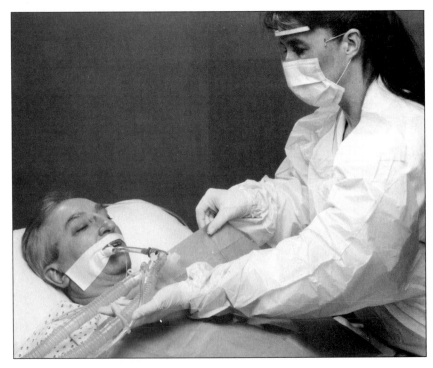

Prepare the hand-held resuscitation bag for use, and place it and the intubation equipment at the bedside. Then give the patient 100% oxygen from the hand-held resuscitation bag, and suction his ET tube.

▶ **Clinical tip:** To help prevent laryngospasm, use an oxygen delivery system that can provide high-humidity oxygen immediately after extubation.

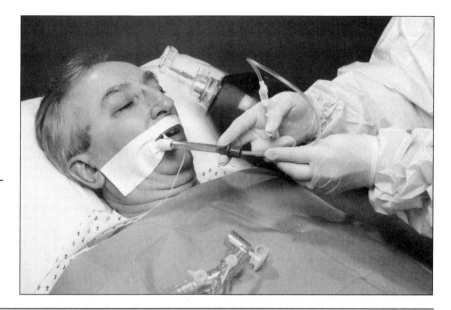

Use the tonsillar suction device to clear the posterior oropharynx (as shown). This will remove any secretions from the top of the ET tube's cuff.

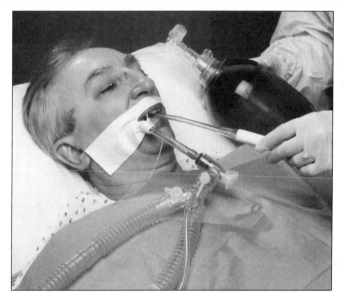

Gently remove the tape or securing straps from the ET tube (near right). Attach the luer-lock syringe to the pilot balloon, and withdraw all the air from the ET tube's tracheal cuff (far right).

▶ **Clinical tip:** Observe the pilot balloon carefully; the tracheal cuff isn't deflated until the pilot balloon completely collapses.

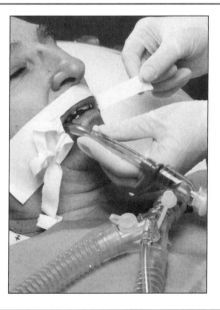
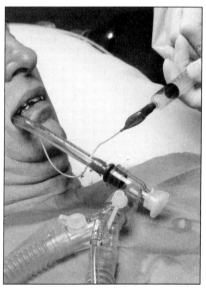

Insert the sterile suction catheter into the ET tube 1″ to 2″ (2.5 to 5 cm) below its distal end. Have the patient take a deep breath. At the peak of inspiration, simultaneously remove the ET tube and the suction catheter (while applying suction) in one smooth outward and downward motion, following the natural curve of the patient's mouth. Suctioning during extubation removes secretions retained at the end of the tube.

Note: Some hospitals permit only a doctor or a nurse anesthetist to remove an ET tube in case immediate reintubation becomes necessary.

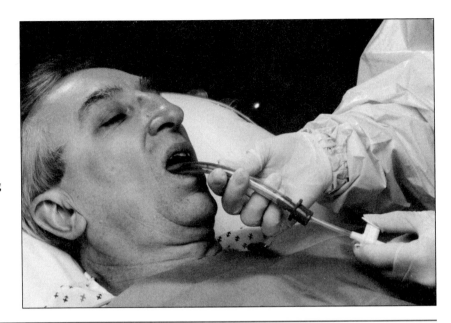

If the patient is able to hold the tonsillar suction device, show him how to use it. Then use this alternative removal method. Grasp the ET tube with the linen-saver pad, and ask the patient to cough. As he does so, gently but firmly pull out the ET tube, wrap it in the linen-saver pad, and discard it in the biohazard container.

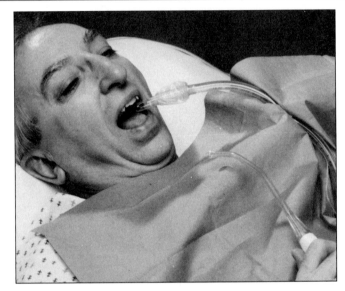

Adjust the flowmeter to the ordered FIO₂ setting, and place the oxygen mask or other ordered oxygen delivery device on the patient's face. Tell the patient to breathe deeply and cough.

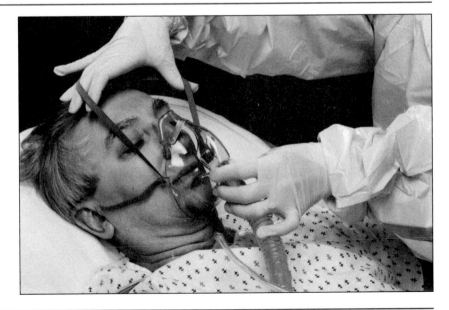

Suction the pharynx as necessary. Instruct the patient to use the tonsillar suction device to suction his throat and mouth as needed to remove oral secretions.

After extubation, monitor the patient for shortness of breath, hoarseness, respiratory fatigue, or other signs of respiratory distress. Evaluate oxygenation by monitoring arterial blood gas levels and pulse oximetry findings as ordered. Document the patient's tolerance of extubation, being sure to record any complications as well as nursing or medical interventions.

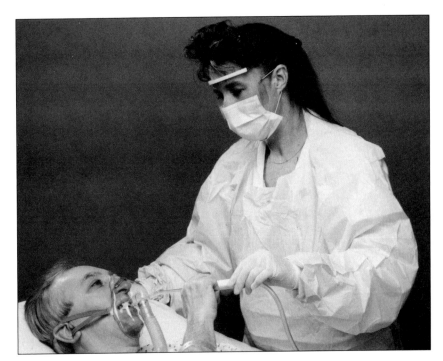

PROVIDING TRACHEOSTOMY TUBE CARE

Created surgically, a tracheostomy is an external opening to the trachea. The insertion of an indwelling tube into this opening prevents the airway from closing. A tracheotomy is performed when a patient has a complete upper airway obstruction and endotracheal (ET) intubation is contraindicated. Usually preferred for long-term intubation, a tracheostomy minimizes the vocal cord damage possible with ET intubation and provides airway access when a patient has unmanageable secretions.

Tracheostomy care includes maintaining airway patency and mucous membrane and skin integrity, preventing infection, and providing psychological support. If the tracheostomy is a permanent measure, the patient and his family may need home care teaching. (See the patient-teaching aid *How to care for your trach tube,* pages 310 and 311.)

Tracheostomy tubes are available in metal and plastic. The metal tube (mainly for long-term therapy) has an outer cannula, an inner cannula, and an obturator that guides insertion of the outer cannula. Some plastic tubes have the same three parts, but most consist of an obturator and a single-walled tube. The single-walled tube is surrounded by an inflatable cuff. (See *Comparing tracheostomy tubes.*)

No matter what type of tube your patient has, using sterile technique when providing care will help prevent infection.

Comparing tracheostomy tubes

Made of plastic or metal, tracheostomy tubes come in uncuffed, cuffed, and fenestrated varieties. Tube selection depends on the patient's condition and the doctor's preference. The following chart lists the advantages and disadvantages of some commonly used tubes.

TYPE	ADVANTAGES	DISADVANTAGES
Uncuffed (plastic or metal) 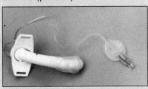	• Permits air to flow freely around the tracheostomy tube and through the larynx • Reduces the risk of tracheal damage • Is a safer choice for children	• Increases the risk of aspiration in adults • May require adapter for mechanical ventilation
Cuffed (plastic) 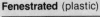	• Disposable • The cuff and the tube won't separate accidentally inside the trachea because the cuff is bonded to the tube. • Doesn't require periodic deflating to lower pressure because the cuff pressure is low and evenly distributed against the tracheal wall • Reduces the risk of tracheal damage	• May cost more than other tubes
Fenestrated (plastic) 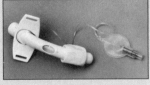	• Permits speech through the upper airway when the external opening is capped and the cuff is deflated • Allows breathing by mechanical ventilation with the inner cannula in place and the cuff inflated • Allows easy removal of the inner cannula for cleaning	• The fenestrations may become occluded. • May allow the inner cannula to dislodge

Kate McGovern, RN, BSN, CCRN, and *Marguerite S. Ambrose, RN, MSN, CCRN,* contributed to this section. Ms. McGovern is a clinical leader in the Surgical Trauma Unit at Abington (Pa.) Memorial Hospital. Ms. Ambrose is an assistant professor at LaSalle University, Philadelphia. The publisher thanks *Grand View Hospital,* Sellersville, Pa., for its help.

Caring for the tracheostomy site

You'll need a tracheostomy care kit (which includes two sterile containers, sterile cotton-tipped applicators, sterile 4″ × 4″ gauze pads, tweezers, and a sterile drape), a container of 0.9% sodium chloride solution, a container of hydrogen peroxide, a suction kit, sterile pre-cut 4″ × 4″ drain sponges, two pairs of sterile gloves, a gown, and a mask and goggles or a face shield. You'll also need a water-proof biohazard container.

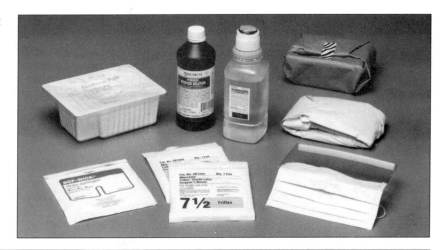

Explain the procedure to the patient, and place her in semi-Fowler's position (unless contraindicated). Place the waterproof biohazard container (in this case, a plastic bag) within easy reach to avoid reaching across the sterile field or the patient's stoma when discarding soiled items.

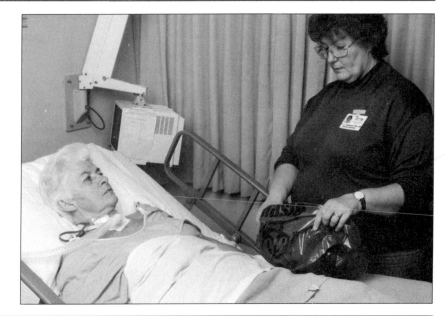

Before opening the sterile tracheostomy care kit and the suction kit, wash your hands. Loosen the caps of the cleaning solution bottles and put on gloves, a mask, and goggles (or a face shield), and a gown.

Disconnect the patient's oxygenation device and place it on a clean area such as the inside of the sterile glove wrapper. Suction the patient (as shown) and then reconnect her to the oxygenation device or the ventilator.

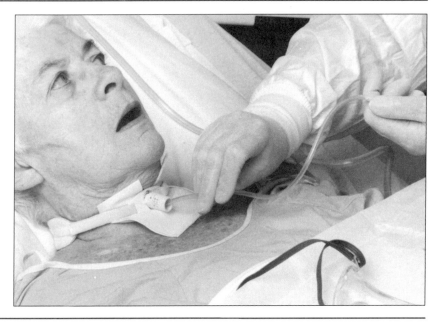

Keeping one hand sterile and one hand clean, separate the basins from the kit and pour about 100 ml of 0.9% sodium chloride solution into one of the sterile containers. Pour about 100 ml of hydrogen peroxide or a mixture of hydrogen peroxide and 0.9% sodium chloride solution (according to hospital protocol) into the other sterile container to make the cleaning solution.

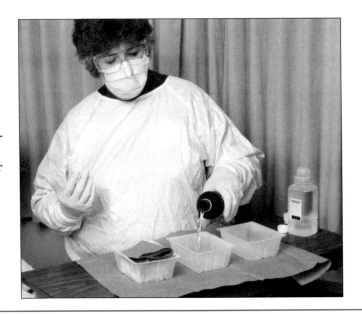

Remove the sterile drape from the package and place it under the tracheostomy tube, remembering to keep one hand sterile and one hand clean.

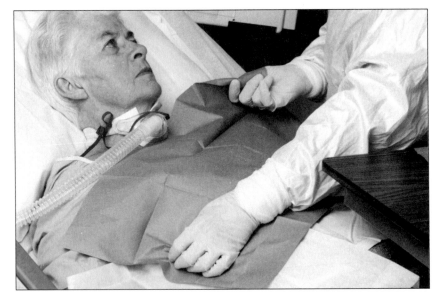

Remove the patient's oxygenation device and place it on a clean surface (as you did when suctioning her).

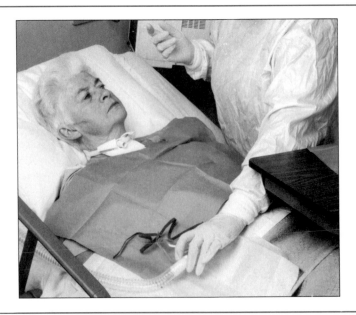

Remove the tracheostomy dressing, and note the color, amount, and consistency of any drainage. Then enclose the dressing in your gloves as you remove them. Discard the soiled items in a biohazard container.

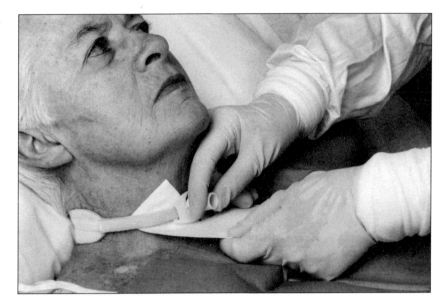

Put on the other pair of sterile gloves. Saturate a sterile gauze pad with the cleaning solution and squeeze out excess liquid. Then wipe the patient's neck under the tracheostomy tube flanges and tracheostomy ties. Repeat until the area is clean, wiping only once with each pad and then discarding the pad.

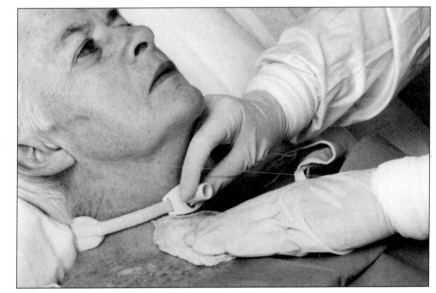

Saturate the cotton-tipped applicators with the cleaning solution. Clean around the stoma site and the tube flanges. Note the condition of the stoma and the surrounding area.

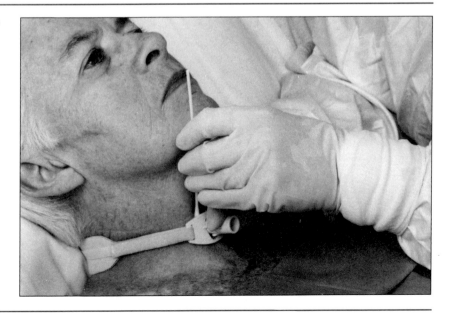

Next, wipe the area with 4″ × 4″ gauze pads dampened in 0.9% sodium chloride solution (near right). Dry the area with additional gauze pads and apply a new tracheostomy dressing (far right).

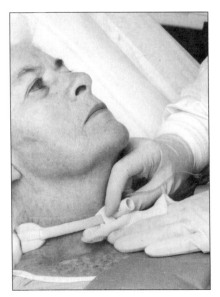 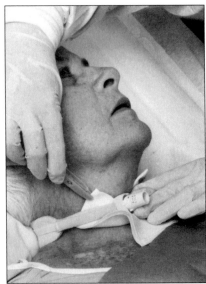

Put the humidification device back in place; then remove and discard your gloves. Document the procedure and your observations of the stoma site and any drainage.

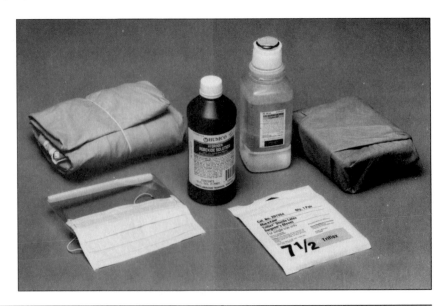

Cleaning and replacing the inner cannula

If your patient has a nondisposable inner cannula, you'll need a prepackaged tracheostomy care kit (including a sterile nylon brush, sterile 6″ pipe cleaners, and two sterile containers), sterile 0.9% sodium chloride solution, hydrogen peroxide solution, sterile gloves, a gown, and a mask and goggles or a face shield.

If your patient uses disposable inner cannulas, you'll need only clean gloves and the disposable cannula. Open the cannula package but leave the cannula inside the wrapper until you're ready to use it.

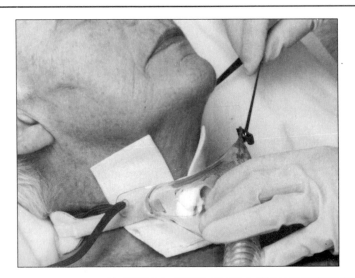

Explain the procedure to the patient and wash your hands. Open the tracheostomy care kit, and loosen the tops of the solution bottles. Put on sterile gloves, a gown, and a mask and goggles or a face shield. Keeping one hand clean and one hand sterile, pour sterile 0.9% sodium chloride solution into one sterile container and hydrogen peroxide into the second sterile container.

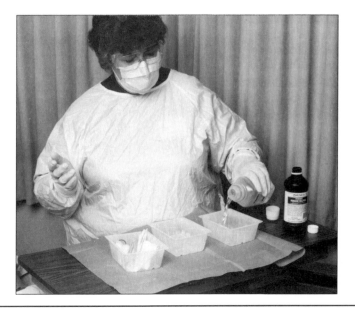

Use your clean hand to disconnect the patient from the ventilator or humidification device.

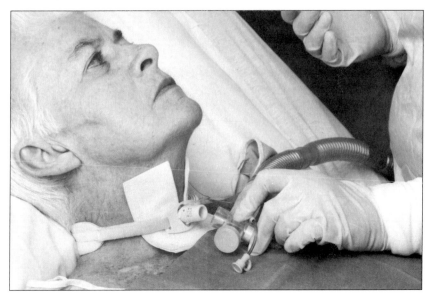

Still using your clean hand, unlock the tracheostomy tube's inner cannula by rotating it counterclockwise (as shown). Remove the cannula and place it in the container of hydrogen peroxide. If the patient can't tolerate being disconnected from the ventilator, replace the cannula with a clean one immediately.

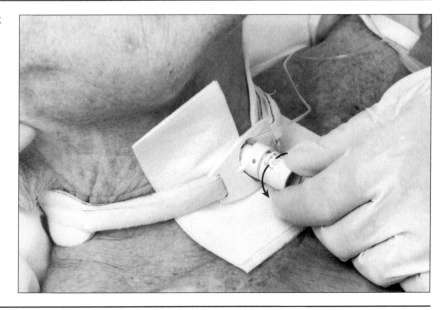

Pick up the cannula with your sterile hand. With your clean hand, scrub the inner cannula with the sterile nylon brush. Use a pipe cleaner if you can't easily slide the brush into the cannula.

▶ *Clinical tip:* Ideally, you should have an alternate inner cannula on hand to replace the soiled device. This isn't always possible, however, so clean the inner cannula quickly because the patient isn't receiving supplemental oxygen during this time.

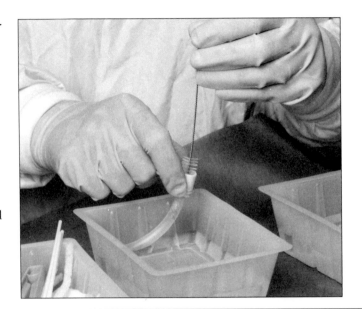

Immerse the cannula in the container of sterile 0.9% sodium chloride solution. Agitate the cannula in the solution for at least 10 seconds to rinse it thoroughly.

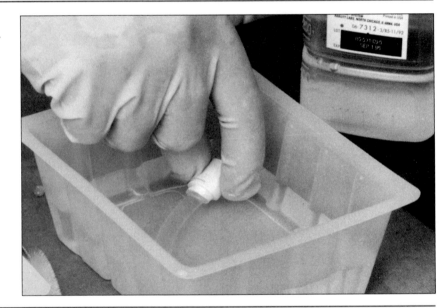

Inspect the cannula for cleanliness and repeat the process if necessary. When the cannula is clean, shake off excess fluid by gently tapping the cannula against the inside of the container.

▶ *Clinical tip:* Don't dry the outer surface of the cannula because the thin film of moisture acts as a lubricant during insertion. However, if you plan to store the cannula, you may dry it with sterile gauze and place it in a sterile container until needed.

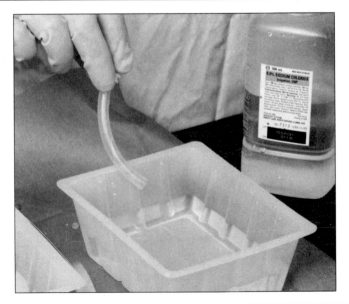

Insert the inner cannula into the patient's tracheostomy tube.

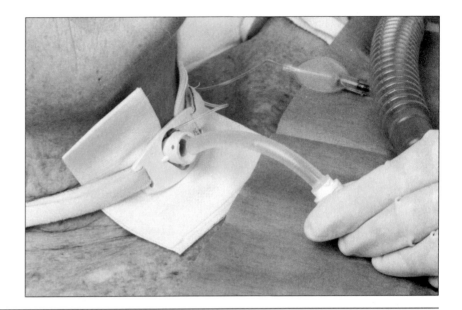

Lock the cannula in place by turning it clockwise until you feel it click snugly into position. Gently tug on it to make sure it's secure. ▶ **Clinical tip:** Some tracheostomy tubes and inner cannulas are marked. When the marks line up, they click, locking the cannula in place.

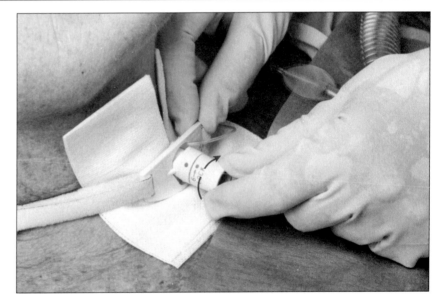

Alternatively, if the patient's tracheostomy tube uses a *disposable inner cannula*, simply remove and discard it. Wash your hands and put on clean gloves. Touching only the outer locking portion, take the new inner cannula from the pre-opened package, and insert it according to the manufacturer's instructions. Be sure to lock it securely in place.

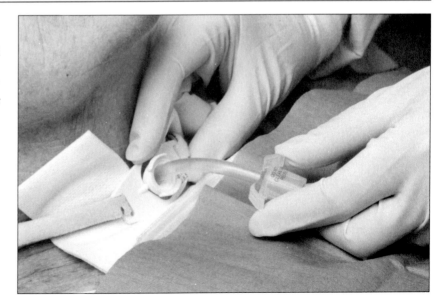

Once you've replaced the reusable or disposable cannula, reconnect the patient to the ventilator or the humidification device.

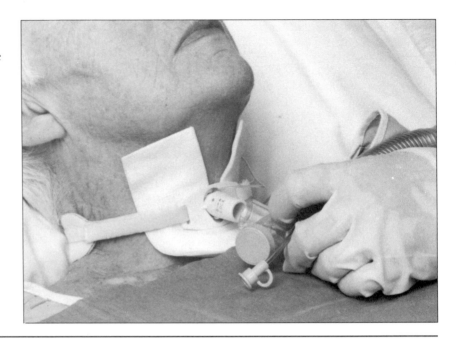

Replacing tracheostomy ties

To change tracheostomy ties, you'll need a 30″ (76-cm) length of twill tape, scissors, sterile gloves, and a hemostat.

▶ *Clinical tip:* Don't change the tracheostomy ties for the first 24 hours after insertion of the tracheostomy tube to avoid dislodging the tube or causing bleeding at the site from manipulation.

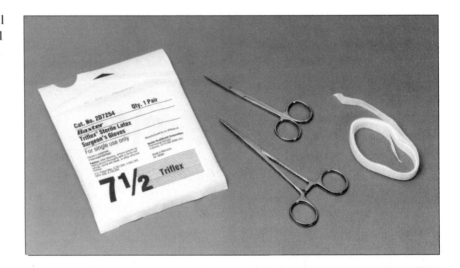

Explain the procedure to the patient and wash your hands. Fold the twill tape into thirds.

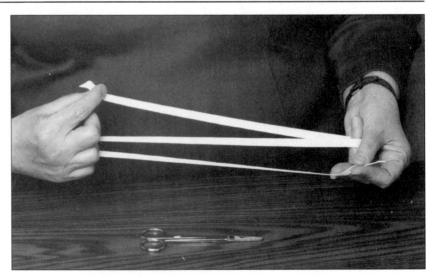

Cut off one-third (10″ or 25 cm) of the twill tape (cut on a slant to make threading the tape through the flange easier).

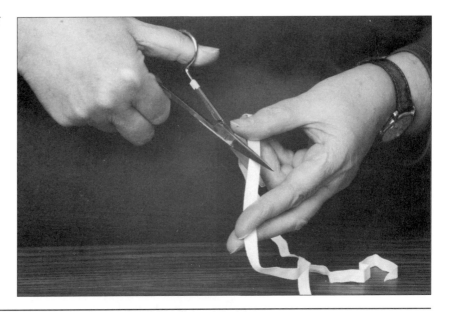

Fold one end of the 10″ piece of tape back 1″ (2.5 cm) on itself. From this folded edge, cut a ½″ slit down the center of the tape. Prepare the longer (20″) piece of tape the same way.

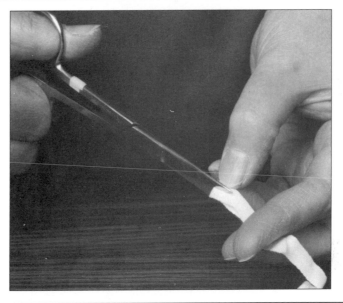

Knot one end of each length of twill tape to prevent fraying.

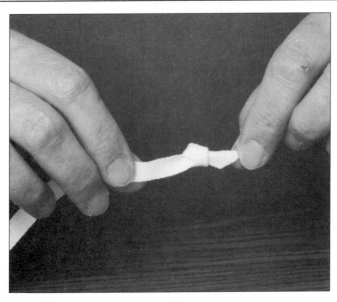

Put on the sterile gloves. Thread the pointed end of the one tie through the eye of one tracheostomy tube flange from the underside (near right), using the hemostat if necessary, until the slit end is near the flange eye. Then thread the pointed end of the tie completely through the slit (far right), and pull it taut so that it loops firmly through the tube's flange. Fasten the second tie to the other side in the same manner.

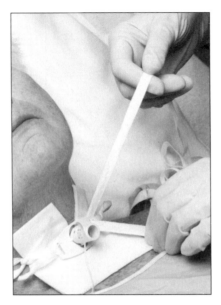
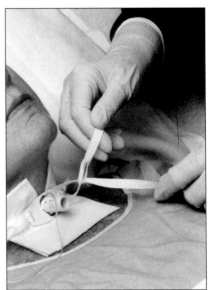

Instruct the patient to flex her neck. Bring the ties around to the side and fasten them with a square knot.

▶ **Clinical tip:** Flexion produces the same neck circumference as coughing and helps prevent an overly tight tie.

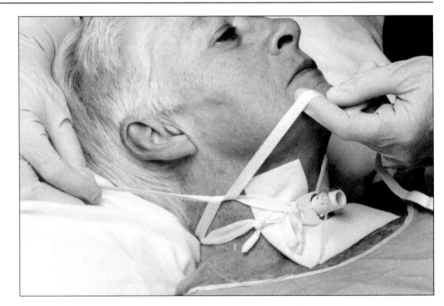

Slip one finger under the ties. They should feel snug, but not tight, over your finger. If they're too tight or too loose, repeat the procedure and check the ties again. Trim off excess tape.

▶ **Clinical tip:** For a patient who has neck trauma or has undergone neck surgery, check the ties frequently to detect any neck swelling.

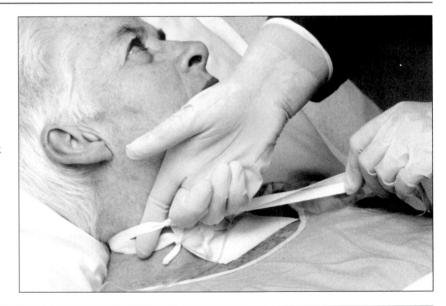

Cut the knot on the old tracheostomy ties, pull the ties through the flanges, and discard them. Be careful not to cut the tube of the pilot balloon.

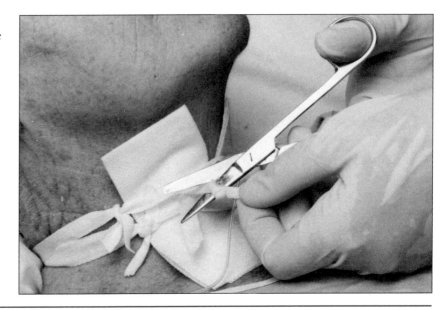

Alternatively, the patient may have a Velcro tube holder securing the tracheostomy tube. To replace soiled Velcro tape, put on gloves and place the center of the new Velcro tape behind the patient's neck. Place the ends of the new tape (unfastened) on either side of the patient's neck.

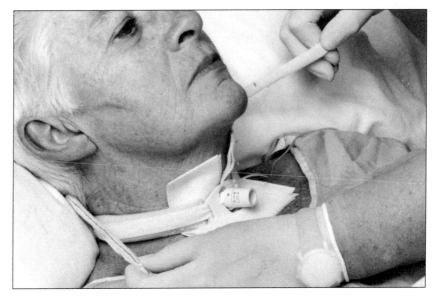

Next, open and remove the Velcro tape from one end of the tracheostomy tube. Pick up the end of the new tape, and insert it into the slit on the tracheostomy tube from the underside to the top side (as shown). Secure the looped side to the soft side of the tape. Repeat the procedure on the other side of the tracheostomy tube.

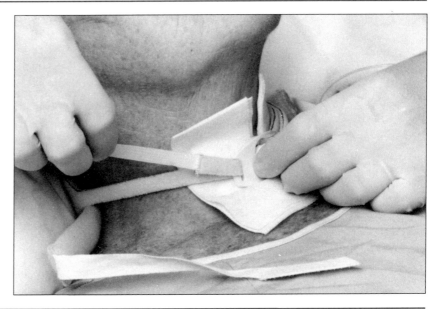

How to care for your trach tube

Dear Patient:

The tracheostomy tube (or "trach tube") that you have in your throat will keep your windpipe open and make your breathing easier. This tube has three parts: an inner cannula, an outer cannula, and an obturator. You'll need to remove and clean the inner cannula regularly to prevent infection. You'll also replace the ties that hold the trach tube in place when they become soiled.

How to clean the inner cannula

Remove and clean the inner cannula regularly, as your doctor directs.

1 Gather this equipment near a sink: a small basin, a small brush, mild liquid dish detergent, a gauze pad, a pair of scissors, and clean trach ties (twill tape).

Or open a prepackaged kit that contains the equipment you need. Now wash your hands. Position a mirror so that you can see your face and throat clearly.

2 Rotate the cannula counterclockwise or pinch the sides to unlock it, and then remove it by pulling steadily outward and downward.

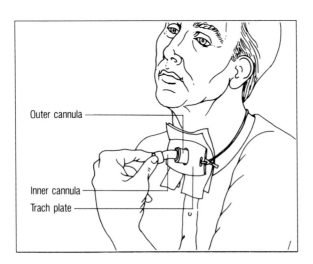

Prepare to clean the soiled cannula immediately for reinsertion. (Or put the soiled cannula aside and slip a clean inner cannula inside the outer cannula.) If you start to cough, cover your stoma with a tissue, bend forward, and relax until the coughing stops.

3 Run water into the basin and add a few drops of mild liquid dish detergent. Swish the water around the basin so that the detergent and water mix thoroughly. Then place the cannula in the basin and let it soak briefly.

4 Clean the cannula with a small brush. If the cannula is heavily soiled, try soaking it in a basin of hydrogen peroxide solution. You'll see foaming as the solution reacts with the secretions coating the cannula. When the foaming stops, scrub the cannula with the brush.

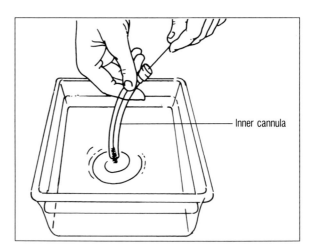

You can obtain a special trach tube brush at a medical supply company or pharmacy. However, the small brushes used to clean coffee pots work just as well. They're inexpensive and available at many hardware stores. Just be sure to use the brush only for your trach tube.

How to care for your trach tube *(continued)*

5 Rinse the inner cannula under running water. Make sure you've removed all of the cleaning solution. Shake off the excess water and reinsert the clean, moist cannula immediately. Don't dry it; the remaining water drops help lubricate the cannula, making reinsertion easier.

6 Reinsert and lock the clean inner cannula in place. (It will click when locked.)

7 Now replace the soiled ties that secure your trach plate. Use scissors to carefully clip and remove one trach tie at a time. Knot the end of each clean trach tie to prevent fraying. Then cut a ½-inch slit near the knotted end of each tie.

8 Thread the end that isn't knotted through the opening on the trach plate. Then feed that end through the slit, and gently pull the tie taut. Do the same for the other tie.

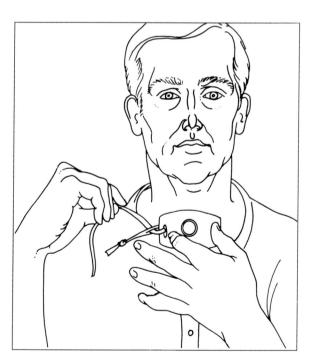

9 Secure the ties at the side of your neck with a square knot. Leave enough room so that you feel comfortable. You should be able to slip two fingers between the side of your neck and the knot.

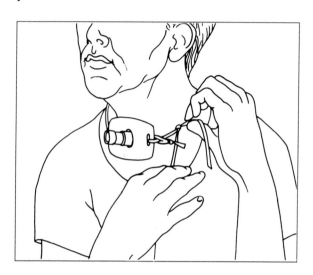

10 Finally, place a 4-by-4-inch gauze pad behind the tube to protect your neck. To do this, make a slit down the middle of the gauze pad until you reach the center. Next, cut a hole in the center just big enough to go around the trach tube. Carefully insert

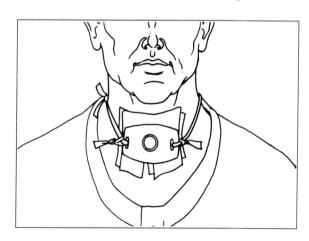

the gauze pad under the trach plate from above the tube. If you have heavy discharge draining from the stoma, insert the gauze pad from below the tube.

MEASURING TRACHEAL CUFF PRESSURE

An endotracheal or tracheostomy cuff provides a closed system for mechanical ventilation, allowing a desired tidal volume to be delivered to the patient's lungs. It also protects the patient's lower respiratory tract from secretions or gastric contents that may accumulate in the pharynx.

To function properly, the cuff must exert enough pressure on the tracheal wall to seal the airway without compromising the blood supply to the tracheal mucosa. The ideal pressure—known as minimal occlusive volume—is the lowest amount needed to seal the airway. Many authorities recommend maintaining a cuff pressure lower than venous perfusion pressure—usually about 16 to 24 cm H_2O. (More than 24 cm H_2O may exceed venous perfusion pressure.) Actual cuff pressure will vary with each patient, however. To keep pressure within safe limits, measure minimal occlusive volume at least once each shift or as directed by hospital policy. Cuff pressure can be measured by a respiratory therapist or by the nurse.

To measure cuff pressure, you'll need a cuff-pressure manometer, gloves, and a stethoscope. You'll also need suctioning equipment.

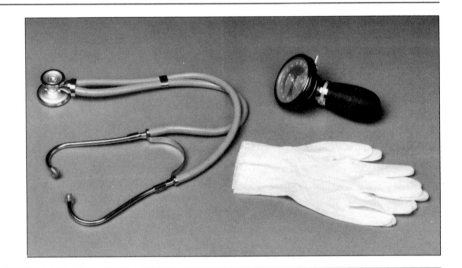

Explain the procedure to the patient. Don gloves and suction the endotracheal or tracheostomy tube and the patient's oropharynx to remove accumulated secretions above the cuff. Then attach the cuff-pressure manometer to the pilot balloon port (as shown).

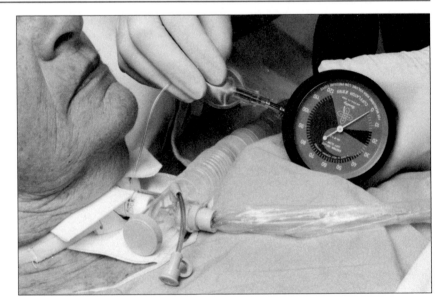

Place the diaphragm of the stetho-scope over the trachea and listen for an air leak. Keep in mind that a smooth, hollow sound indicates a sealed airway; a loud, gurgling sound indicates an air leak.

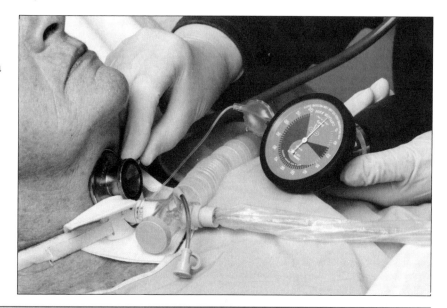

If you don't hear an air leak, press the red button under the dial of the cuff-pressure manometer to slowly release air from the balloon on the tracheal tube. Auscultate for an air leak.

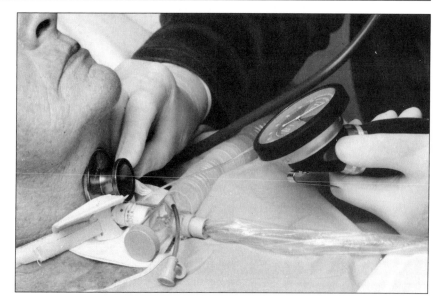

As soon as you hear an air leak, release the red button and gently squeeze the handle of the cuff-pressure manometer to inflate the cuff. Continue to add air to the cuff until you no longer hear an air leak.

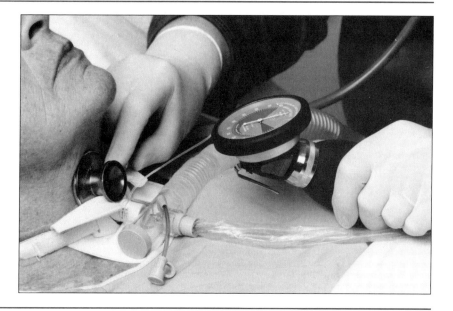

When the air leak ceases, read the dial on the cuff-pressure manometer. This is the minimal pressure required to effectively occlude the trachea around the tracheal tube. In many cases, this pressure will fall within the green area (16 to 24 cm H_2O) on the manometer dial.

Keep in mind that some patients require less pressure, whereas others—for example, those with tracheal malacia (an abnormal softening of the tracheal tissue)—require more pressure. Maintaining the cuff pressure at the lowest possible level will minimize cuff-related problems.

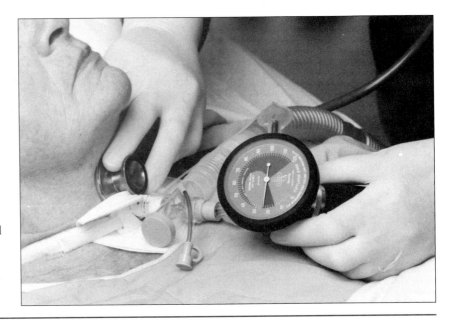

Disconnect the cuff-pressure manometer from the pilot balloon port. Document the pressure value.

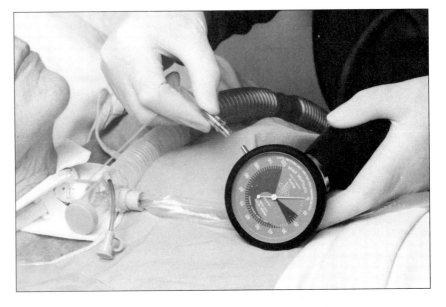

Mechanical Ventilation

LEARNING ABOUT MECHANICAL VENTILATION

When your patient suffers respiratory failure, he'll need treatment to supply him with oxygen, to reduce dyspnea, and to rest and recondition his fatigued ventilatory muscles so that his normal respiratory function can resume. Mechanical ventilation does this by artificially controlling or supporting his breathing efforts. To meet this patient's needs, you'll need to know how to manage his care and breathing equipment effectively and efficiently.

To begin, you'll need to understand the ventilator you'll work with. Available in various types (volume-cycled or pressure-cycled, for example), mechanical ventilators are engineered to deliver ventilations in various modes, such as continuous mandatory and intermittent mandatory ventilations. (See *Comparing mechanical ventilation modes,* pages 318 and 319.) Besides supporting a patient's breathing, the ventilator helps prevent alveolar collapse by supplying adjunctive therapies, such as continuous positive airway pressure (CPAP) and positive end-expiratory pressure (PEEP).

INDICATIONS FOR MECHANICAL VENTILATION

If your patient can't generate a spontaneous respiration or if his respiratory efforts fail to expand his chest and deliver oxygenated gas to his lungs, the doctor may order mechanical ventilation based on such signs as accessory muscle use, labored breathing, a rapid respiratory rate, and airway obstruction. Typically, he won't wait for the results of an arterial blood gas analysis or pulmonary function tests.

Two types of disorders that respond to mechanical ventilation include gas exchange and extrapulmonary disorders. In gas exchange disorders, mechanical ventilation increases oxygenation; in extrapulmonary disorders, mechanical ventilation helps control or support respiratory mechanics.

Gas exchange disorders
Conditions that alter gas exchange affect ventilation or perfusion or both. For instance, a respiratory tract infection fills alveoli with secretions, thereby interfering with ventilation. Pulmonary emboli reduce the amount of blood available for diffusion at the alveolocapillary membrane. And adult respiratory distress syndrome (ARDS) disrupts both ventilation and perfusion and causes changes in the

alveolocapillary space. These changes impede diffusion across the alveolocapillary membrane even if ventilation and perfusion remain adequate.

In a patient with any of these disorders, mechanical ventilation increases the amount of oxygen that's available while the patient receives treatment for the underlying problem.

Extrapulmonary disorders
Instead of directly affecting ventilation or perfusion, extrapulmonary disorders interfere with normal neurologic or neuromuscular mechanics. Central nervous system disorders—a brain stem injury, for instance—typically disrupt neural control of respiration. Neuromuscular diseases, such as Guillain-Barré syndrome, stop stimuli from being transmitted to the respiratory muscles. Flail chest and other musculoskeletal disorders lower tidal volume by inhibiting adequate chest expansion. In these situations, mechanical ventilation controls or supports respiratory mechanics.

VENTILATOR CHOICES

Mechanical ventilators come in four basic types: negative-pressure, volume-cycled, pressure-cycled, and high-frequency. You'll usually work with volume-cycled or pressure-cycled ventilators, but you'll need to understand how all types work because the ventilator will vary with the patient's condition.

Negative-pressure ventilators
The original ventilators, negative-pressure machines work by alternately removing and replacing gas from one of two kinds of chambers: one that encloses the entire body except for the head (the Drinker respirator, or iron lung) or one that encloses just the front and sides of the chest and upper abdomen (the chest shell).

As the mechanism drives gas from the chamber, the resulting negative pressure forces the chest wall to expand, pulling gas into the lungs. Then the device's diaphragm returns to its normal position, allowing the chest wall to fall, thereby causing exhalation.

Although these machines don't require you to insert an artificial airway (an important advantage), they do have several drawbacks. They are noisy and

Judith S. McCann, RN, BSN, a clinical editor with Springhouse Corp., wrote this section. The publisher also thanks the following organizations for their help: *Bird Products Corp.,* Palm Springs, Calif.; *Bunnell, Inc.,* Salt Lake City, Utah; *Grand View Hospital,* Sellersville, Pa.; and *Puritan-Bennett Corp., Boston Division,* Wilmington, Mass.

Comparing mechanical ventilation modes

In mechanical ventilation, a mode determines how much inspiratory effort a patient will need to trigger a ventilation cycle from the ventilator. The doctor bases mode selection on the patient's condition and ventilatory needs. The following chart presents common modes and describes features, advantages, and disadvantages of each.

The actual pressure waveforms show the point at which inspiration starts. Where applicable, arrows point to the beginning of patient-initiated breaths that trigger the ventilator to deliver a breath. Graph features also include the relative duration of inspiration (shaded) and expiration (colored). The numbers to the left of the graphs indicate pressure in cm H_2O.

MODE	FEATURES	ADVANTAGES	DISADVANTAGES
Continuous mandatory ventilation (CMV) 	• Appropriate for patients with apnea caused by central nervous system (CNS) or neuromuscular dysfunction, a drug overdose, or status asthmaticus • Completely controls respiration by delivering preset tidal volume at a set rate regardless of patient's attempt to breathe independently	• Decreases work of breathing, which decreases oxygen consumption and carbon dioxide (CO_2) production	• Doesn't allow patient to compensate when CO_2 level increases • Causes respiratory muscle atrophy, making weaning difficult • Causes decreased venous return and decreased cardiac output • Fosters anxiety and agitation by preventing patient from breathing independently
Assist-control ventilation (ACV) 	• Used for patients with normal respiratory drive but weak respiratory muscles • Augments breathing without completely controlling it • Has adjustable sensitivity setting to alter amount of negative pressure needed to initiate ventilation (usual setting range: −1 to −3 cm H_2O)	• Keeps respiratory muscles from atrophying, making weaning easier • Allows patient to respond to changes in CO_2 level	• May decrease venous return and cardiac output
Intermittent mandatory ventilation (IMV) 	• Provides partial ventilatory support by delivering a preset tidal volume (typically, 10 to 15 ml/kg of ideal body weight) at a preset rate (to allow some independent breathing while maintaining normal arterial blood gas and pH levels) • Allows patient to breathe independently between machine ventilations • Delivers humidified oxygenated air from a separate circuit to support independent breaths	• Keeps respiratory muscles from atrophying, making weaning easier • Allows patient some control over breathing, thereby decreasing anxiety • Carries lower risk of cardiovascular problems than do CMV and ACV modes • Carries lower risk of barotrauma with positive end-expiratory pressure (PEEP) than does CMV	• Contraindicated in patients who must have low oxygen concentration and who must perform minimal work when breathing
Synchronized intermittent mandatory ventilation (SIMV) 	• Synchronizes machine-delivered breaths with spontaneous breathing • Delivers a mandatory breath if patient doesn't breathe within a preset time	• Has same advantages as IMV but is more efficient	• Increases work of breathing because of time lag in machine-delivered ventilations

Comparing mechanical ventilation modes (continued)

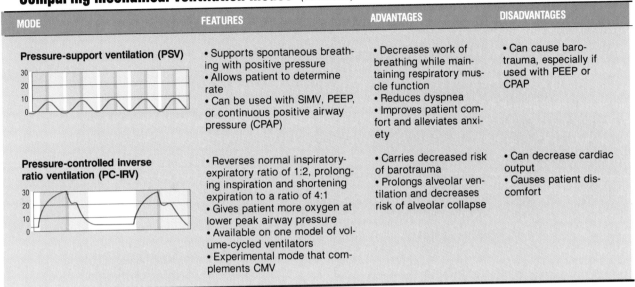

MODE	FEATURES	ADVANTAGES	DISADVANTAGES
Pressure-support ventilation (PSV)	• Supports spontaneous breathing with positive pressure • Allows patient to determine rate • Can be used with SIMV, PEEP, or continuous positive airway pressure (CPAP)	• Decreases work of breathing while maintaining respiratory muscle function • Reduces dyspnea • Improves patient comfort and alleviates anxiety	• Can cause barotrauma, especially if used with PEEP or CPAP
Pressure-controlled inverse ratio ventilation (PC-IRV)	• Reverses normal inspiratory-expiratory ratio of 1:2, prolonging inspiration and shortening expiration to a ratio of 4:1 • Gives patient more oxygen at lower peak airway pressure • Available on one model of volume-cycled ventilators • Experimental mode that complements CMV	• Carries decreased risk of barotrauma • Prolongs alveolar ventilation and decreases risk of alveolar collapse	• Can decrease cardiac output • Causes patient discomfort

restrictive—especially the iron lung. And their design makes nursing care difficult to provide and the air seal difficult to maintain.

Volume-cycled ventilators

These machines stop inspiration after delivering a preset tidal volume of gas, regardless of the pressure needed to deliver it. Then they allow passive expiration. A volume-cycled ventilator is ideal for a patient with ARDS or bronchospasm because it will deliver a preset tidal volume of air despite increased airway resistance caused by changes in airway pressure or compliance.

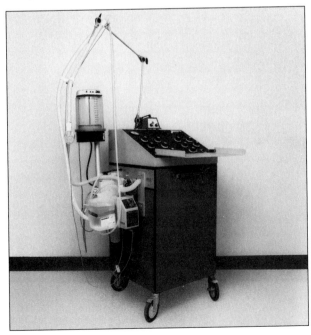

Used most commonly, these ventilators have several features and modes of operation. As ordered, you can set the tidal volume, respiratory rate, inspiratory-expiratory (I:E) ratio and, by adjusting the flow rate, inspiratory time. To maintain an adequate partial pressure of oxygen in arterial blood (PaO_2), you can also set the oxygen concentration—measured as the fraction of inspired oxygen (FIO_2)—anywhere from 0.21 (room air) to 1.0.

Volume-cycled ventilators have several features you won't find on other ventilators, including an automatic sigh mechanism (usually set to sigh one to three times a minute). The sigh mechanism promotes alveolar reexpansion to prevent atelectasis. These machines also have pressure limit alarms to alert you to high peak airway pressures, which can cause lung damage. Another feature on some machines, a high-pressure relief valve, relieves excessive pressure. This is particularly useful when high pressure is needed to deliver a preset volume.

Pressure-cycled ventilators

Just as volume-cycled ventilators deliver a preset volume of gas, pressure-cycled ventilators deliver inspiratory gas at a preset pressure. Then they stop the inspiration to allow passive expiration. Used mainly for short-term therapy (less than 24 hours), pressure-cycled ventilators reduce the risk of lung damage from high inspiratory pressure. For this reason, they may be used for neonates, who have a small lung capacity.

Pressure-cycled ventilators have an important drawback, however. Because they deliver gas at a preset pressure, airway resistance and poor lung compliance can decrease the tidal volume that the patient receives. At the same pressure setting, a patient with stiff lungs or mucus plugs will receive a lower tidal volume than a patient whose lungs have normal elasticity.

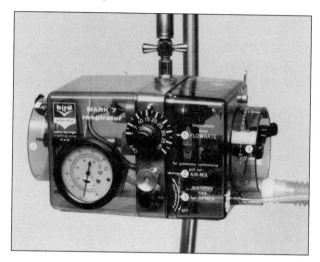

Combining ventilator functions

Current advances in ventilators are evident in models that combine the benefits of volume-cycled and pressure-cycled operation. An example is the Puritan-Bennett 7200 microprocessor ventilator system shown here.

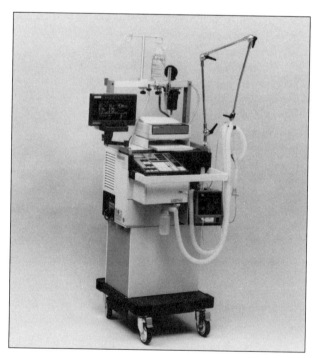

Having all the features of the volume-cycled ventilator, this device also permits pressure-cycled ventilation. It relies on a computer program to control the ventilator, to extensively monitor the patient and ventilator, and to perform all calculations.

To operate the ventilator, you activate desired functions by pressing the appropriate keys on the keyboard display panel (a single membranous sheet rather than multiple knobs and dials). This allows you to set ventilatory patterns to meet the patient's needs and decreases the chance for accidents, such as liquid leaking into the ventilator. Instead of one general alarm, this ventilator has a hierarchy of alarms that give specific information about operating conditions. As ordered, you can set the I:E ratio anywhere from 1:4 to 4:1. This system can be upgraded as needed.

High-frequency ventilators

All high-frequency ventilators use high respiratory rates (usually four times the normal rate) and low tidal volumes (less than or equal to the patient's dead space volume) to maintain alveolar ventilation. The low tidal volume minimizes the risk of barotrauma and cardiovascular changes.

Of the three kinds of high-frequency ventilation—high-frequency positive-pressure ventilation (HFPPV), high-frequency oscillation (HFO), and high-frequency jet ventilation (HFJV)—HFJV (shown below) is the most common.

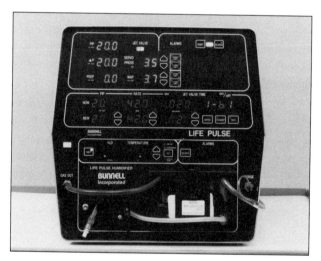

The infrequently used HFPPV generates a breath when a volume of compressed gas is delivered by a pneumatic valve. The FIO_2 that the patient receives matches that of the compressed gas.

HFO vibrates the delivered gas at a rate ranging from 690 to 3,000 cycles/minute. It's best suited for infants with severe neonatal respiratory distress syndrome.

In HFJV, gas moves at a pressure of 10 to 50 psi through a fluid or electromechanical control system that has a flow interrupter and an electric timer. This type of ventilation can be used alone or with a volume-cycled ventilator that is set on the CPAP mode. Traveling through a transtracheal catheter or the extra lumen of an endotracheal tube, small, pulsed jets of gas with a tidal volume of only 50 to 400 ml enter the patient's airway at a rate of 100 to 600 breaths/minute.

ADJUNCTS TO MECHANICAL VENTILATION

Many patients who need mechanical ventilation also need adjunctive therapy, such as PEEP or CPAP. Both of these therapies keep the alveoli expanded. And both deliver pressure at the end of expiration: PEEP for patients receiving machine-delivered breaths and CPAP for patients breathing spontaneously.

PEEP and CPAP therapy can help patients who have inadequate surfactant, the naturally occurring substance that interrupts the lungs' surface tension and enables them to expand. A surfactant deficiency may result from neonatal respiratory distress syndrome, ARDS, smoke inhalation, or lung damage caused by toxic substances.

In keeping the alveoli expanded, PEEP and CPAP can help some patients who have pulmonary edema. Here's how: If the alveoli become larger and the amount of fluid stays the same, the area available for gas exchange increases—promoting oxygenation. And some clinicians think the positive pressure pushes fluid back into the alveolar capillaries. (See *Effects of PEEP and CPAP,* page 322.)

Both PEEP and CPAP are contraindicated, however, for patients with untreated hypovolemia caused by hemorrhage; dehydration; neurogenic, anaphylactic, or septic shock; or drug-induced decreased cardiac output or compromised circulation. Because these patients already have compromised circulatory systems, the extra pressure generated by PEEP or CPAP would only aggravate the problem. Similarly, PEEP and CPAP are contraindicated for patients with injury or disease affecting only one lung because these therapies would heighten the difference in blood distribution and ventilation between the two lungs.

Both therapies also are contraindicated for patients with chronic obstructive pulmonary disease complicated by hypoxemia, pulmonary hyperinflation, or elevated functional residual capacity (FRC) with increased or normal compliance. Because high FRC already causes excessive pressure in the lungs, these adjuncts would only lead to further vascular compression and shunting, venous admixture, and hypoxemia.

Understanding PEEP

First used in the early 1970s, PEEP lets the patient exhale while maintaining a preset positive pressure at the end of expiration. Maintaining positive airway pressure in the lungs increases FRC and helps inflate and keep open alveoli that previously collapsed. This increases the number of alveoli that are available for ventilation. PEEP also improves arterial oxygenation, decreases intrapulmonary shunting, and lessens the respiratory effort needed to expand collapsed alveoli.

Who needs PEEP

A doctor may order PEEP for a patient with hypoxemic respiratory failure caused by acute diffuse restrictive lung disease that doesn't respond to supplemental oxygen therapy alone.

Occasionally, PEEP may be ordered to increase intrapulmonary pressure in patients with intrathoracic bleeding. The resulting increase in pressure decreases venous return and may lessen bleeding. But decreased venous return also may require you to provide extra fluids to prevent hypovolemic shock.

Using high-level PEEP in patients with increased intracranial pressure (ICP) raises central venous pressure, which further increases ICP. Such patients shouldn't receive PEEP unless they also receive adjunctive therapy to decrease carbon dioxide levels and decrease vasoconstriction.

Patients with bronchopulmonary fistula or those recovering from lung surgery may receive PEEP if they have a chest tube. Monitor these patients carefully for related complications, such as barotrauma.

Understanding CPAP

Used to correct oxygenation failure and to wean patients from mechanical ventilation, CPAP oxygenates by decreasing FRC and lung compliance. The patient must be awake and alert, with a PEEP of less than 12 cm H_2O, good tidal volume and vital capacity, a respiratory rate under 24 breaths/minute, a normal to low $PaCO_2$, and a normal pH—all indicators that he can maintain the work of breathing. CPAP works only for patients who can breathe spontaneously.

You'll need a continuous flow system to provide CPAP. (Some ventilators have such a system, but you can deliver CPAP without a ventilator.) Intubated patients can receive CPAP through ventilator circuitry attached to the endotracheal, nasotracheal, or tracheostomy tube. Others can receive CPAP through a tight-fitting, continuous-flow face mask.

Who needs CPAP

The doctor will order CPAP for a patient who can ventilate adequately but can't oxygenate effectively because of decreased FRC. Like PEEP, CPAP can help a patient who has secretions blocking his airway, fluid-filled alveoli, or refractory hypoxemia resulting from atelectasis—a condition that's common among postoperative patients.

Effects of PEEP and CPAP

Review these illustrations showing changes caused by positive end-expiratory pressure (PEEP) and continuous positive airway pressure (CPAP) on lung pressure and the alveoli.

Lung pressure changes

Compare the waveforms below. The waves on the left side of the waveform represent the baseline normal airway pressure of a patient receiving assist-control ventilation (ACV) without PEEP. The waves on the right side of the same waveform represent the baseline normal airway pressure of a patient on ACV with PEEP of 5 cm H_2O. Note how the waveforms fluctuate with inspiration (I) and expiration (E).

Pressure exerted in PEEP

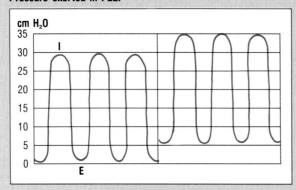

Similarly, pressure exerted in CPAP appears in the waveform below. Waves on the left side represent the intrathoracic pressure of a patient breathing normally; waves on the right side represent the intrathoracic pressure of a patient breathing spontaneously while receiving CPAP of 5 cm H_2O.

Pressure exerted in CPAP

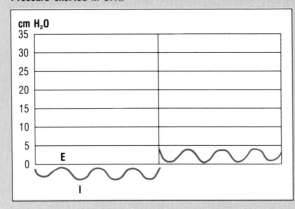

Alveolar changes

These illustrations represent the effects of PEEP and CPAP on an alveolus.

In a normal alveolus, functional residual capacity (FRC) provides the gas volume that keeps the alveolus open for gas exchange.

Normal alveolus

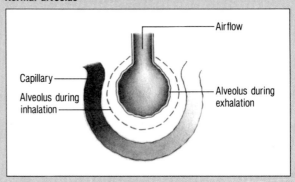

A deflated alveolus, however, has less area for gas exchange. The dark shading indicates a lower PaO_2 in the capillary.

Alveolus with decreased FRC

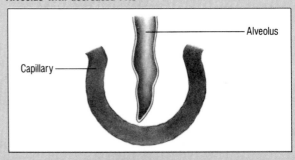

With PEEP or CPAP, the positive pressure exerted keeps the alveolus expanded, thereby increasing FRC.

Alveolus expanded using PEEP or CPAP

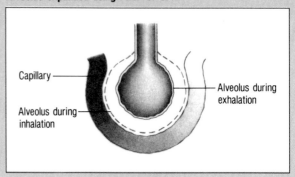

INITIATING MECHANICAL VENTILATION

Successful mechanical ventilation depends on good organization and skillful care. Before starting ventilation, prepare the equipment—and the patient—carefully. Although in most hospitals the respiratory therapist sets up the equipment and starts ventilation, you may encounter special or emergency situations in which you must perform this task. If so, you'll need to respond quickly and efficiently.

Before mechanical ventilation can begin, the patient must have an endotracheal (ET) or a tracheostomy tube in place. If he doesn't, prepare him for intubation, and assist the doctor or anesthetist with the procedure as necessary.

Preparing the patient and the ventilator

Prepare a mechanical ventilator, such as the one shown here (the Puritan-Bennett 7200 microprocessor ventilator), in the storage area or at the patient's bedside. Be sure to have a manual resuscitation bag close by whenever you use a ventilator.

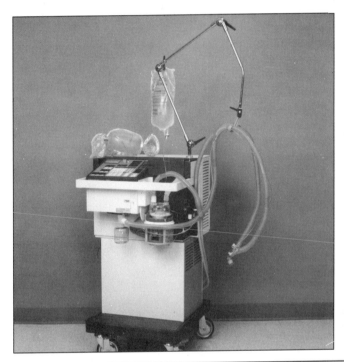

You'll need gloves, suction equipment, sterile water (if it's not in the suction kit), and a stethoscope. You may also need linen-saver pads and a kit for obtaining a sample for arterial blood gas (ABG) analysis.

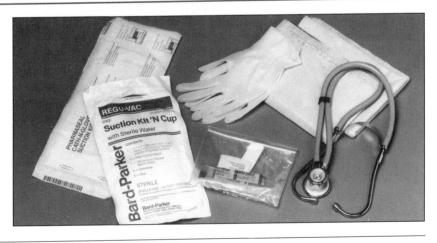

Contributors to this section include *Yvonne Jo Robbins, RRT, MEd*, director of the Respiratory Care Program of West Chester (Pa.) University and Bryn Mawr (Pa.) Hospital, and *Paulette Dorney, RN, MSN, CCRN*, an instructor in Critical Care Staff Development at North Penn Hospital, Lansdale, Pa. The publisher thanks *Abington (Pa.) Memorial Hospital* and *Puritan-Bennett Corp.*, Overland Park, Kan., for their help.

When mechanical ventilation becomes necessary, draw a sample for ABG analysis. Also assess the patient's vital signs, breathing patterns, skin color, character of lung secretions, and level of consciousness and responsiveness. Record the ABG levels and your assessment findings.

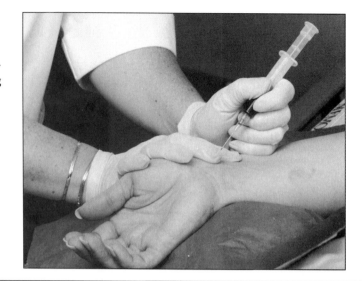

If the patient doesn't have an ET tube or a tracheostomy tube in place, provide additional oxygen by compressing a manual resuscitation bag in front of her nose and mouth. This may also help her relax and breathe more easily.

Explain the procedure—even in an emergency—and inform the patient that she'll need an ET tube or a tracheostomy tube, which will prevent speech. Reassure her that you'll show her another means of communication and that you or another nurse will be nearby. Also explain the purpose of ventilation and the expected sensations during machine-controlled breathing.

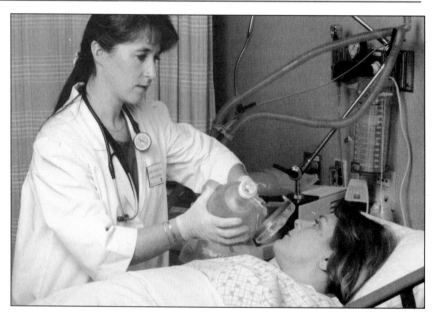

Once the patient has an ET tube or a tracheostomy tube in place, suction the tube to ensure airway clearance. Then auscultate for bilateral breath sounds, and observe chest movement.

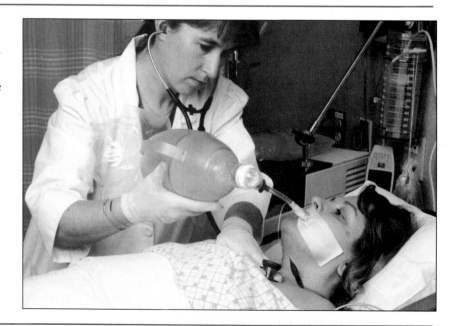

Attaching ventilator components

Begin preparing the ventilator by attaching the humidifier to its base.

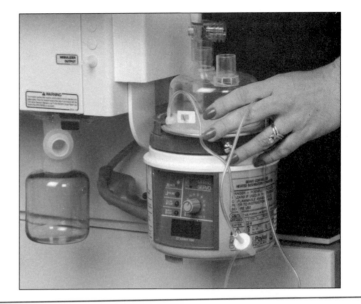

Next, attach the temperature sensor cable to the humidifier base.

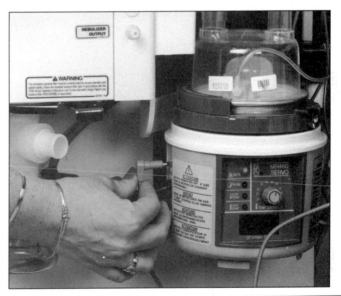

Open the bacteria filter door on the ventilator, and connect the short piece of flexible ventilator tubing (without the swivel-elbow adapter) to the bacteria filter and to the humidifier port marked IN. Then close the bacteria filter door.

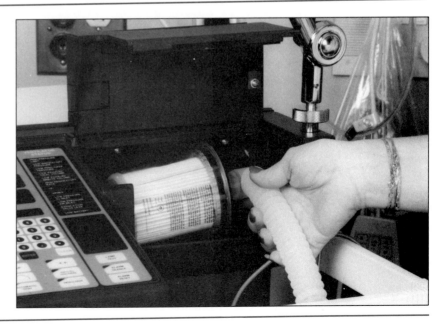

Attach the tube hanger to the flexible arm of the ventilator.

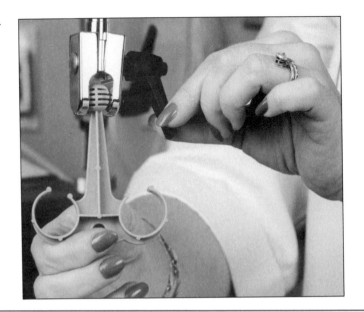

Place the flexible ventilator tubes, used for inspiration and expiration, on the tube hanger about 24″ (61 cm) from the patient's wye. (This hollow, Y-shaped apparatus couples the ventilator tubes with the swivel-elbow adapter that attaches to the patient's ET tube or tracheostomy tube.)

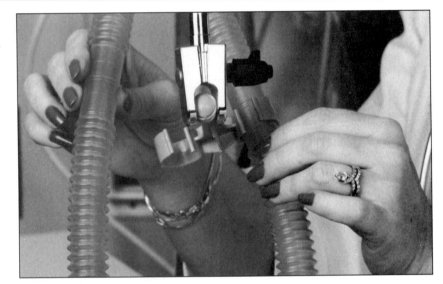

Connect the inspiration tube (leading from the wye) to the humidifier port labeled OUT.

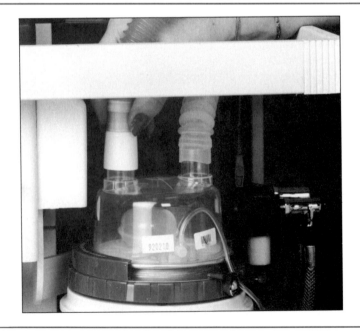

Attach the expiration tube (leading from the other side of the wye) to the adapter on the expiration collector vial (the water bottle).

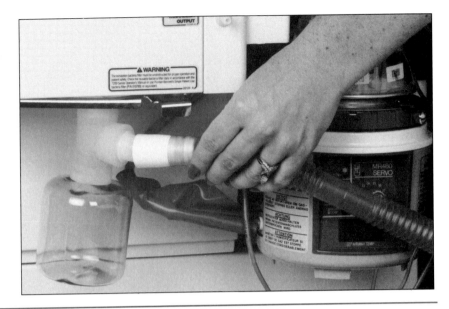

Attach the temperature sensor to the adapter that connects the ventilator tubing to the wye. Be sure that the adapter's opening is on the inspiration side of the tubing; if it isn't, reverse the wye.

▶ **Clinical tip:** To make the temperature sensor cable easier to manage, wrap it around the inspiration tube.

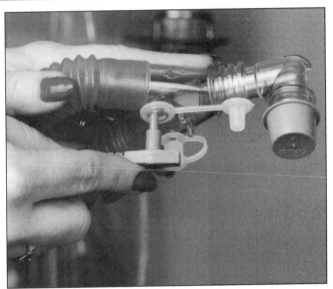

If the doctor orders additional dead space, put a short piece of ventilator tubing between the wye and the swivel-elbow adapter that attaches to the patient's ET (or tracheostomy) tube.

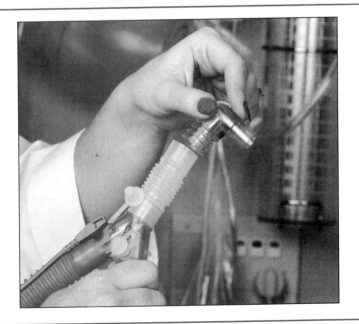

Hang the bag labeled STERILE WATER FOR INHALATION on the ventilator's arm. Open the bag and attach the tubing from the humidifier to the bag. If desired, lay the bag on top of the ventilator.

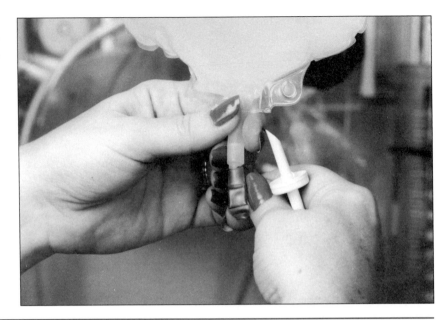

Double-check the security of all connections. One loose connection could interrupt the circuit, activating the alarms and, subsequently, causing the ventilator to fail.

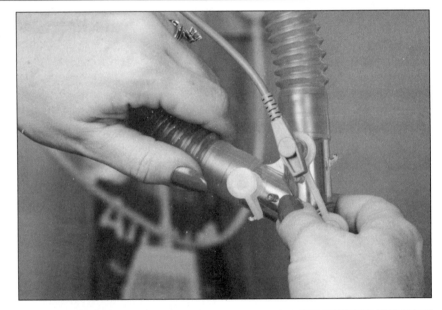

Plug the ventilator into a properly grounded, three-pronged, emergency outlet (near right). Then plug the air and oxygen hoses into the appropriate outlets (far right).

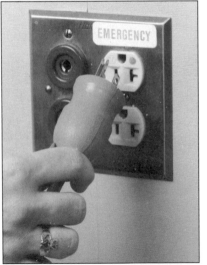
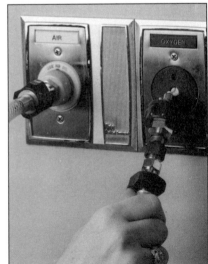

Checking ventilator functions

Turn on the power. On the Puritan-Bennett 7200 microprocessor, you'll need to lift a protective cover on the utility panel to reach the switch. Before this ventilator begins working, it runs a 10- to 15-second self-test. During this test, the message POWER ON SELF-TEST appears in the message window. Not all ventilators have this feature, but those that have it run the test when power stops momentarily and also when an extended self-test (EST) begins.

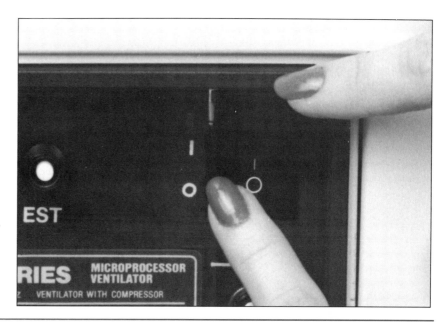

To check the system for leaks, activate the 90-second EST (leak test). Use a cap to occlude the wye (near right). Then, if you're using the ventilator shown here, press the EST button on the utility panel. The ventilator will automatically check for leaks.

▶ *Clinical tip:* If the ventilator doesn't have the automatic EST feature, press the MANUAL INSPIRATION key (after capping the wye). Wait for the high-pressure alarm to sound, which also indicates an airtight system.

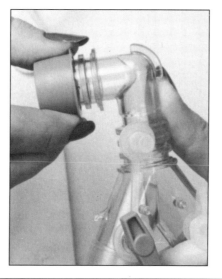

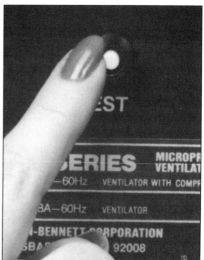

Once you're confident that the system is intact and secure, check the electronic function by activating the 40-second lamp test. This feature tests all visual displays, meters, keyboard lights, audible alarms, and the analogue output signal connector. On the ventilator shown here, press the LAMP TEST key first, then the ENTER key. The test will run twice. If all visual displays, meters, alarms, and lights function properly, you can safely use the ventilator on the patient.

▶ *Clinical tip:* You can test some ventilators manually if they don't have an automatic lamp test feature. Follow the manufacturer's directions.

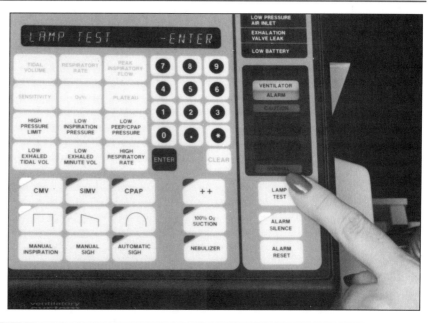

Selecting ventilator settings

Before connecting the ventilator to the patient, select the ordered ventilator settings. On the equipment shown here, you'll choose most settings by pressing the appropriate keys. But first, you need to silence the alarms. Do this by pressing the ALARM SILENCE key.

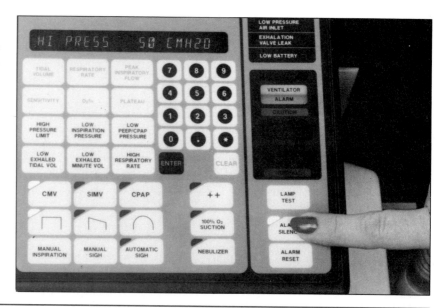

Set the tidal volume, which is the amount of air inspired or expired during normal breathing. (This value reflects 10 to 15 ml of air per kilogram of body weight.) To do this, press the TIDAL VOLUME key, select the ordered tidal volume on the control panel's numeric keypad, and then press the ENTER key.

▶ *Clinical tip:* The ventilator shown here computes tidal volume in liters, *not* milliliters. If you wish to set a tidal volume in milliliters—say, 700 ml—press the decimal symbol on the numeric keypad, followed by 700. Then press ENTER.

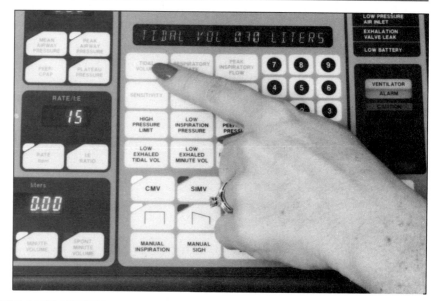

Next, set the respiratory rate ordered by the doctor. (The desired adult respiratory rate ranges between 10 and 15 breaths/minute.) To do this, press the RESPIRATORY RATE key, select the ordered respiratory rate on the numeric keypad, and then press ENTER.

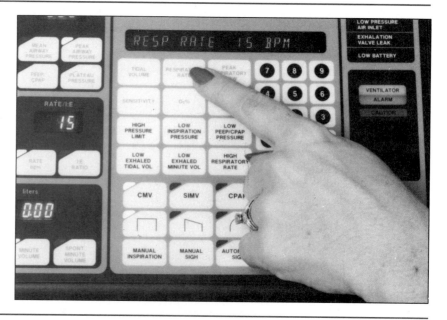

Keep in mind that the peak inspiratory flow rate usually isn't decided in advance. It's set to meet the demand of a patient who can breathe on her own. The doctor bases the rate on tidal volume, respiratory rate, and patient effort. He aims for a setting that's high enough to prevent the patient from fighting the ventilator.

A normal rate ranges between 40 and 60 liters/minute (lpm), but this varies among patients. To choose the setting, press the PEAK INSPIRATORY FLOW key, select the ordered rate on the keypad, and press ENTER.

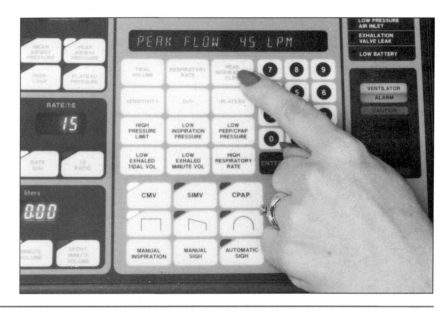

To set sensitivity (the effort required to trigger an inspiration), press the SENSITIVITY key. To change the preset value (shown here), select the ordered sensitivity on the numeric keypad and press ENTER. The pressure will be displayed in the message window. Usually you'll set the sensitivity at -0.5 cm H_2O to ensure that the ventilator responds easily to the patient's respiratory efforts.

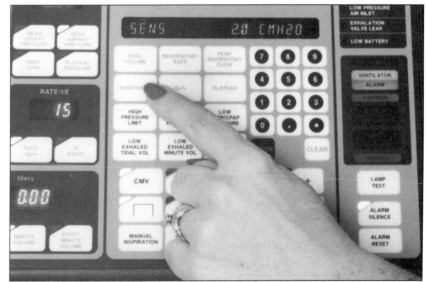

Enter the oxygen percentage ordered by the doctor by pressing the O_2% key, selecting the appropriate numbers on the numeric keypad and pressing ENTER. To ensure adequate oxygenation for the patient, the doctor or hospital may require you to monitor ABG levels while the patient is on the ventilator.

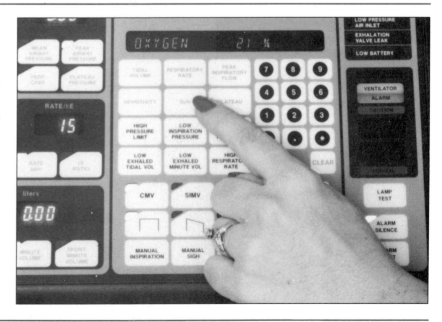

If the doctor orders it, select a plateau. A plateau sustains inspiration for a specified time, which may be useful for increasing oxygenation. To set this limit, press the PLATEAU key, select the appropriate time in seconds on the numeric keypad, and press ENTER. If the doctor doesn't order a plateau, be sure that this setting remains at zero.

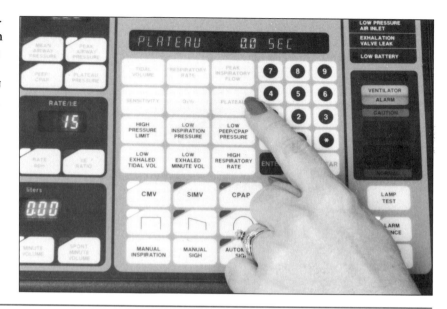

Once you've selected the settings, press the key for the ordered ventilation mode: continuous mandatory ventilation (CMV), synchronized intermittent mandatory ventilation (SIMV), or continuous positive airway pressure (CPAP). The selected key will light up.

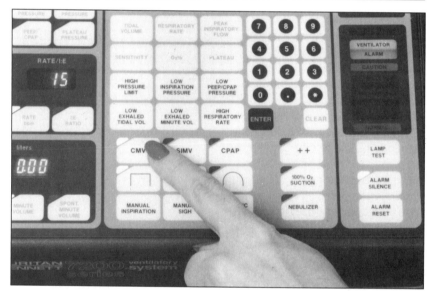

Select the patient's flow pattern by pressing the appropriate waveform key and then pressing ENTER. The ventilator will beep twice, and the key will light up. Consult the doctor or a respiratory therapist about choosing this setting, which is determined by the patient's condition.

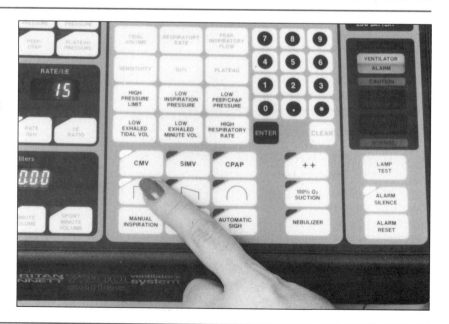

To set the sigh volume, first press the AUTOMATIC SIGH key. The parameter prompt will appear in the message window. Select each parameter value on the numeric keypad, pressing ENTER after every selection. When the update prompt appears in the message window, press ENTER again. Then press ENTER a third time to activate the automatic sigh. The AUTOMATIC SIGH key will light up.

▶ **Clinical tip:** Sighs prevent atelectasis, which may result from monotonous tidal ventilation. Sighs aren't necessary in the SIMV mode.

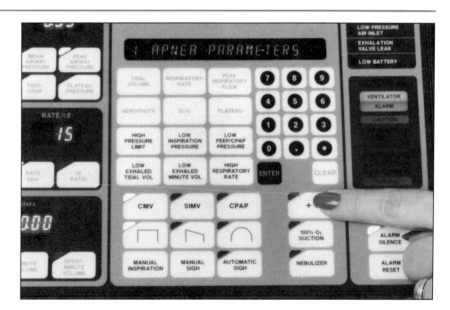

Set the apnea parameters. On the ventilator shown here, press the key marked with a double plus sign (+ +) until APNEA PARAMETERS appears in the message window. Then press ENTER to scroll through the parameter prompts.

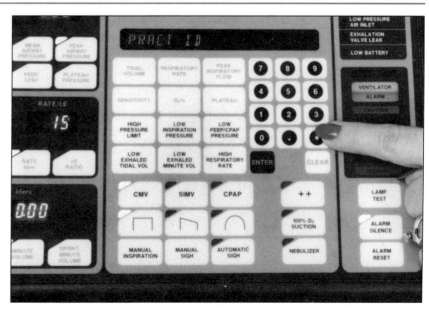

To adjust certain settings, press CLEAR or ENTER, select the desired value, then press ENTER. To retain the current value, also press ENTER. This will continue the scroll through the various settings. Use the asterisk (*) key to scroll backward. When the UPDATE PARAMETERS message appears, press ENTER only. On the ventilator shown here, the preprogrammed apnea parameters serve as a backup in case the ventilator malfunctions or the patient doesn't breathe adequately.

Now you've chosen all the required settings. But before connecting the patient to the ventilator, first adjust or check the alarms to be sure that they're set correctly. To adjust alarms on the ventilator shown here, press the appropriate keys (which also act as alarm threshold keys), use the numeric keypad to enter the desired value for each alarm, and press ENTER.

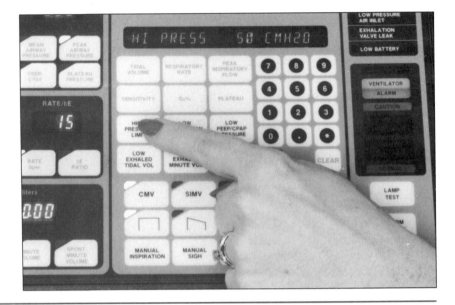

Connecting the ventilator to the patient

When you're ready to make the connection between the ventilator and the patient, tell the patient what you're about to do. Then attach the wye of the ventilator tubing to the patient's ET tube. Once the tubes are secure, listen to the patient's breath sounds, and confirm bilateral ventilation. Double-check the flow rate and alarm settings.

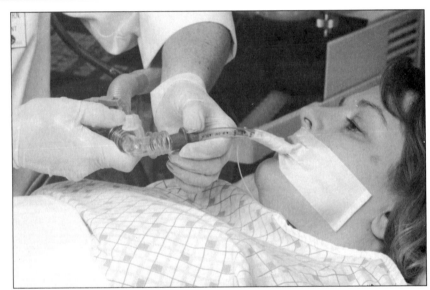

If the doctor orders positive end-expiratory pressure (PEEP) or continuous positive airway pressure (CPAP), select this setting next. Turn the PEEP-CPAP knob to the desired amount while observing the pressure manometer or digital display.

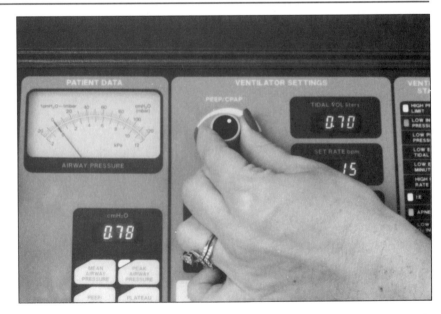

Finally, attach the manual resuscitation bag to an oxygen source, and place it at the patient's bedside. This is an important step. If the ventilator fails, you'll use this apparatus to help the patient breathe.

You will need to monitor ABG levels and vital signs about 15 to 20 minutes after ventilation starts. Additional measures involve checking ventilatory function, settings, and tube cuff pressure.

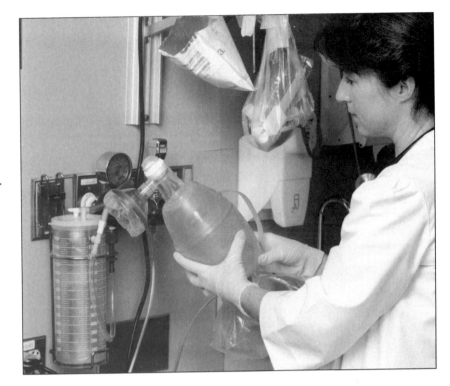

Setting ventilator alarms

Because you'll adjust the ventilator's alarms and monitor the patient's condition, you need to keep in mind the usual and safe ranges for ventilator alarm settings. Use the information below as a guide. Remember that normal ranges vary according to the patient and his condition.

ALARM SETTING	USUAL LIMIT
Low inspiratory pressure	10 to 15 cm H_2O below the pressure needed to ventilate the patient
High inspiratory pressure	10 to 15 cm H_2O above the pressure needed to deliver a breath
Low exhaled tidal volume (V_T)	100 ml below the set V_T (volume of air inhaled and exhaled normally)
Low exhaled minute volume	The set V_T minus 100 ml multiplied by the actual respiratory rate (breaths/minute)
High respiratory rate	5 to 10 breaths/minute above the actual respiratory rate
Low PEEP-CPAP	2 to 3 cm H_2O below the set positive end-expiratory pressure (PEEP) or continuous positive airway pressure (CPAP)

Responding to ventilator alarms

Most ventilators have alarms to warn you of hazardous situations—for instance, when inspiratory pressure rises too high or drops too low. Use the chart below to help you respond quickly and effectively to a ventilator alarm.

ALARM	POSSIBLE CAUSE	INTERVENTIONS
Low pressure	• Tube disconnected from ventilator • Endotracheal (ET) tube displaced above vocal cords, or tracheostomy tube extubated • Leaking tidal volume from low cuff pressure (from an underinflated or ruptured ET cuff or a leak in the cuff or one-way valve) • Ventilator malfunction • Leak in ventilator circuitry (from loose connection or hole in tubing, loss of temperature-sensing device, or cracked humidification container)	• Reconnect the tube to the ventilator. • If extubation or displacement has occurred, manually ventilate the patient and call the doctor. • Listen for a whooshing sound (an air leak) around the tube; check cuff pressure. If you can't maintain pressure, the doctor may insert a new tube. • Disconnect the patient from the ventilator and manually ventilate him if necessary. Get another ventilator. • Make sure that all connections are intact. Check the humidification container and the tubing for holes or leaks, and replace if necessary.
High pressure	• Increased airway pressure or decreased lung compliance caused by worsening disease • Patient biting on ET tube • Secretions in airway • Condensate in large-bore tubing • Intubation of right mainstem bronchus • Patient coughing, gagging, or trying to talk • Chest wall resistance • Malfunctioning high-pressure relief valve • Bronchospasm, pneumothorax, or barotrauma	• Auscultate the lungs for evidence of increasing lung consolidation, barotrauma, or wheezing. Call the doctor if indicated. • If needed, insert a bite guard. • Use suction or have the patient cough. • Remove any condensate. • Check the tube's position. If it has slipped, call the doctor, who may need to reposition it. • If the patient is fighting the ventilator in any way, he may need sedation or a neuromuscular blocker, as ordered. • Reposition the patient if his position limits chest expansion. If ineffective, give a prescribed analgesic. • Have the faulty equipment replaced. • Assess the patient for the cause. Report the disorder to the doctor, and provide treatment as ordered.
Spirometer or low exhaled tidal volume, or low exhaled minute volume	• Power interruption • Loose connection or leak in delivery system • Leaking cuff or inadequate cuff seal • Leaking chest tube • Increased airway resistance in patient on pressure-cycled ventilator • Disconnected spirometer • Any change that sets off high- or low-pressure alarms and prevents delivery of full air volume • Malfunctioning volume measuring device	• Check all electrical connections. • Make sure that all connections in the delivery system are secure; check for leaks. • Listen for a leak with a stethoscope. Reinflate the cuff according to hospital policy. Replace the cuff if necessary. • Check all chest tube connections. Be sure that the water seal is intact; then notify the doctor. • Auscultate the lungs for signs of an airway obstruction, barotrauma, or lung consolidation. • Make sure that the spirometer is connected. • See the interventions for high- and low-pressure alarms. • Alert the respiratory therapist to replace the device.
High respiratory rate	• Anxious patient • Patient in pain • Secretions in airway	• Assess the patient for the cause. Dispel the patient's fears as possible; sedate, if necessary. • Position the patient comfortably. Administer medication for pain as ordered. • Suction the patient.
Low PEEP-CPAP	• Leak in system • Mechanical failure of PEEP mechanism	• Check that all connections are secure. Check for holes in the tubing and replace if necessary. • Discontinue PEEP and call the respiratory therapist.

Maintaining mechanical ventilation

To detect or avoid infection and other complications in a patient receiving mechanical ventilation, you'll need to provide continuous monitoring and frequent, thorough assessment. You'll monitor her vital signs, neurologic status and level of consciousness, psychological state, breathing effort, respiratory secretions, and general skin appearance. You'll also assess her overall system status, checking especially for cardiopulmonary and hemodynamic changes.

You'll monitor airway pressure and ventilator function regularly and, sometimes, continuously. You'll also provide care to keep the patient as comfortable as possible. Ultimately, your care will support the patient until she can breathe independently.

USING ACCESSORY EQUIPMENT

You may use several monitoring devices continuously or intermittently. Continuous monitoring is an intrinsic feature of the ventilator. For example, the Puritan-Bennett 7200 microprocessor, featured on these pages, continuously measures and displays the patient's exhaled tidal volume, respiratory rate, and airway pressures. If the patient is acutely ill, a cardiac monitor can provide immediate and continuous measurements of her heart rate and rhythm.

For intermittent assessment, the most commonly used tools are a sphygmomanometer and a stethoscope. Depending on the patient's hemodynamic stability and arterial blood gas (ABG) levels, a pulmonary artery catheter or a peripheral arterial line may also be used. Accompanying pressure tracings can give additional information about the patient's hemodynamic status. Pulse oximetry and ABG measurements are invaluable for determining oxygenation and acid-base status.

Airway access in the patient requiring mechanical ventilation will be through either an endotracheal (ET) tube or a tracheostomy tube. Generally, an acute respiratory problem necessitates ET tube insertion. A tracheotomy may be required in an emergency. Usually, though, it's performed only if the patient needs mechanical ventilation for an extended period or if she has chronic airway problems.

Maintaining the ventilator

Check the ventilator settings at least hourly. Make sure that all settings coincide with the doctor's orders and are documented. Check the set tidal volume, the fraction of inspired oxygen (FIO_2), and the respiratory rate. Compare the set respiratory rate with the actual number of breaths per minute the patient takes. Check the peak flow for consistency. Record airway pressures to establish a trend, and report any consistent peak pressure over 60 cm H_2O.

Note: If peak airway pressure increases, watch for a buildup of secretions in the airway, a pneumothorax, or stiffening lung tissue. If peak airway pressure decreases, suspect a leak in the airway system.

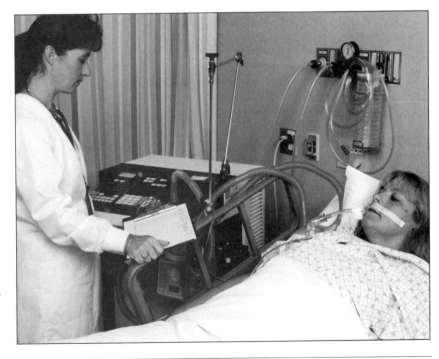

Kathy Yandle, BA, RRT, CPFT, and *Denise Salvo, RN,C, MSN, CCRN,* contributed to this section. Ms. Yandle is a clinical educator in Cardio-Respiratory Services at Grand View Hospital, Sellersville, Pa. Ms. Salvo is an instructor at Widener University, Chester, Pa. The publisher thanks the following organizations for their help: *Abington (Pa.) Hospital; Grand View Hospital,* Sellersville, Pa.; and *Puritan-Bennett Corp.,* Carlsbad, Calif.

Check that the ventilator mode is set as ordered. Modes available are continuous mandatory ventilation (CMV), synchronized intermittent mandatory ventilation (SIMV), or continuous positive airway pressure (CPAP). If ordered, set and adjust positive end-expiratory pressure (PEEP). Change the mode as ordered.

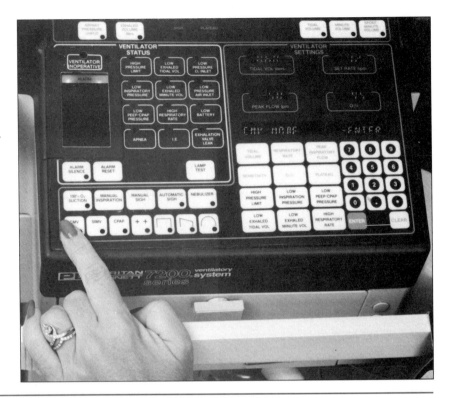

Empty any water (condensate) that collects in the ventilator tubing. To do this, disconnect the tubing quickly and drain the water into a nearby basin or biohazard container. Never drain the water into the humidifier—this contaminates the humidified air supplied to the patient.

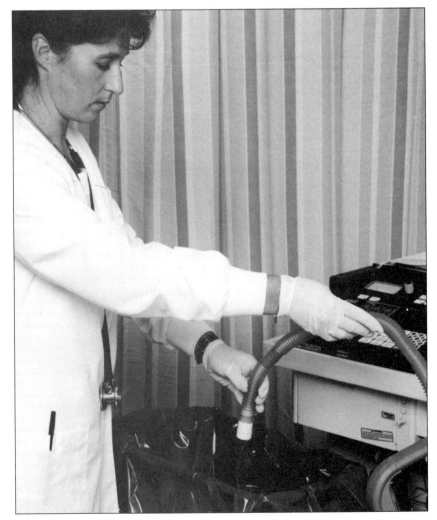

Reconnect all tubing. Take care to ensure tight connections.

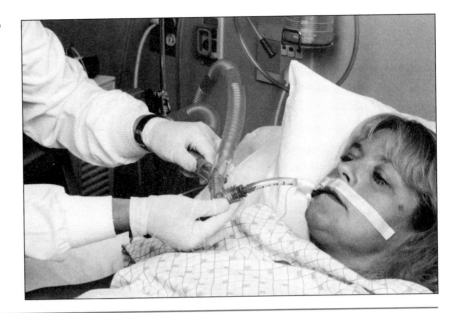

If the ventilator alarm sounds, silence it quickly to avoid upsetting the patient unnecessarily. Reassure her as you investigate the situation, and reset the alarm to ensure her safety.

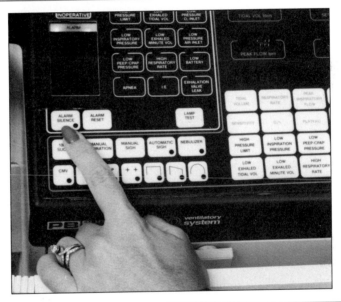

If you can't readily correct the problem or if the patient is in respiratory distress, call for help and manually ventilate her until the problem is resolved.

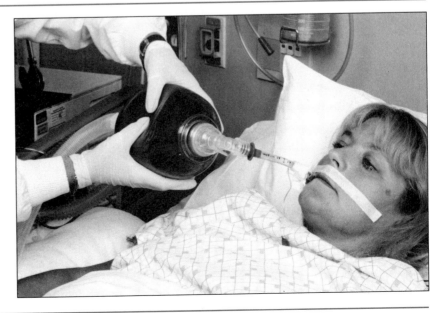

Managing the patient's care

Check that the equipment you'll need for general care is available. Your equipment may include a stethoscope; a sphygmomanometer; an ABG kit; gloves; a hand-held resuscitation bag; a cuff pressure manometer; a sputum specimen trap, a gown, and a face mask or shield; and tape. If needed, a pulse oximeter should also be available.

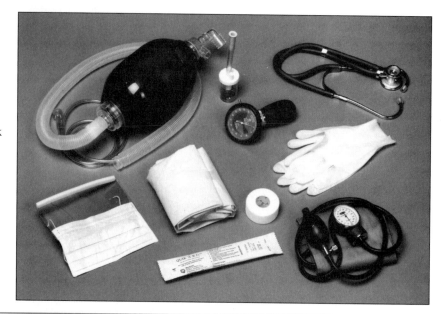

Begin by assessing the patient's condition. Check her breathing pattern and respiratory status. Evaluate her chest expansion, noting symmetry and breathing depth. Watch for use of accessory muscles during respiration—a sign of labored breathing. Be alert also for anxiety, diaphoresis, pallor, and cyanosis, which point to respiratory distress. Also observe the patient closely for changes in level of consciousness.

▶ *Clinical tip:* If anxiety contributes to the patient's respiratory distress, try to reassure and calm her. If necessary, provide sedation.

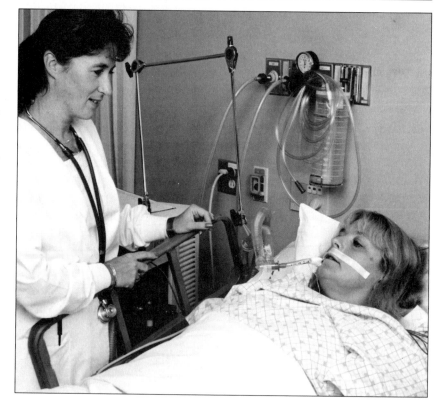

Assess the patient's blood pressure, heart rate, and respiratory rate every 2 hours and whenever a change occurs in her condition or treatment. Document your findings. Take and record her temperature every 4 hours (more frequently if it's elevated). If her vital signs change significantly, report them to the doctor immediately.

Fever, for example, may be the first sign of infection. Other changes in vital signs may indicate the body's attempts to compensate for respiratory insufficiency.

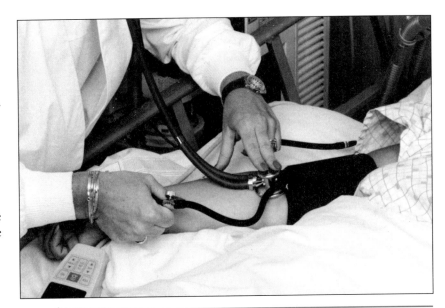

Observe the patient's heart rhythm on the cardiac monitor, noting any changes that occur as you provide care. Immediately report arrhythmias and any significant increase or decrease in heart rate.

▷ *Clinical tip:* Remember that patient movement may cause artifacts on the monitor screen and fluctuations in the recorded heart rate. So don't rely solely on the heart rate displayed on the monitor screen when assessing vital signs.

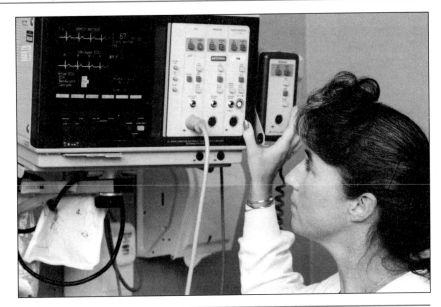

Evaluating oxygenation

Draw blood for ABG analysis as ordered, usually at least daily. Also draw a blood sample whenever the patient has evident respiratory distress.

▷ *Clinical tip:* Wait 20 to 30 minutes after suctioning or ventilator changes to obtain an ABG sample.

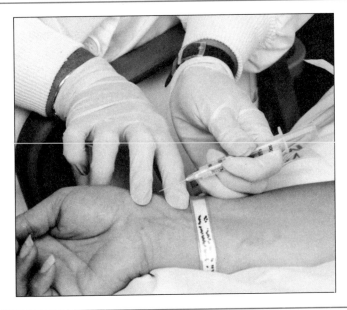

Assess arterial oxygen saturation (SaO_2) by using pulse oximetry, if available. Compare the SaO_2 level recorded by the oximeter with the oxygen saturation obtained from ABG analysis.

Note: Pulse oximetry readings alone may be misleading or inaccurate, especially if the patient has poor peripheral perfusion or if her activity causes fluctuations or artifacts in the waveform.

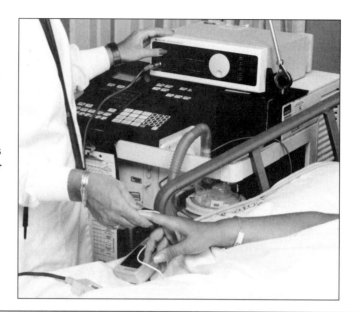

Evaluating pulmonary condition

Auscultate the patient's anterior and posterior chest every 2 to 4 hours and whenever her condition changes. Listen carefully. Breath sounds should be equal and bilateral. Listen also for adventitious sounds. If you hear breath sounds on only one side of the chest, alert the doctor immediately. The patient may have unilateral atelectasis, consolidated fluid, or pneumothorax. If the patient has an oral or a nasal ET tube, the sounds you hear may result from the tube's incorrect positioning in the bronchus rather than in the trachea.

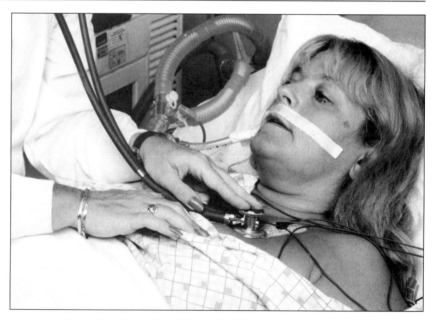

Ensuring airway patency

Retape the ET tube daily. When you retape the tube, check that it's positioned correctly. To do this, check that the mark or tape on the ET tube is at the point where the tube exits the nose or mouth (as shown). Then auscultate for equal, bilateral breath sounds. If necessary, resecure the ET tube with adhesive tape or a Velcro fastener. Notify the doctor if the tube needs repositioning.

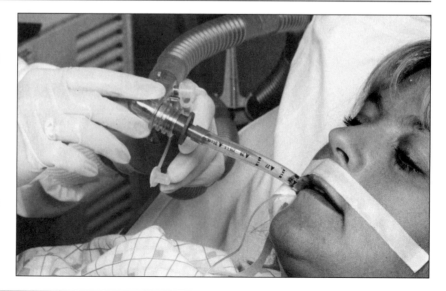

Check the ET tube's cuff for leakage if you can hear escaping air during inspiration or if the tidal volume alarm on the ventilator sounds. Do this by auscultating the patient's trachea. A smooth hollow sound indicates a sealed airway; a loud gurgling sound indicates an air leak.

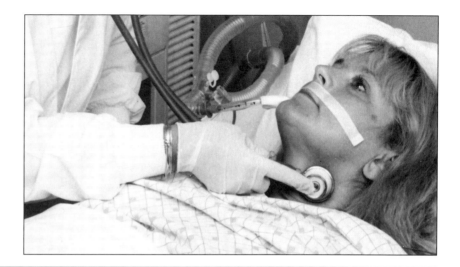

Next, attach a cuff pressure manometer to the cuff's air inlet. Increase the cuff pressure gradually until no leaks are heard. Note the reading on the pressure gauge, and keep in mind that cuff pressures should be 25 mm Hg or less. If leaks occur, add air to the cuff using the pumping device attached to the manometer and take another reading.

▷ *Clinical tip:* If you can't maintain adequate cuff pressure to administer the prescribed tidal volume, call the doctor. The ET tube may need to be replaced.

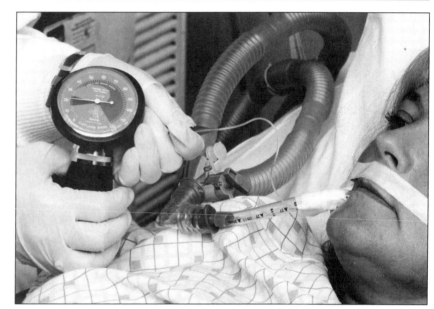

Controlling infection

To identify infection early, collect sputum specimens for culture and sensitivity studies, as ordered, if you note a color change in respiratory secretions, if secretions develop an odor or increase in amount, or if the patient's temperature rises above 101.5° F (38.6° C). Collect the sputum by placing a specimen trap in the suction catheter line. Document your actions and observations.

▷ *Clinical tip:* If you might be exposed to contaminated body fluids when collecting a sputum specimen, wear gloves, a mask, eyewear, and a gown.

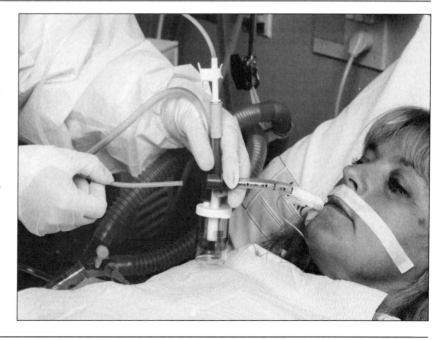

Providing supportive care

Your plan of care for the patient receiving mechanical ventilation will include maintaining his airway, meeting his medication and nutrition needs, sustaining mobility and communication, and providing oral hygiene.

Suctioning the patient's airway
• Clear the patient's airway as needed. Indications for suctioning include frequent coughing, secretions in the endotracheal (ET) tube, and activation of the equipment's high-pressure alarm.
• Explain the procedure to the patient first. Warn him that suctioning will cause breathlessness and a feeling that he needs to cough. Reassure him that these sensations are temporary and that he'll receive extra oxygen during the procedure.
• Note the amount, color, and consistency of the secretions and document your findings.
• If the patient is alert enough, teach him to remove his oral secretions himself with a rigid, plastic Yankhauer catheter and basin. Remind him to be careful not to dislodge the ET tube.

Providing medications and nutrition
• Administer prescribed drug therapy to relieve bronchial constriction caused by lung disease or accumulated secretions.
• Place the medication into a small-volume nebulizer, and insert the nebulizer into the inspiratory line of the ventilator circuit. Connect the administration tubing to the nebulizer port of the ventilator.
• Monitor the patient for adverse reactions, such as tachycardia, bronchospasm, or anxiety. After treatment, suction the patient because bronchodilation usually mobilizes secretions.
• Assess the patient's nutritional status when he first begins mechanical ventilation and then throughout treatment. Depending on his condition, provide parenteral or enteral nutrition, as ordered.
• Weigh the patient initially to establish a baseline weight. Then weigh him daily if he's receiving parenteral nutrition and every 2 to 3 days if he's receiving enteral feedings.

• Document your findings and compare them with previous records.
• Keep in mind that an inability to wean the patient from the ventilator may be caused by nutritional deficiency.

Promoting mobility and communication
• Reposition the patient every 2 hours to help mobilize respiratory secretions and to make him comfortable. Whenever possible, help him sit in a chair near the ventilator.
• Encourage the patient who can turn himself to change positions frequently. Repositioning prevents pressure ulcers and improves lung aeration.
• Perform chest physiotherapy, as ordered, on patients with copious or tenacious respiratory secretions. This therapy helps move secretions to the larger airways where they can be removed through suctioning.
• Maintain the patient's muscle tone by performing range-of-motion exercises. Explain each exercise and encourage the patient to participate, if possible. Plan exercises related to his specific needs and tolerance.
• If the patient is well enough, set up a writing board or other communication tool so that he can convey his questions and concerns. Place the call button within easy reach, and reassure him that you'll answer his calls promptly.
• Explain that the patient's equipment (the ventilator, cardiac monitor, and pulse oximeter) has alarms that will immediately alert the health care team to any situation needing attention.

Maintaining oral hygiene
• Move the ET tube from one side of the patient's mouth to the other as necessary to help prevent mucosal breakdown or lesions.
• Brush the patient's teeth or rinse his mouth at least every 4 hours.
• Sponge the patient's oral mucosa to keep his mouth clean and moist and to make him more comfortable, as needed.

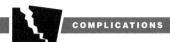
COMPLICATIONS

Coping with problems from mechanical ventilation

Mechanical ventilation can save your patient's life, but it can also cause serious complications. The chart below will help you recognize and manage such problems.

PROBLEM	SIGNS AND SYMPTOMS	INTERVENTIONS
Acid-base and fluid and electrolyte imbalance Results from positive water balance created by secretion of antidiuretic hormone; also caused by reduced insensible losses from respiratory tract	Probable change in arterial blood gas (ABG) measurements (decreased vital capacity), weight gain, ankle edema, moist crackles in lower lobes of lungs, pulmonary edema confirmed by X-ray studies	• Carry out the doctor's orders to restrict fluid intake and administer diuretics. • Give medications (or, rarely, apply rotating tourniquets) to control pulmonary edema or to correct acid-base or electrolyte imbalance as ordered.
Airway obstruction Caused by secretions, incorrect tube position, or bronchospasm	Cyanosis, bradycardia or tachycardia, anxiety, increased airway pressures	• Suction frequently. • Perform chest physiotherapy. • If the doctor orders bronchoscopy, prepare the patient for the procedure. • Use a pulse oximeter to monitor the patient's oxygen level. • Adjust the endotracheal (ET) tube's position. • Administer nebulizer treatments as ordered.
Atelectasis Caused by insufficient deep breathing, pneumothorax, retained secretions, or a combination of these	Transient fine crackles, diminished breath sounds over the affected lung segment, bronchial sounds over the peripheral lung fields, decreased compliance, possible change in ABG values	• Turn the patient frequently. • Suction and hyperinflate the patient's lungs periodically. • Have the patient cough and take deep breaths every 2 hours. • Perform chest physiotherapy, as ordered. • If the doctor orders bronchoscopy, prepare the patient for the procedure.
Barotrauma Occurs as pneumothorax, subcutaneous emphysema, or mediastinal emphysema; usually caused when volume and pressure settings are too high or during administration of positive end-expiratory pressure (PEEP)	Sudden cyanosis, sudden drop in blood pressure, sudden decrease in lung compliance, increased anxiety • With pneumothorax, diminished or absent breath sounds over the affected lung, acute pain on the affected side, and a trachea deviated away from the pneumothorax • With subcutaneous emphysema, crepitus of the face, abdomen, and extremities • With mediastinal emphysema, reduced cardiac output and crepitus over the heart	• Call the doctor immediately. He may insert a chest tube. • Use pulse oximetry to monitor the patient's oxygen levels.
Cardiovascular impairment Occurs when positive intrathoracic pressure reduces venous return to the right side of the heart and compresses pulmonary circulation	Decreased blood pressure and cardiac output, possible decreased urine output, increased central venous pressure and pulmonary artery pressure, increased heart rate	• Carry out the doctor's orders to reduce intrathoracic pressure by decreasing PEEP, inspiratory flow rate, or tidal volume. • Administer additional I.V. fluids or plasma expanders, such as albumin or colloidal substances, as ordered.
Gastrointestinal distress Occurs as GI bleeding, gastric distention, paralytic ileus, or stress ulcer; usually caused by stress or swallowing air	Abdominal distention, steady decrease in hemoglobin and hematocrit values, positive Hematest results on nasogastric (NG) drainage and stools, tarry stools	• As ordered, insert NG tube for drainage. • Replace lost blood. • Use NG tube to provide antacids or other medications to decrease acid production.

(continued)

Coping with problems from mechanical ventilation *(continued)*

PROBLEM	SIGNS AND SYMPTOMS	INTERVENTIONS
Oxygen toxicity Caused by high oxygen concentrations (over 60%) administered over prolonged period (8 hours or more); may cause fibrotic tissue changes in lungs, possibly leading to death	Retrosternal pain; sore throat; nasal congestion; burning chest pain on inspiration; dry, hacking cough; dyspnea; decreased compliance; decreased arterial oxygen levels despite the same oxygen concentration; decreased vital capacity; and changes seen on X-ray films	• Monitor oxygen levels carefully, and report signs of oxygen toxicity immediately.
Respiratory tract infection Occurs from ventilator equipment bypassing the upper airway and thereby eliminating the body's natural defense mechanisms against infection; also caused by flawed aseptic technique	Elevated temperature and white blood cell count, increased respiratory secretions and change in secretion color or odor	• Notify the doctor. • Change the patient's position frequently, and perform chest physiotherapy as indicated. • Use aseptic technique for tracheostomy care and for suctioning. • Administer prescribed antibiotics.
Tracheal trauma Caused by constant pressure of cuffed ET tube or tracheostomy tube on the patient's trachea or by injury related to intubation	Decreased tidal volume (because of air leak), bleeding from trachea	• Depending on the type of damage, help the doctor insert a new tracheostomy tube, thereby changing the position of the ET tube's cuff and allowing the injured area to heal. • Provide meticulous cuff care until you can remove the ET tube.

LEARNING ABOUT VENTILATOR WEANING

Easing a patient from mechanically supported ventilation to independent breathing is called weaning. Some patients make the transition effortlessly; others don't—especially if they've had prolonged mechanical ventilation or developed pulmonary complications. Nursing responsibilities during weaning include closely assessing, monitoring, and supporting the patient. In many facilities, the respiratory therapist obtains the weaning parameters and weans the patient from the ventilator. Even a tiny change in physical status may speed or delay the patient's progress to spontaneous ventilation.

Although the doctor usually decides exactly when to wean the patient from ventilation therapy, the nurse has the information on hand to determine the patient's readiness. Obviously, the decision to wean the patient focuses on his respiratory function (see *Understanding weaning parameters*). Arterial blood gas (ABG) analysis should show that he can maintain a partial pressure of arterial oxygen at an acceptable level (usually 55 mm Hg) without more than 5 cm H_2O of positive end-expiratory pressure and without a fraction of inspired oxygen greater than 50%. Other ABG levels also should stay within an acceptable range (depending on the patient and his disorder). The patient's overall condition, strength, level of consciousness, and psychological preparedness are additional considerations.

(continued)

Understanding weaning parameters

To help identify your patient's readiness to breathe on his own, check his pulmonary function against the respiratory parameters below. Keep in mind that these values are only guides and may not be reliable for all patients.

PULMONARY FUNCTION	DEFINITION	WEANING PARAMETER
Respiratory frequency (f)	Number of respirations per minute	The patient's f value should be less than 25 breaths/minute.
Tidal volume (V_T)	Volume of air inspired and expired during a normal respiratory cycle	During spontaneous respiration, the patient's V_T should measure 4 to 5 ml/kg.
Minute volume ($\dot{V}_E$) also called minute ventilation	Total volume of air inhaled or exhaled in 1 minute	The patient's $\dot{V}_E$ should measure less than 10 liters/minute; a greater $\dot{V}_E$ suggests that the patient must work too hard to breathe independently.
Vital capacity (VC)	Maximum expiratory volume	The patient's VC should measure between 10 and 15 ml/kg to ensure enough airflow for adequate gas exchange and secretion mobilization.
Negative inspiratory pressure also called negative inspiratory force	Ability to take a deep breath and generate a cough strong enough to clear secretions	The patient's negative inspiratory pressure should measure at least −20 cm H_2O.
Maximum voluntary ventilation (MVV) not routinely measured	Ability to sustain ventilation under stress	The patient's MVV should measure between 10 and 20 liters/minute.

Contributors to this section include *Denise Salvo, RN,C, MSN, CCRN,* and *Joanne Dimitriadis, RN.* Ms. Salvo is an instructor at Widener University, Chester, Pa. Ms. Dimitriadis is a clinical leader in the intensive care unit at Abington (Pa.) Memorial Hospital. The publisher thanks *Abington (Pa.) Memorial Hospital* for its help.

CHOOSING A WEANING METHOD

The type of weaning method selected depends on several factors—among them, the patient's physical condition, how long he's been on the ventilator, and his mental outlook. Possible choices include intermittent mandatory ventilation, synchronized intermittent mandatory ventilation, continuous positive airway pressure, pressure support ventilation, and assist-control ventilation (see *Comparing weaning methods*). With all of these methods, the patient continues to receive ventilatory support, which allows weaning to proceed slowly and safely. And the alarms remain active to alert you to problems.

Another weaning method involves using a T-piece. This method is used without ventilatory support.

MONITORING THE PATIENT

Monitor the patient's response to his increased respiratory workload. If signs reveal that he isn't ready to be weaned (such as arrhythmias or significantly increased blood pressure, heart rate, or respiratory rate), stop weaning and return him to the ventilator.

REMOVING THE BREATHING TUBE

Once the patient requires minimal ventilatory assistance, extubation completes weaning. This reduces airway resistance and the work of breathing.

If the patient has a tracheostomy tube, the doctor may leave it in place to avoid repeated insertion if the patient needs the tube later. While he waits for the tube to be removed, he may use a tracheostomy collar, a tracheostomy button, or a T-piece.

Comparing weaning methods

METHOD	INDICATIONS	FEATURES
Intermittent mandatory ventilation or synchronized intermittent mandatory ventilation	• Older or debilitated patients • Chronic pulmonary or muscle disorders • Difficulty weaning • Fear of being off the ventilator	• Delivers a preset tidal volume (V_T) at a fixed rate regardless of the patient's efforts, although the patient can initiate an independent breath and receive support for that breath • Gradually increases the interval between ventilator-delivered breaths until all ventilations are spontaneous • At lower settings, allows air to be dispersed in the lungs more evenly • Helps prevent muscle atrophy and incoordination
Continuous positive airway pressure	• Prolonged continuous mandatory ventilation • Difficulty weaning • Respiratory muscle reconditioning needed • Effective ventilation but inability to oxygenate because of decreased functional residual capacity (FRC) • Fluid-filled alveoli or excessive secretions • Refractory hypoxemia resulting from atelectasis	• Allows mechanically supported breaths if the patient's inspiratory effort fails • Ensures positive airway pressure during spontaneous ventilations (inspiration and expiration) • Promotes oxygenation by increasing FRC and lung compliance • Allows progression from continuous ventilatory support to intervals during which the patient breathes through a T-piece
Pressure support ventilation	• Long-term ventilatory support • Muscle atrophy • Psychological dependence on the ventilator	• Augments spontaneous ventilations with positive pressure (most often used with synchronized intermittent mandatory ventilation or continuous positive airway pressure) • Sustains preset inspiratory pressure throughout the inspiratory cycle, then gradually decreases the level of pressure
Assist-control ventilation	• Prolonged continuous mandatory ventilation • Difficulty weaning • Respiratory muscle reconditioning needed	• Delivers preset V_T triggered by patient's inspiratory effort. If the patient doesn't initiate a breath, the ventilator takes over, guaranteeing minimum ventilation. • Provides positive pressure to augment the patient's spontaneous breaths
T-piece ventilation	• Ventilatory support received for less than 2 days • Long-term therapy but no psychological dependence on the ventilator	• Allows delivery of oxygen and humidity past breathing tube • Permits periodic removal of the patient from the ventilator until spontaneous breathing resumes • Patient's spontaneous breathing is the only source of ventilation

PREPARING FOR VENTILATOR WEANING

Be aware that for some patients, the change from mechanical ventilation to spontaneous breathing may induce excessive anxiety. To help your patient adjust to the change safely, prepare her physically and emotionally. As you prepare her physically, by suctioning her and connecting her to a cardiac monitor and pulse oximeter, reassure her that you or another nurse will be nearby if she has a problem. Take any necessary steps to relieve her fears because anxiety poses a major barrier to successful weaning.

Assemble the following equipment at the bedside: a stethoscope, suction equipment, gloves, a gown, a face shield, a pulse oximeter sensor, a hand-held resuscitation bag with connecting tubing, and an appropriate-size face mask.

Additional equipment includes a sphygmomanometer, a thermometer, a pulse oximeter monitor, and an oxygen source and a flowmeter. You may also need a cardiac monitor.

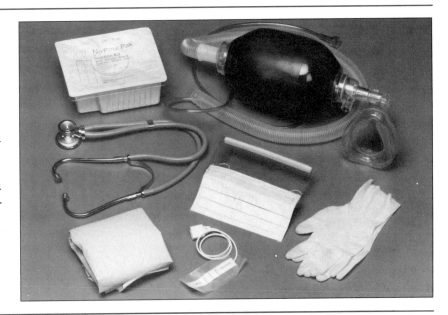

Wash your hands and explain weaning to the patient. Observe her level of consciousness and assess whether she can cooperate. Inform her that you'll stay with her after weaning begins. Later, reassure her that she can summon you quickly by using the call button. Elevate the head of the bed between 45 and 60 degrees. Obtain baseline vital signs (as shown) and watch for a fever (which may cause excessive fatigue during weaning).

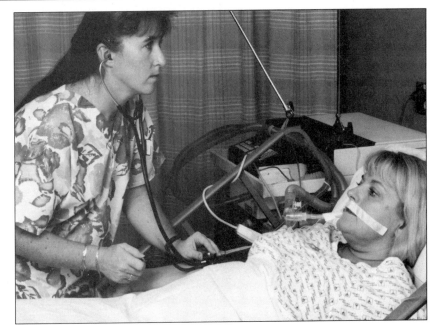

Put on gloves, a gown, and a face shield, and suction any secretions from the patient's endotracheal or tracheostomy tube and mouth. Doing so ensures an open airway and decreases airway resistance. Then auscultate the patient's chest for adequate breath sounds. Remove your gloves, gown, and face shield.

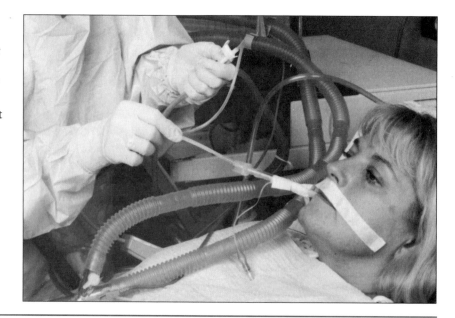

Connect the patient to a cardiac monitor (if you haven't already done so), and obtain a baseline rhythm strip.

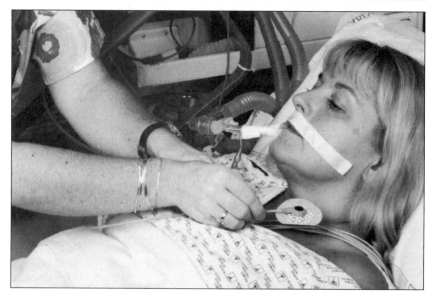

Attach the pulse oximeter sensor to the patient's ear or finger (as shown). Then attach the distal end of the hand-held resuscitation bag's connecting tubing to the flowmeter. Test the bag to make sure that it works properly, and place it within easy reach in case you need it quickly.

▶ *Clinical tip:* Using a pulse oximeter can help you detect decreasing oxygenation at an early stage. Just remember to obtain a doctor's order for its use (if your hospital, like most, requires this).

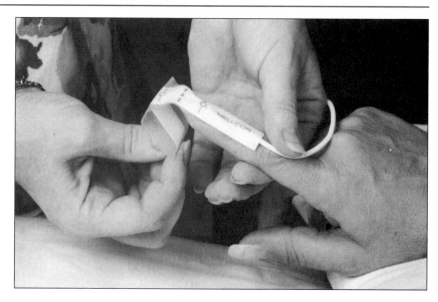

WEANING A PATIENT USING VENTILATORY SUPPORT

To breathe adequately on her own, the patient should meet certain criteria, including respiratory parameters that measure her pulmonary function. Once the patient meets these criteria, the doctor will order the weaning method that best meets the patient's needs in the transition from mechanical to spontaneous ventilation.

Measuring pulmonary function with the ventilator

For a patient on a ventilator (such as the Puritan-Bennett 7200 microprocessor shown on the following pages), you'll need a ventilation worksheet and a calculator. You may also need suction equipment, a gown, gloves, a face shield, and an arterial blood gas kit.

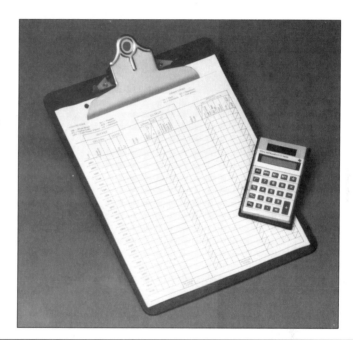

Begin assessing pulmonary function by noting the patient's respiratory frequency (f). Inform the patient that she'll be breathing on her own for the next 2 to 3 minutes. Reassure her that she'll continue to receive oxygen through the ventilator during that time but that the ventilator won't breathe for her. Press the CPAP key on the ventilator first (as shown) and then press ENTER. Observe the patient's breathing pattern.

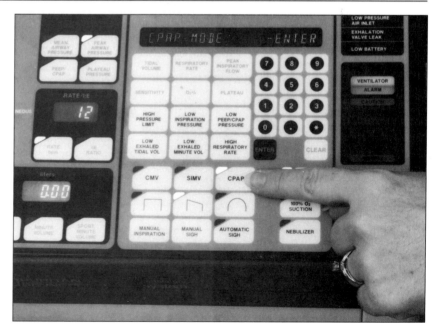

As soon as the patient's breathing becomes rhythmic, begin counting her respirations for 1 minute. Then return her to the previous ventilation mode; this will allow her to rest between pulmonary function assessments.

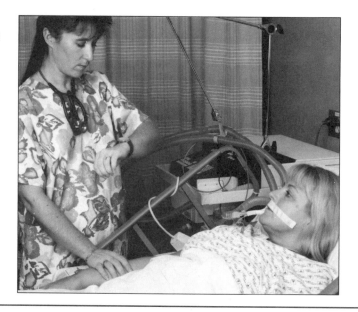

To measure minute volume (V̇E), again tell the patient that she'll be breathing on her own for the next 2 to 3 minutes but that she'll continue to receive oxygen. Press the CPAP and ENTER keys. Then press the SPONT. MINUTE VOLUME key (as shown).

Wait 1 minute after the patient begins breathing rhythmically. Then read the digital display denoting liters: This is the V̇E. After noting the value, return the patient to her previous ventilation mode. Once you know the f and V̇E values, calculate mean tidal volume (VT) as follows:

$$VT = \dot{V}E \div f$$

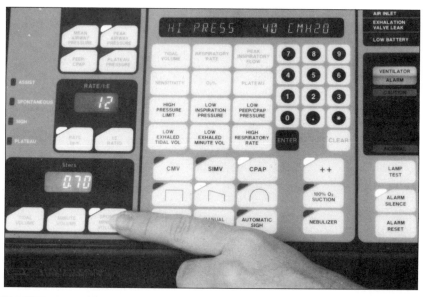

To measure vital capacity (VC), press the key with the double plus signs (+ +), and read the function prompt in the message window. Keep pressing the + + key until the words "32 VITAL CAPACITY" appear. (The number 32 is the function number for VC.)

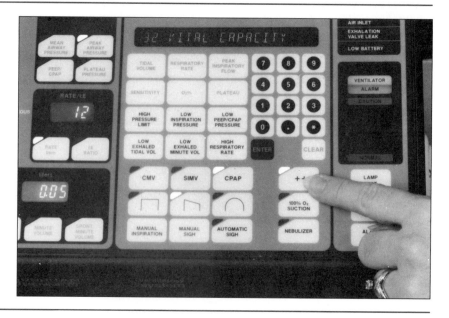

To continue measuring VC, instruct the patient to exhale, to inhale as deeply as possible, and then to exhale again as completely as possible without forced effort. As soon as the patient exhales *the second time*, press ENTER. Read the digital display appearing in the message window.

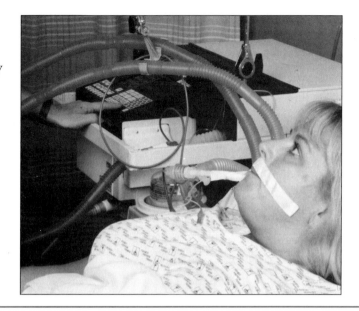

To measure negative inspiratory pressure, press the + + key and watch for the function prompt in the message window. Continue to press the + + key until "31 NEG INSP PRESSURE" appears in the message window. (The number 31 is the function number for negative inspiratory pressure.)

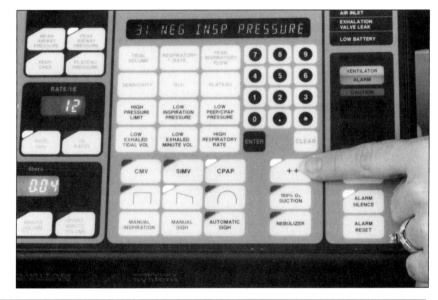

Before measuring negative inspiratory pressure, inform the patient that you'll ask her to take a deep breath. Explain that when she does, she'll feel like she can't get enough air. Reassure her that this sensation will last only a few seconds.

Once she takes the deep breath, press the ENTER key. Read the measurement that appears in the message window.

▶ *Clinical tip:* A negative inspiratory pressure below -20 cm H_2O suggests that the patient may not tolerate weaning.

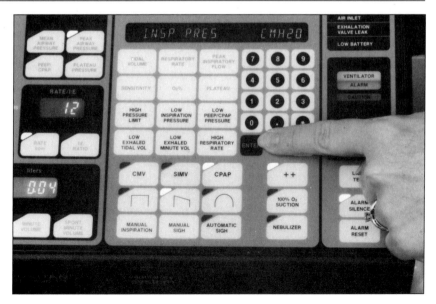

Setting the weaning mode

Once the pulmonary function test results indicate that the patient may be weaned successfully, the doctor will order the method—intermittent mechanical ventilation (IMV), synchronized intermittent mandatory ventilation (SIMV), continuous positive airway pressure (CPAP), pressure support ventilation (PSV), or assist-control ventilation (ACV), for example. Although the equipment used here doesn't perform ACV (SIMV would be used instead), some ventilators do offer this option.

Put on gloves and drain any fluid from the large-bore ventilator tubing into a glove attached to the proximal portion of the ventilator tubing (as shown) or into a waste receptacle. Secretions and condensate increase air resistance and the work of breathing.

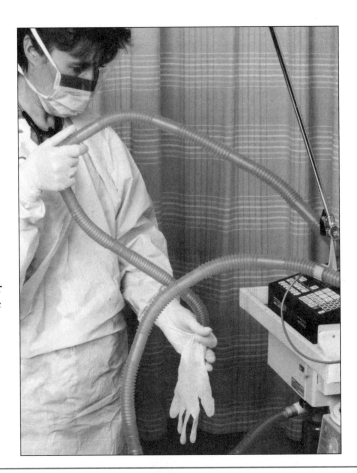

To select the IMV or SIMV modes

If you'll be using the IMV or SIMV mode, inform the patient that she'll begin breathing on her own but that she'll also receive some breathing assistance from the ventilator. Check her chart to verify the ordered respiratory rate, V_T, and fraction of inspired oxygen (FIO_2). Press the SIMV key and then press ENTER. Select the ordered respiratory rate, V_T, and FIO_2. Record all settings on the ventilator worksheet.

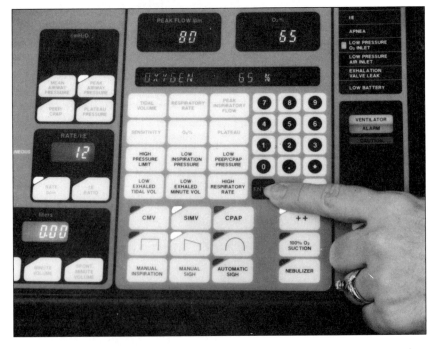

To select the CPAP mode

If the doctor also orders CPAP, tell the patient that she'll be breathing on her own but that an alarm will go off if she begins having difficulty. Press the CPAP key on the ventilator and then press ENTER.

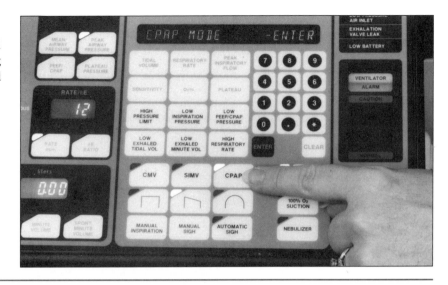

Next, press the PEEP/CPAP key located on the left side of the ventilator (near right).

Turn the PEEP/CPAP knob to the desired amount while observing the digital display in the window labeled "cm H$_2$O" above the PEEP/CPAP key (far right). Now check the analog meter to confirm the setting. The display needle should return to the ordered CPAP after the patient exhales. For example, if the patient should receive 5 cm H$_2$O of CPAP, the needle should remain at the number 5 after the patient exhales.

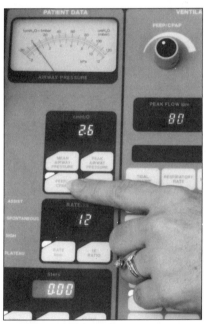

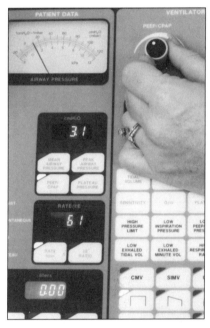

To select the PSV mode

If the doctor orders PSV, you'll usually set the ventilation mode for CPAP (PSV is more commonly used with CPAP than SIMV). Then press the + + key and watch the message display for "APNEA PARAMETERS." Again press the + + key until the message "10 PRESS SUPPORT" appears. (The number 10 is the function number for PSV.) Press ENTER and then select the ordered PSV value on the number keypad. Press ENTER again. The + + key light should remain illuminated, indicating that PSV is active.

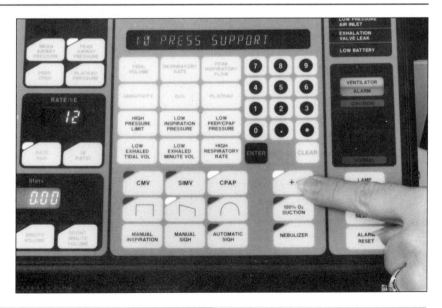

Monitoring patient response

To ensure that you're alerted to a problem promptly, check the alarms to make sure they're set correctly. To adjust the alarms, press the appropriate keys in the ventilator settings panel. Use the number keys to enter the desired value for each alarm, and then press ENTER.

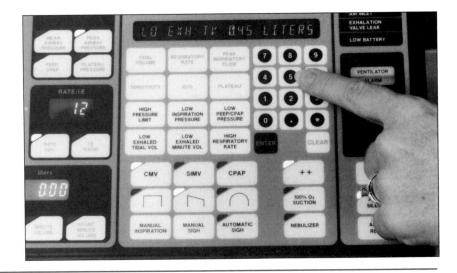

If needed, suction the patient after delivering several breaths of 100% oxygen through the ventilator.

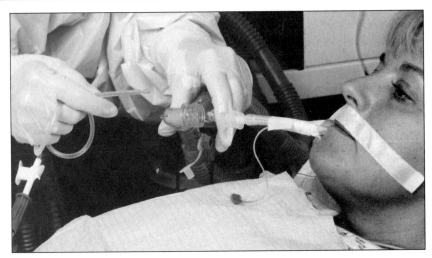

Wait 30 minutes and then draw a a blood sample for arterial blood gas (ABG) analysis. As ordered, make ventilator adjustments, such as decreasing the respiratory rate. Document the patient's response to weaning. Reassure her as necessary about her progress.

▶ *Clinical tip:* Be alert for such complaints as dyspnea, fatigue, abnormal breathing patterns, a heart rate exceeding 10% of baseline, arrhythmias, diaphoresis, pallor or cyanosis, confusion, restlessness, or agitation. If the patient exhibits any of these signs or symptoms, assess vital signs, draw blood for ABG analysis, return the patient to her original ventilator settings, and notify the doctor.

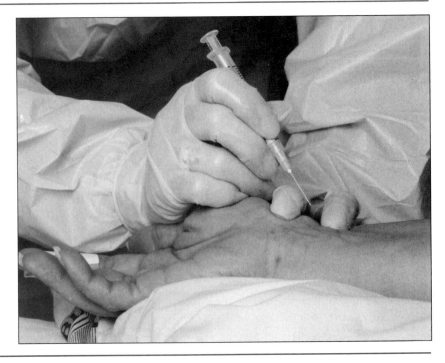

WEANING A PATIENT USING A T-PIECE

For some patients, the doctor may order weaning with a T-piece. This method is often used in the recovery room after anesthesia. Because weaning by this method doesn't have the advantage of the ventilator as a safety net, monitor your patient carefully throughout the procedure. Prepare her physically and emotionally as you would if you were using ventilatory support, but use other means (such as a respirometer and a negative inspiratory pressure meter) to measure pulmonary function.

You'll need a one-way T-piece circuit (which includes a T-piece, 6' [2 m] of large-bore, corregated tubing, and 3" to 6" of large-bore, corregated extension tubing—shown assembled), a pulse oximeter sensor, a suction kit, an arterial blood gas (ABG) kit, two sterile drapes, a rubber band, and several face shields, gowns, and pairs of gloves.

Additional equipment includes a respirometer, a negative inspiratory pressure meter, a mechanical jet nebulizer containing sterile distilled water or another device for delivering heated aerosolized oxygen, an oxygen source, a flowmeter, a pulse oximeter monitor, and the patient's ventilation worksheet.

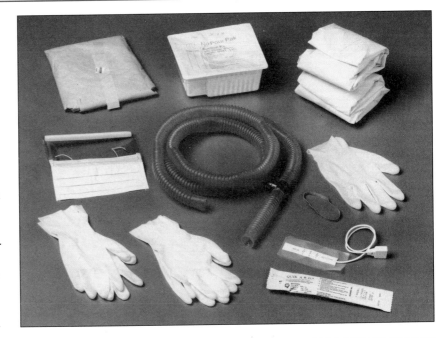

Measuring pulmonary function

Assess your patient's readiness for weaning by checking her pulmonary function with a respirometer and a negative inspiratory pressure meter. Put on a gown, gloves, and a face shield. Then place a sterile drape over the patient's upper chest. You may want to connect the patient to a cardiac monitor if she's not already being monitored.

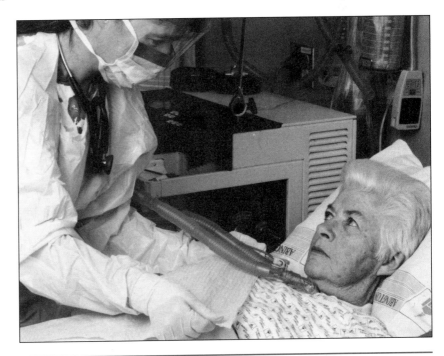

Attach the inspiratory port of the respirometer to the expiratory port of the T-piece circuit.

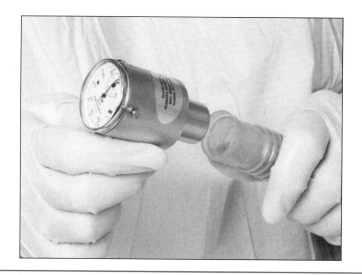

Disconnect the patient from the ventilator (as shown), and place the ventilator tubing on the sterile drape. Then connect the T-piece circuit to the patient's tracheostomy or endotracheal (ET) tube.

▶ *Clinical tip:* Placing the T-piece circuit between the respirometer and the patient's airway helps to prevent contamination of the respirometer with airway secretions.

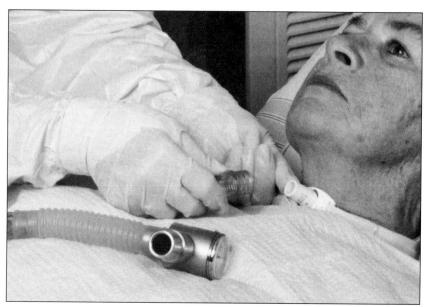

Zero the respirometer (as shown). As soon as the patient begins breathing rhythmically, measure respiratory frequency (f) by counting her respirations for 1 minute. After noting this value, turn the respirometer off and note the total number of liters and milliliters registered on the gauge. This is the minute volume ($\dot{V}E$) — also called minute ventilation.

▶ *Clinical tip:* You can also calculate $\dot{V}E$ by using this formula:

$$\dot{V}E = f \times VT$$

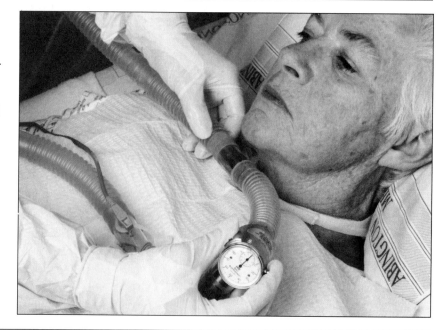

To measure tidal volume (VT), ask the patient to breathe normally. As she does so, watch the needle on the respirometer as it moves with each breath. Note the readings for several breaths, and use the average reading (in milliliters) to determine VT.

▶ **Clinical tip:** To determine mean VT, use this formula:
mean $VT = \dot{V}E \div f$

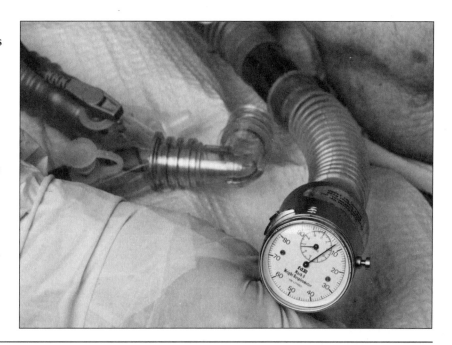

Because the patient usually doesn't receive supplemental oxygen during these tests, reconnect her to the ventilator as soon as possible. Let her rest and receive oxygen before repeating the tests. Repeat them only if the results don't match the patient's clinical condition or if you suspect that the patient misunderstood your directions. Record the measurements that are closest to normal.

▶ **Clinical tip:** If the doctor orders supplemental oxygen for the patient, first attach a piece of oxygen tubing to the flowmeter. Then place the other end near the inspiratory port of the T-piece. Blowing supplemental oxygen through the oxygen tubing and into the T-piece may give the patient enough oxygen to complete the pulmonary function tests without returning to the ventilator.

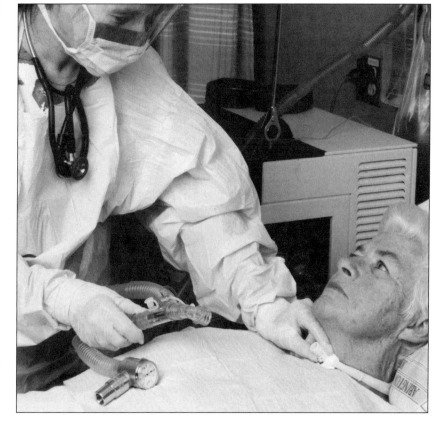

To measure vital capacity (VC), re-connect the respirometer to the expiratory port of the T-piece and again zero the instrument. Instruct the patient to exhale normally and then to inhale as deeply as possible. Tell her to hold her breath for 1 second.

While she holds her breath, turn on the respirometer so that maximum expiratory volume can be measured. Have her exhale as completely as possible without forced effort. Note the total number of liters and milliliters recorded on the respirometer. Again, reconnect the patient to the ventilator and allow her to rest.

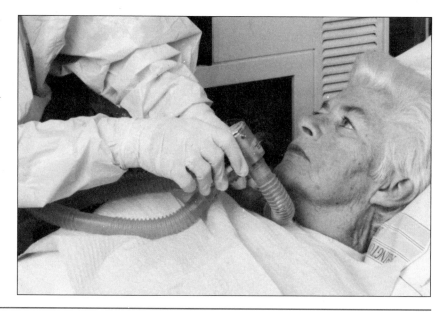

To measure maximum voluntary ventilation (MVV), disconnect the ventilator tubing and lay it on the sterile drape. Connect the T-piece to the tracheostomy or ET tube, and connect the respirometer to the T-piece. Zero the meter. Ask the patient to breathe as deeply and as quickly as possible for 15 seconds. Note the total number of liters and milliliters on the respirometer gauge. Multiply this number by 4 to obtain the patient's MVV over the course of 1 minute.

▶ *Clinical tip:* Don't be surprised if a patient with a tracheostomy opens her mouth when you ask her to take a deep breath. This is a common reflex action in tracheostomy patients.

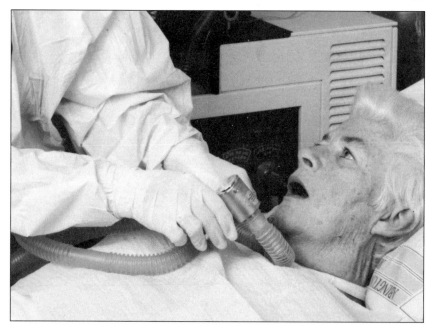

To measure negative inspiratory pressure, attach the negative inspiratory pressure meter to the inspiratory port of the T-piece. Position both the black and red needles at the zero mark on the gauge.

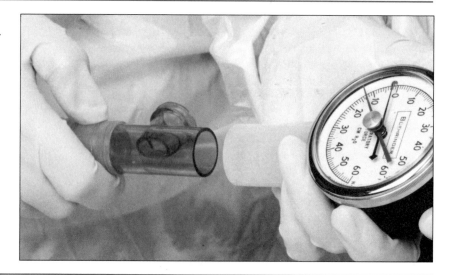

Disconnect the ventilator tubing and place it on the drape. Connect the T-piece to the patient's ET or tracheostomy tube (as shown). Warn the patient that she won't be able to inhale while you're performing this test. Reassure her that you'll complete the test within 10 seconds.

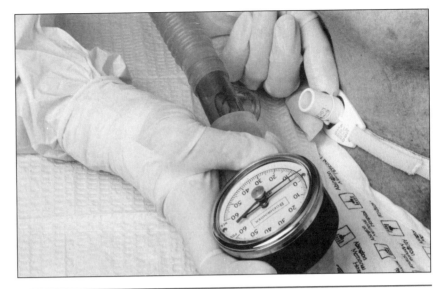

Ask the patient to exhale and then inhale as deeply as possible. The black needle on the gauge will move with inspiratory effort and then return to zero. The red needle will register and remain at the greatest negative pressure reading achieved. If the patient tolerates the test, repeat it twice more. Note the position of the red needle.

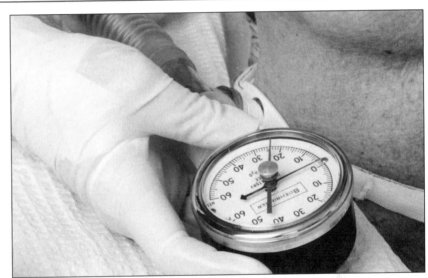

Initiating weaning

Before disconnecting the patient from the ventilator, explain the procedure. Put on another gown, gloves, and face shield. Then unscrew the lid from the nebulizer, and attach it to the oxygen source (as shown).

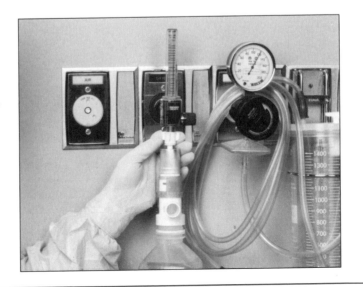

Attach the large-bore, corrugated extension tubing to the gas outlet of the nebulizer (as shown). Then place the T-piece at the opposite end.

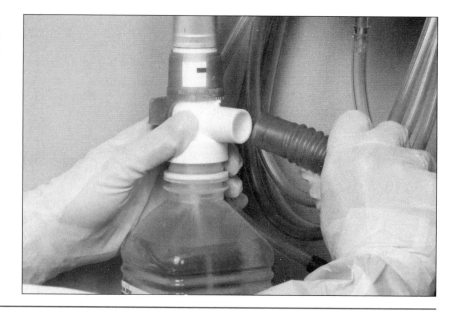

Finally, connect a piece of 3″ to 6″ extension tubing to the expiratory port of the T-piece. (This will act as an oxygen reservoir.)

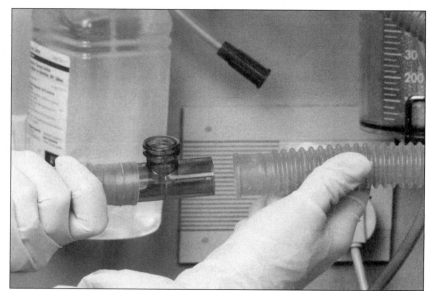

Turn on the oxygen flowmeter to the ordered level for fraction of inspired oxygen (FIO_2).

▶ **Clinical tip:** You'll usually need to increase the FIO_2 by 10% when using a T-piece. Doing so offsets the patient's additional breathing workload and his drop in VT.

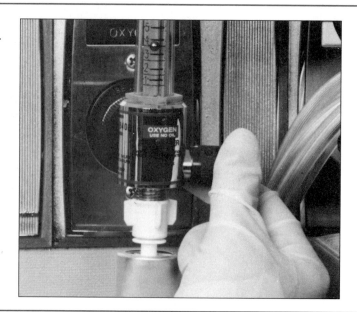

Place a new sterile drape across the patient's chest. Remove the ventilator circuit from the artificial airway, and place the ventilator tubing on the sterile drape. Attach the T-piece to the tracheostomy or ET tube. Then place a clean glove over the opening on the ventilator tubing or wrap the ventilator tubing with the sterile drape, and secure the drape in place with a rubber band to maintain the tubing's cleanliness.

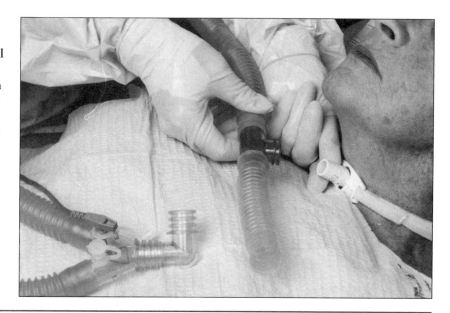

Instruct the patient to breathe normally. Look at the monitor and note the patient's respiratory frequency and pattern, heart rate, and cardiac rhythm (as shown). Also monitor the patient's breath sounds, pulse oximetry findings, and general appearance. Record your findings on the ventilation worksheet.

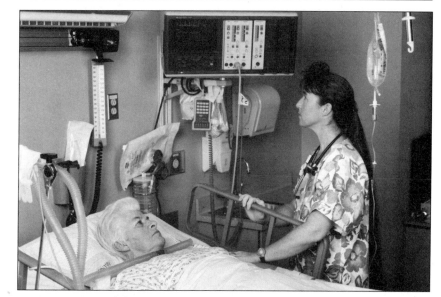

If necessary, suction the patient. Be sure to use the hand-held resuscitation bag and 100% oxygen to deliver additional oxygen before and after suctioning.

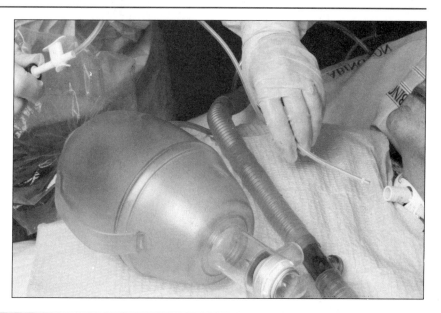

After the patient has been breathing spontaneously for 30 minutes with the T-piece, obtain an ABG analysis as ordered.

▷ *Clinical tip:* Be alert for dyspnea, fatigue, abnormal breathing patterns, a heart rate more than 10% above baseline, arrhythmias, diaphoresis, pallor or cyanosis, confusion, restlessness, or agitation. If the patient exhibits any of these signs or symptoms, draw a blood sample for ABG analysis, return the patient to her original ventilator settings, and notify the doctor.

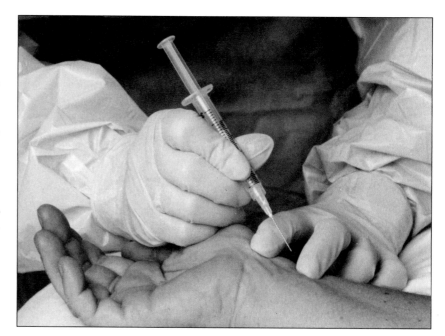

Return the patient to the ventilator after the prescribed weaning time elapses. Document her response to the weaning trial. Reassure her about her progress as appropriate.

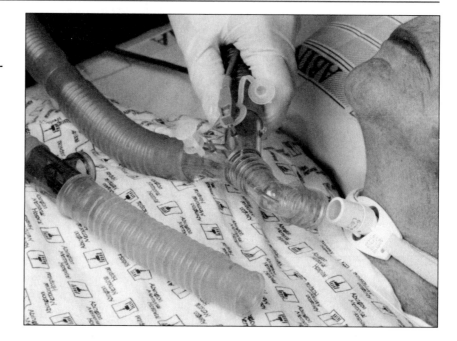

When to stop weaning

Discontinue weaning and resume mechanical ventilation if the patient experiences any of the following:
• blood pressure elevation of more than 20 mm Hg systolic or more than 10 mm Hg diastolic
• heart rate more than 10% above baseline or a rate above 120 beats/minute
• respiratory rate increase of more than 10 breaths/minute or a rate above 30 breaths/minute

• arrhythmias
• reduced tidal volume
• elevated partial pressure of arterial carbon dioxide
• anxiety
• dyspnea
• accessory muscle use in breathing or an otherwise deteriorating breathing pattern.

PERFORMING EXTUBATION

Once the patient achieves successful spontaneous ventilation, you may remove her endotracheal (ET) tube. (If the patient has a tracheostomy tube, the doctor may direct that it stay in place for awhile.) Before removing any breathing tube, however, make sure that the patient has a patent upper airway, that she can clear secretions, and that she has adequate spontaneous tidal volume, vital capacity, minute volume (also called minute ventilation), and negative inspiratory pressure.

Take the following equipment needed to remove the ET tube to the patient's bedside: a suction kit, tonsillar suction equipment, a 10-ml luer-lock syringe, a hand-held resuscitation bag with an appropriate-sized face mask, gloves, a gown, a face shield, an oxygen delivery system (usually a face mask), and a linen-saver pad.

You'll also need an oxygen flowmeter attached to an oxygen source.

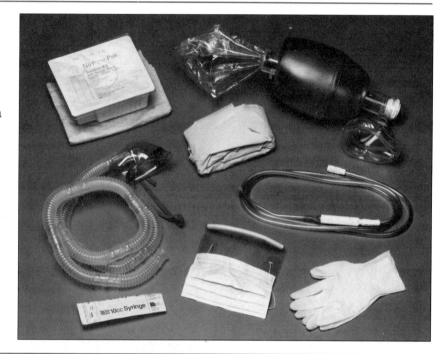

Wash your hands, explain the procedure to the patient, and put on the gown, gloves, and mask. Place her in an upright position, and lay the linen-saver pad across her upper chest.

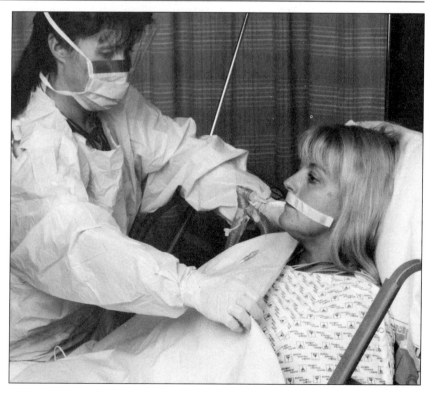

Set up the oxygen delivery system that the patient will use after extubation (as shown). Be sure the hand-held resuscitation bag and intubation equipment are nearby.

▷ *Clinical tip:* To help prevent laryngospasm, use an oxygen delivery system that can provide high-humidity oxygen immediately after extubation.

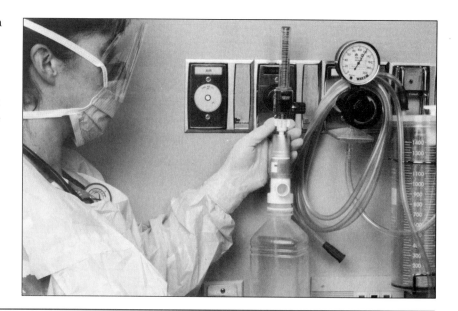

After giving the patient 100% oxygen from the hand-held resuscitation bag, suction her ET tube.

Then use the tonsillar suction device to clear the posterior oropharynx (as shown). This will remove any secretions from the top of the ET tube's cuff.

Again give the patient several breaths of 100% oxygen via the hand-held resuscitation bag.

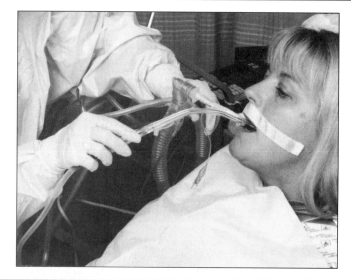

Gently remove the tape or securing straps from the ET tube (near right). Attach the luer-lock syringe to the pilot balloon, and withdraw all the air from the ET tube's tracheal cuff.

▷ *Clinical tip:* Observe the tracheal cuff carefully; it isn't deflated until the pilot balloon completely collapses (far right).

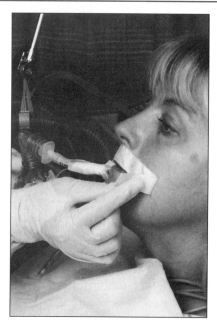
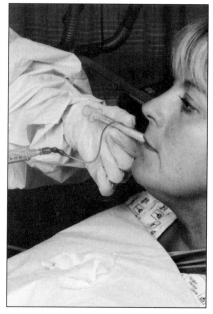

Grasp the ET tube, and ask the patient to cough. As she does, gently but firmly pull out the ET tube, wrap it in the linen-saver pad, and discard it in a biohazard container.

Note: Some hospitals permit only a doctor or a nurse anesthetist to remove an ET tube in case immediate reintubation becomes necessary.

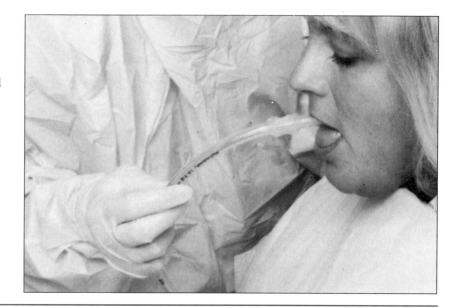

Alternatively, insert a sterile suction catheter into the ET tube 1″ to 2″ (2.5 to 5 cm) below the distal end of the ET tube. Have the patient take a deep breath. At the peak of inspiration, remove the ET tube and the suction catheter (while applying suction) simultaneously, in one smooth, outward and downward motion. Follow the natural curve of the patient's mouth. Suctioning during extubation removes secretions retained at the end of the tube.

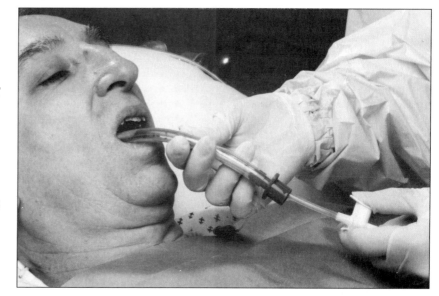

Adjust the flowmeter to the ordered FIO₂ setting, and place the oxygen mask or other ordered oxygen delivery device on the patient's face.

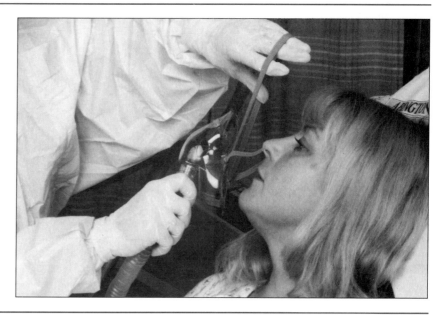

If the patient can use a tonsillar suction device, give her the device and explain how to use it. Instruct her to suction her throat and mouth as needed to remove oral secretions.

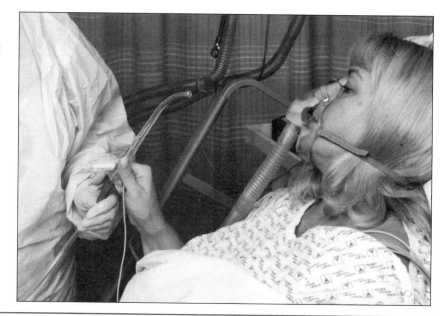

After extubation, monitor the patient for shortness of breath, hoarseness, respiratory fatigue, or other signs of respiratory distress. Evaluate oxygenation by monitoring ABG levels and pulse oximetry findings as ordered. Document the patient's tolerance of extubation, being sure to record any complications as well as nursing or medical interventions.

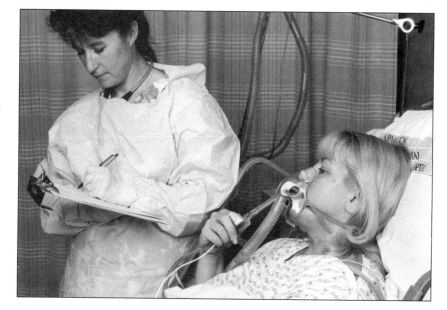

Understanding terminal weaning

Some patients never recover adequate spontaneous ventilation because of a primary respiratory problem or a nonrespiratory condition, such as a disease, sepsis, or malnutrition. In such situations, an informed patient who is competent to make medical decisions or a designated family member may choose to discontinue life-sustaining ventilation. This is known as terminal weaning.

Life-sustaining ventilation may also be discontinued if further treatment is medically futile or will only prolong the patient's pain and suffering.

Whatever the reason, terminal weaning should be carried out with utmost sensitivity to the patient's and family's emotional needs. Schedule the withdrawal of ventilatory support according to the patient's and family's wishes. Administer ordered analgesics as necessary to ensure patient comfort. Also, keep in mind that although the expected outcome is death, death may not occur immediately or at all.

Neurologic Monitoring

LEARNING ABOUT NEUROLOGIC MONITORING

With the availability of such powerful diagnostic tools as computed tomography scanning and magnetic resonance imaging, identifying and treating neurologic disorders has become faster, less invasive, and more accurate. Besides promising better health care for today's patients, these and other technological advances have made the nurse's role more challenging and crucial than ever.

Assisted by sophisticated monitors, computers, and related equipment, today's nurse can contribute to faster, more precise medical diagnosis, anticipate potential complications, and act to offset secondary or permanent effects.

However, with the increasing array of equipment and monitoring techniques, the nurse must continually refine her skills and update her knowledge. Just to implement the skills needed to evaluate cerebral function, cranial nerves, sensory and motor functions, or reflexes may seem overwhelming.

On the whole, however, assessing neurologic status is reasonably straightforward. In fact, most daily nursing routines already include several parts of the neurologic examination. For example, simply talking to a patient tests his orientation, level of consciousness (LOC), and ability to form and execute speech. Mastering more complex techniques, such as intracranial pressure (ICP) monitoring, may be less difficult than you anticipate—especially with the help you'll find on the following pages.

ASSESSING NEUROLOGIC VITAL SIGNS

Called a neurocheck, the assessment of neurologic vital signs is a quick and simple way to detect and evaluate nervous system changes in your patient. This evaluation becomes especially important if your findings include subtle changes that point to serious complications, such as increasing ICP, an expanding infarction, or increasing pressure on the spinal cord.

Because the central nervous system (CNS) does not regenerate and the peripheral nervous system heals slowly and incompletely, you need to recognize signs of neurologic complications as soon as possible. Prompt detection may spare your patient irreversible damage, such as hemiparesis, aphasia, or impaired cognitive function.

A neurocheck supplements a routine vital signs assessment. It usually includes an evaluation of LOC, degree of orientation, pupillary activity, and muscle strength and tone.
• An evaluation of LOC checks the patient's response to stimuli, which reflects brain stem function. Changes in the LOC may well be the first sign of CNS deterioration.
• Evaluating the patient's degree of orientation (to place, time, date, situation, and person) helps check his higher cerebral function and thought-processing abilities.
• Alterations in pupillary activity (pupil size, shape, equality, and reactivity) may indicate changes in ICP.
• Muscle strength and tone, reflexes, and posture are all indicators of a patient's neurologic condition.

EVALUATING FURTHER

Depending on the patient's condition and the doctor's orders, you may perform neurologic assessments every 15 minutes to every 2 hours. Typically, you'll do frequent neurologic assessments to detect early complications from diagnostic or neurosurgical procedures. Frequent neurologic assessments also may be done before or after certain emergency interventions, such as cardiopulmonary resuscitation.

Some patients, such as those with spinal cord injuries or a cerebrovascular accident, will need more extensive neurologic assessment. For example, if your patient has a spinal cord injury, detailed information about his muscle tone and strength may help you identify a condition that preceded or followed the injury (for example, misalignment from a halo vest). Remember that patients with spinal cord injuries require frequent sensory assessment also.

But if your patient was admitted with a cerebrovascular accident, a head injury, or a tumor, you may need detailed information on cranial nerve function. With a head injury, for example, you'll evaluate cranial nerves VII (facial), IX (glossopharyngeal), and XII (hypoglossal) in depth.

Julie Tackenberg, RN, MA, CNRN, who contributed to this section, is a clinical nurse specialist for the Arizona Comprehensive Epilepsy Program, University Medical Center, Tucson. The publisher thanks *Doylestown (Pa.) Hospital* and *Hill-Rom*, Batesville, Ind., for their help.

PERFORMING A NEUROCHECK

A neurocheck helps you evaluate a patient's condition and stability quickly, identify signs of neuro-logic problems, and establish a firm base for your plan of care.

Assessing LOC and orientation

Explain the procedure to the patient, even if she appears unresponsive. Then measure her responses to various stimuli. Does she respond to auditory stimuli? If she doesn't, try a light tactile stimulus, such as a touch on her shoulder. Use standard test devices, such as the Glasgow Coma Scale, to score your findings.

▶ *Clinical tip:* When assessing LOC, remember that you are providing the stimulus.

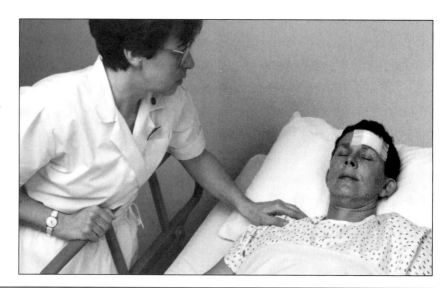

If neither sound nor touch arouses the patient, apply a painful stimulus. Using moderate pressure, squeeze the nail beds of her fingers. Assess the response. Then observe whether she maintains her LOC. The greater the stimulus needed to elicit a response, the greater the neurologic compromise.

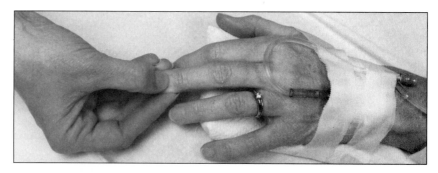

If the patient can speak or write a response, proceed with assessing her orientation. First, ask her to say her full name. If she responds, ask her where she is, then the day, season, and year. Assess her replies. Garbled words indicate problems with the motor nerves that govern speech. Rambling responses suggest difficulty with processing thoughts. Time the interval needed by the patient to respond. A prolonged interval suggests difficulty with thought processing and higher cognitive function.

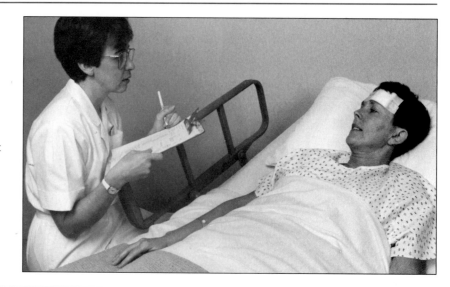

Evaluate how well the patient understands and follows one-step commands that require a motor response. For example, ask her to open and close her eyes and to stick out her tongue. Note whether she maintains her LOC, and check motor responses bilaterally to rule out monoplegia (paralysis of a single area) and hemiplegia (paralysis of one side of the body).

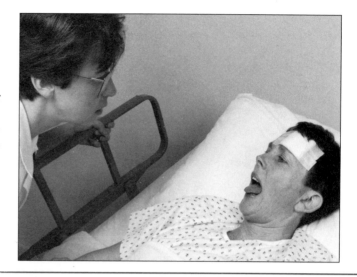

If possible, ask the patient to grip your hand—first with one hand, then the other. This quickly tests bilateral motor responses of the upper extremities.

▷ **Clinical tip:** If you rouse the patient from a deep sleep, be sure that she is fully awake and can give her full effort before you proceed. If you must gently shake her to keep her focused on your commands, suspect neurologic compromise.

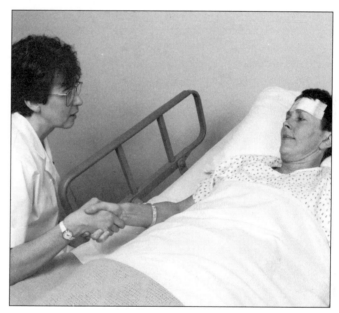

Examining pupillary response and eye movement

How the pupils respond and the eyes move tells you about cranial nerves II (optic), III (oculomotor), IV (trochlear), and VI (abducens) and, consequently, about brain stem function. To assess pupillary response and eye movement, you'll need a penlight and a pupil gauge. A pencil or pen is optional.

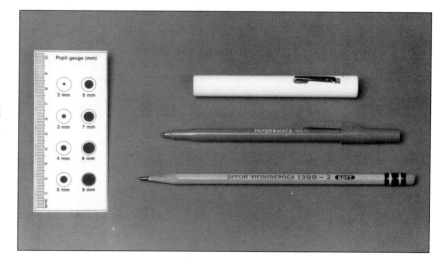

Begin by explaining the procedure to the patient. Then ask her to open her eyes. If she doesn't respond, gently lift her upper eyelids. In the room light, observe each pupil's size and shape. Compare both pupils for equality. As shown, use a gauge to evaluate pupil size more precisely. Remember that pupil sizes vary considerably, and some patients have normally unequal eyes (anisocoria). Also observe whether the pupils deviate from the eye's midline.

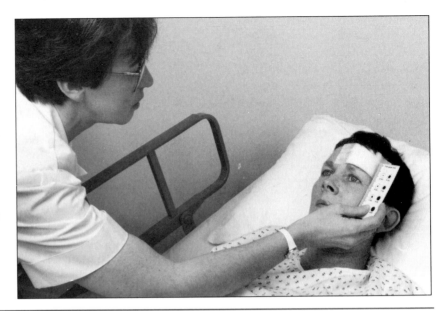

Test the patient's response to direct light. Darken the room slightly. Then hold one eyelid open and keep the other eye covered. Turn on the penlight, and swing the beam from the patient's ear toward the facial midline. Shine the light directly into the open eye. Normally, the pupil constricts immediately. When you turn off the penlight, the pupil should dilate. Wait about 20 seconds to repeat the test on the other pupil. This lets the eye recover from reflex stimulation.

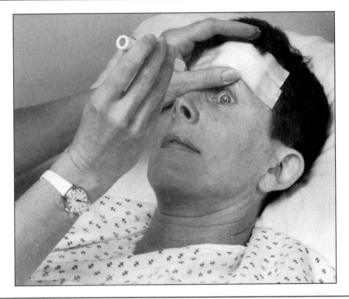

Test the consensual light response. Holding both eyelids open, shine the light into one eye only. Watch for constriction in the unlighted pupil, which indicates proper function of the branch of the optic nerve that crosses the optic chiasm.

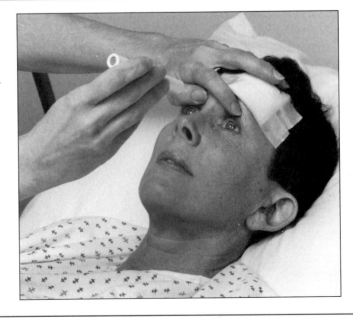

Brighten the room and have the conscious patient open her eyes. Observe the eyes for ptosis (drooping). To check extraocular movements, hold up a pencil (or your finger). Ask the patient to watch the pencil as you move it up, down, laterally, and obliquely. Ask her to move only her eyes—not her head. Watch carefully to see if her eyes move together as they track the pencil. Be alert for an eye that doesn't travel fully in the direction of the pencil or one that jerks or oscillates (nystagmus) involuntarily.

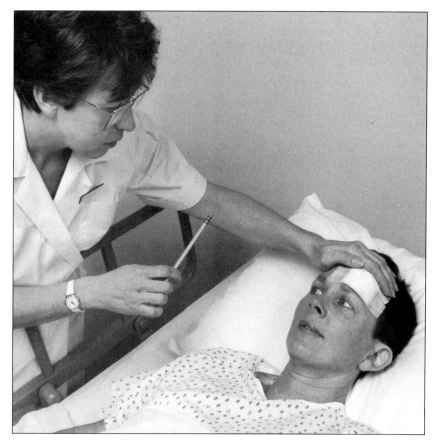

Next, check accommodation. Hold the pencil (or your finger) midline and a few feet from the patient's face. Have the patient focus on the pencil while you gradually move it toward her nose. Normally her eyes should converge, with both pupils constricting equally.

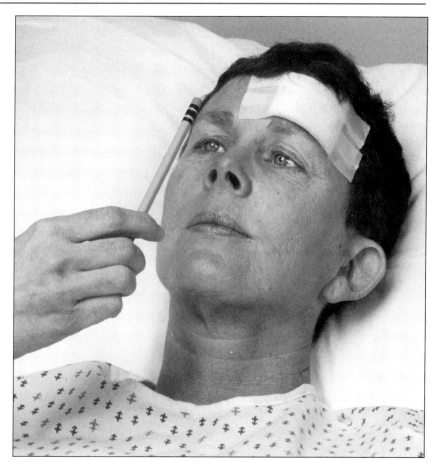

In an *unconscious patient,* test the oculocephalic (doll's eye) reflex. First be sure that the patient is lying flat. Remove the pillow. Then stand at the head of the bed. Hold the eyes open, using your hand nearest the patient.

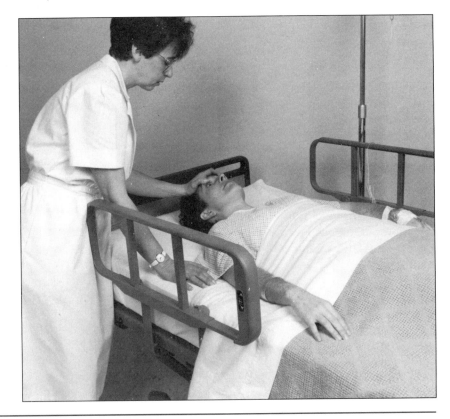

Rapidly turn the patient's head to one side, then the other. If the eyes move in the direction opposite the side to which you turned her head (for example, if her eyes move right when you turn her head left), the reflex is intact. In comatose patients, the eyes usually don't move or they move from side to side very slowly.

▶ *Clinical tip:* Never perform this procedure if you suspect that the patient has an injured cervical spine.

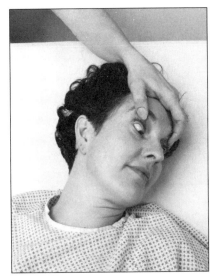

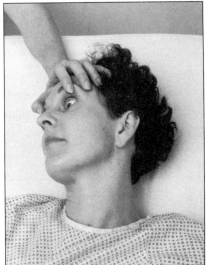

Evaluating muscle strength and tone

If your patient is conscious, test her grip strength in both hands at the same time. Extend your hands, ask the patient to squeeze your fingers as hard as she can, and compare the strength of each hand. The patient's dominant hand usually has a stronger grip.

▶ *Clinical tip:* Extend only two or three fingers for the patient to squeeze. An over-zealous patient may hurt you unintentionally.

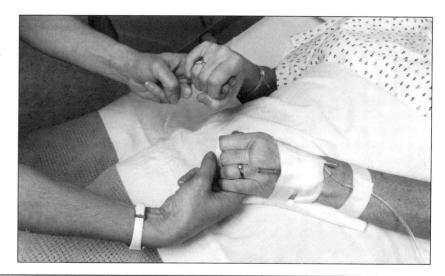

Test the patient's arm strength by having her flex one arm at a time. Ask her to try to bring her fist to her chest while you provide resistance by pulling her arm toward you. Note the strength in each arm and the equality of effort in both arms.

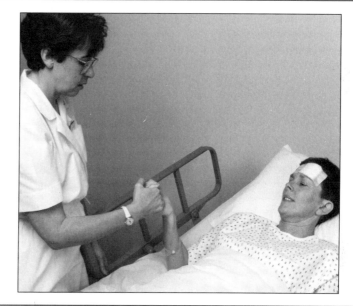

To test leg strength, have the patient raise her legs, one at a time, against gentle downward pressure from your hand. Gently push down on the anterior aspect of the lower leg below the shin to evaluate muscle strength (as shown). Or have the patient push down into your hand with her foot, then move her toes toward her head while you provide resistance by pulling her toes toward you.

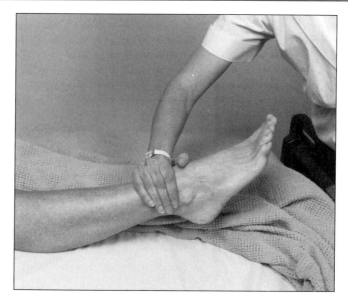

To assess muscle tone and abnormal responses, flex and extend the patient's arms, first on one side and then on the other side. Observe and palpate the muscles during this activity (as shown) to identify normal, rigid, or flaccid tone.

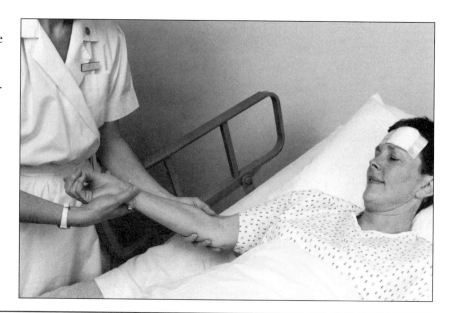

Next, flex and extend one leg and then the other, again observing and palpating for muscle tone.

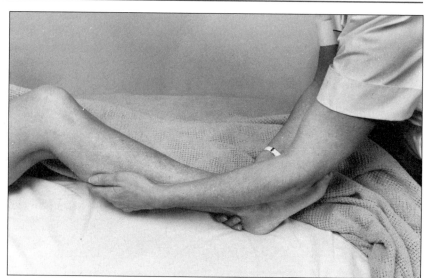

If your patient is unconscious, judge muscle strength and tone by the vigor of her spontaneous and reflex movements. To do so, apply a strong painful stimulus (as shown) to elicit movement. If the patient draws away, compare the rapidity and strength of her response to her baseline response. If she fails to respond or assumes a decorticate or a decerebrate posture, notify the doctor at once.

Whether the patient is conscious or unconscious, complete the assessment by measuring vital signs. Note the pulse pressure—the difference between systolic and diastolic pressures—because widening pulse pressure suggests increasing ICP.

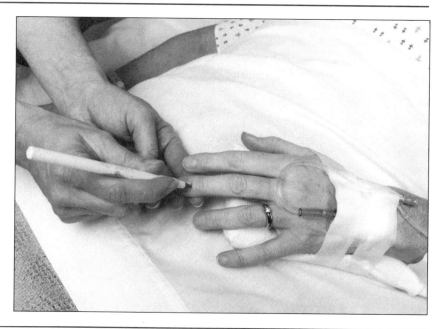

INSIGHTS AND INTERPRETATIONS

Understanding pupil size and reaction to light

As a nurse, you know that observing pupillary activity is an important part of a neurologic screening. You know, too, that the ongoing record of your patient's pupil size and reaction to light allows you to quickly recognize possible neurologic disorders and complications. Use the responses and indications described below as a guide when you assess your patient's pupil responses.

Note: Although this chart describes pupil size generally as small and large, you'll need to document pupil size by exact measurement whenever you assess your patient's pupillary changes.

PUPIL DESCRIPTION	REACTION TO LIGHT	SIGNIFICANCE
Large, unilateral	Nonreactive	Uncal herniation with oculomotor nerve damage or brain stem compression resulting from any expanding mass or lesion or from an aneurysm
Large, bilateral	Nonreactive	Midbrain damage. (Parasympatholytic drugs, such as atropine or scopolamine hydrobromide, may also cause this response.)
Midposition, bilaterally fixed	Nonreactive	Midbrain damage caused by edema, hemorrhage, infarctions, lacerations, or contusions
Small (pinpoint), usually bilateral but may be unilateral	Nonreactive	Lesion of the pons, usually after a hemorrhage; may result in blocked sympathetic impulses. Expect this response in a patient receiving opiates, such as morphine.
Small, bilateral	Reactive	Expect this response in certain toxic or metabolic conditions, such as phenothiazine toxicosis.

Using the Glasgow Coma Scale

The Glasgow Coma Scale provides a standard reference for assessing or monitoring a patient with suspected or confirmed brain injury. The scale measures three responses to stimuli—eye opening, verbal response, and motor response—and assigns a number to each possible response within the categories. The lowest total score is 3; the highest, 15. A score of 7 or less indicates coma.

Note: If your patient's eyes are closed by swelling, mark his chart with a "C." If he can't speak because he has an endotracheal or tracheostomy tube, don't attempt to score his verbal response. Rather, record "E" if he has an endotracheal tube or "T" for a tracheostomy tube.

CHARACTERISTIC	RESPONSE	SCORE
Eye opening	• Spontaneous	4
	• To verbal command	3
	• To pain	2
	• No response	1
Best verbal response (Arouse patient with painful stimuli, if necessary)	• Oriented and converses	5
	• Disoriented and converses	4
	• Uses inappropriate words	3
	• Makes incomprehensible sounds	2
	• No response	1
Best motor response	• Obeys commands	6
	• To painful stimuli: Localizes pain, pushes stimulus away	5
	• Flexes and withdraws	4
	• Abnormal flexion	3
	• Extension	2
	• No response	1
		Total: 3 to 15

COMPLICATIONS

Recognizing warning postures

If your patient is unconscious and assumes either decorticate or decerebrate posturing, alert the doctor immediately. These are ominous signs of central nervous system deterioration.

Decorticate posture
In this abnormal flexion, the patient's arms lie adducted and flexed, with the wrists and fingers flexed on the chest. The legs may extend stiffly and turn inward. The feet are in plantar flexion. Decorticate posture usually indicates a lesion—of the frontal lobe, internal capsule, or cerebral peduncles.

Decerebrate posture
In this position marked by abnormal extension, the patient's arms are adducted and stiffly extended with the wrists pronated and the fingers flexed. One or both legs extend stiffly with the feet in plantar flexion. Typically, decerebrate posture indicates upper brain stem lesions.

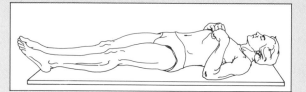

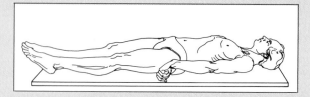

LEARNING ABOUT I.C.P. MONITORING

Intracranial pressure (ICP) results from the brain and related cranial contents exerting pressure against the inside of the skull. Normally, ICP ranges from 0 to 15 mm Hg. It rises when the volume of any component in the cranial vault—brain tissue, blood, or cerebrospinal fluid (CSF)—increases without an equivalent decrease in another component.

In your practice, you'll need to monitor ICP for various reasons—for instance, if your patient undergoes a craniotomy, sustains severe head trauma, or has an intracranial hemorrhage. Monitoring can detect elevated ICP early, before danger signs develop. Early detection and prompt intervention may avert or minimize neurologic damage.

Because ICP monitoring is an invasive procedure, it carries risks, such as infection, hemorrhage, increased cerebral edema, and meningeal irritation. Besides assessing your patient for these and other complications, you'll observe the equipment for occlusions in the intracranial catheter or the monitor's sensing device and other problems.

REVIEWING MONITORING METHODS AND DEVICES

ICP monitoring requires a catheter, a subarachnoid bolt, or an epidural, an intraparenchymal, or a subdural pressure monitoring device. Some of these systems can also be used to drain CSF and relieve pressure.

Intraventricular catheter monitoring

This type of monitoring measures ICP directly. It also allows evaluation of brain compliance and drainage of significant amounts of CSF. First the surgeon drills a burr hole in the skull and inserts a small polyethylene or silicone rubber catheter into the lateral ventricle. Then he connects the catheter to a fluid-filled line that has an external transducer. (Or he may use a fiber-optic transducer-tipped catheter, which doesn't require a fluid-filled transducer.)

Because the monitoring catheter penetrates the cerebrum, the catheter insertion procedure carries the risk of infection and brain damage. Contraindications typically include stenotic cerebral ventricles, cerebral aneurysm in the path of catheter placement, and suspected vascular lesions.

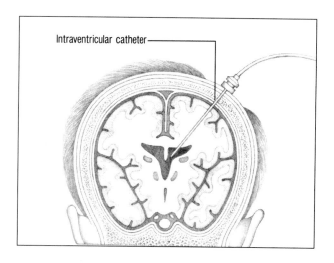

Intraventricular catheter

Subarachnoid bolt monitoring

In this procedure, a special bolt is inserted into the subarachnoid space through a twist-drill burr hole in the front of the skull. The bolt connects to a fluid-filled line that has an external transducer. Monitoring with a subarachnoid bolt carries less risk of infection and parenchymal damage than monitoring with the intraventricular catheter because the bolt doesn't penetrate the cerebrum. The system allows collection of small amounts of CSF for culture.

Disadvantages of this system include its inability to drain large amounts of CSF and its tendency to become occluded more readily than the intraventricular catheter. This system can be used only in patients with intact skulls.

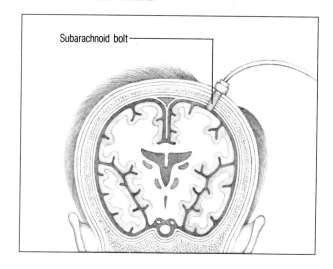

Subarachnoid bolt

Contributors to this section include *Julie Tackenberg, RN, MA, CNRN*, clinical nurse specialist, University Medical Center, Tucson, Ariz.; *Ellie Franges, RN, MSN, CCRN, CNRN*, director of patient care services, CNS Unit, Lehigh Valley Hospital, Allentown, Pa.; and *Marie Wilson, RN, BSN, CCRN*, clinical nurse III, Thomas Jefferson University Hospital, Philadelphia. The publisher thanks *Pudenz-Schulte Medical Corporation*, Goleta, Calif.; *Camino Laboratories*, San Diego; *Delcrest Medical Products*, Blue Bell, Pa.; *Hill-Rom*, Batesville, Ind.; *Lehigh Valley Hospital*, Allentown, Pa.; and *Doylestown (Pa.) Hospital*.

Epidural sensor monitoring

The least invasive procedure with the lowest incidence of infection, this ICP monitoring method uses a tiny fiber-optic sensor inserted into the epidural space through a burr hole. A cable connects the sensor to a monitor.

Unlike an intraventricular catheter or a subarachnoid bolt, the sensor can't become occluded by blood or brain tissue. The system's main disadvantage is its questionable accuracy, because the epidural sensor doesn't measure ICP directly from a CSF-filled space. This method is contraindicated in patients who don't have an intact skull.

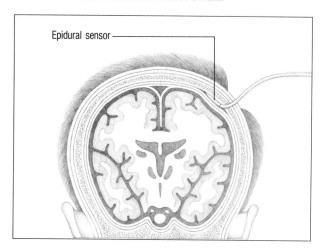

Epidural sensor

Intraparenchymal pressure monitoring

In this procedure, the surgeon inserts a fiber-optic transducer-tipped catheter through a small subarachnoid bolt. After puncturing the dura mater, the surgeon advances the catheter a few centimeters into the brain's white matter. There's no need to balance or calibrate the equipment after insertion.

Although this method doesn't provide direct access to CSF, measurements of ICP are accurate because brain tissue pressures correlate well with ventricular pressures. Intraparenchymal monitoring

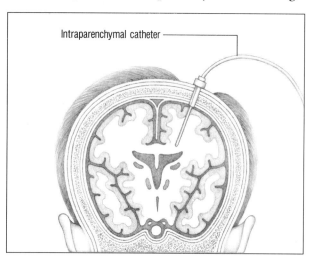

Intraparenchymal catheter

may be used to obtain ICP measurements in patients with compressed or dislocated ventricles.

The main drawback of this method is its inability to drain CSF. Also, accurate measurement of pressure increases exceeding 20 mm Hg is difficult.

Subdural sensor monitoring

After performing a craniotomy, the surgeon inserts a fiber-optic transducer-tipped catheter. He tunnels the catheter through a burr hole and places its tip on brain tissue under the dura mater. The tip must be placed under intact skull—not under a bone flap—to avoid measurement distortions caused by pressure changes from flap movement. The main drawback of this method is its inability to drain CSF.

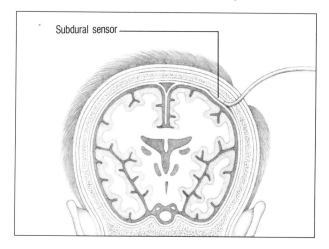

Subdural sensor

Regardless of the method used for your patient, the monitoring device is always inserted by a neurosurgeon in the operating room, emergency department, or critical care unit. The insertion always requires strict sterile technique to reduce the risk of central nervous system infection. Also, you'll use strict sterile technique while setting up the monitoring system.

Although ICP monitoring system designs vary, most work similarly. A fluid-filled line connects the catheter or bolt to a disposable transducer. This fluid-filled catheter system communicates the patient's ICP to the external transducer. The transducer then transmits pressure readings to a monitor for display.

When a fiber-optic transducer-tipped catheter is used, a fluid-filled transducer isn't required. Instead, the device uses optical fibers and a specialized diaphragm to transmit light impulses produced by pressure changes inside the cranium. An amplifier converts the light impulses to electrical signals, which are then displayed on a monitor screen. Another monitor can be connected to display an ICP waveform.

INITIATING I.C.P. MONITORING

Various preassembled ICP monitoring systems are available. Each has its own setup protocol, and each aims to reduce the risk of infection by eliminating the need for multiple stopcocks, manometers, and transducer assemblies. Review your hospital's guidelines and the manufacturer's instructions for your particular system.

Once you've set up the equipment for monitoring ICP, you'll prepare the patient for surgical insertion of the monitoring catheter or subarachnoid bolt. You'll also assist the surgeon with the procedure and dress the site afterward.

Typically, you'll use a preassembled external drainage and monitoring system when you're monitoring ICP by an intraventricular catheter, a subarachnoid bolt, or another intracranial device. The Becker system (shown here) can monitor ICP as well as drain CSF. To begin using the system, you'll need a preassembled and packaged external monitoring system, a disposable transducer and a sterile luer-lock cap, preservative-free 0.9% sodium chloride solution (two vials or a 50-ml bag), a 30-ml luer-lock syringe, a 20G needle, a level, two sterile drapes, sterile gloves and a plastic gown, and sterile surgical masks (optional). In addition, you'll need an I.V. pole and clamp.

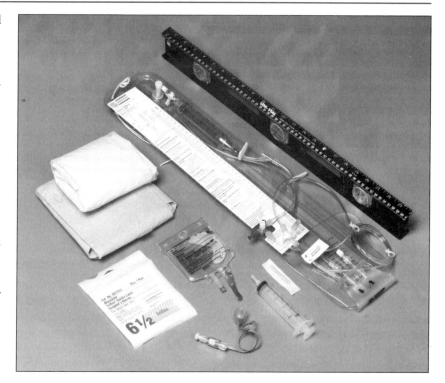

To insert an ICP monitoring device, gather the following equipment: precut sterile 4″ × 4″ gauze pads, linen-saver pads, skin preparation trays, hair scissors, sterile drapes, povidone-iodine solution, sterile gowns, two or more surgical masks, sterile gloves, povidone-iodine ointment, and head dressing supplies (two rolls of sterile 4″ elastic gauze and adhesive tape). You may also need to obtain a fenestrated drape and have suction equipment on hand.

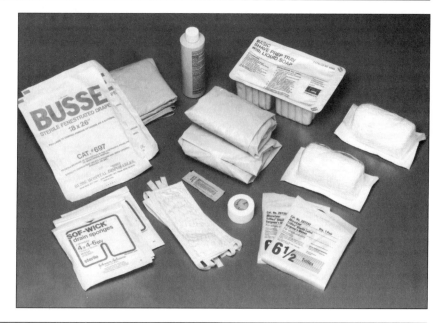

Setting up a preassembled monitoring system

Explain the procedure to the patient or his family, and find out if he's allergic to iodine preparations. Ensure that the patient or a responsible family member has signed a consent form.

Obtain baseline vital signs (routine and neurologic). These will help you to promptly detect any changes in the patient's condition during the procedure. Place the patient in the supine position, and elevate the head of the bed about 30 degrees or as ordered. Use the degree marker on the bed.

Use strict sterile technique to prepare the system. Begin by placing a sterile drape on the overbed table.

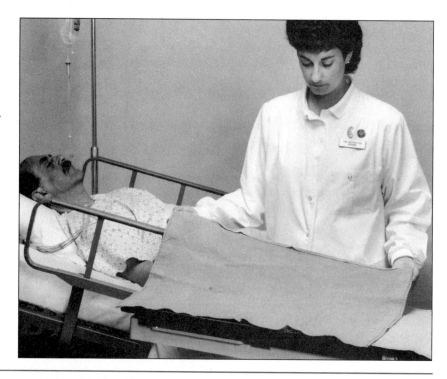

Remove the Becker system from its outer wrapper, and drop it onto the sterile field. Check to make sure that all the components are correctly preassembled and intact according to the manufacturer's description. Also place the luer-lock syringe, the 20G needle, and the two vials or 50-ml bag of preservative-free 0.9% sodium chloride solution (outer wrapper removed) on the sterile field. If you must delay the procedure for any reason, cover the equipment with the second sterile drape.

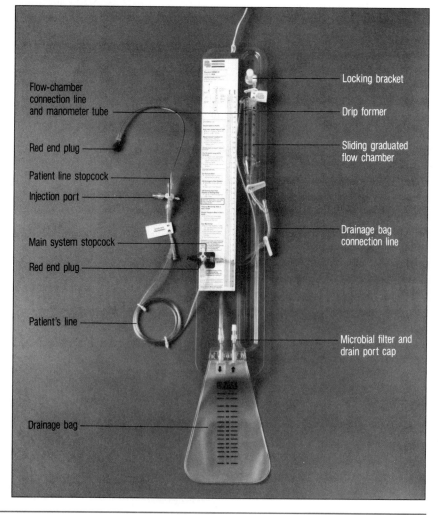

Flow-chamber connection line and manometer tube

Red end plug

Patient line stopcock

Injection port

Main system stopcock

Red end plug

Patient's line

Drainage bag

Locking bracket

Drip former

Sliding graduated flow chamber

Drainage bag connection line

Microbial filter and drain port cap

Don a gown and gloves. Fill the syringe with 30 ml of 0.9% sodium chloride solution from the I.V. bag or the two vials. Remove the needle from the syringe.

▶ *Clinical tip:* Some hospitals also require a mask for this procedure so be sure to check your hospital's policy.

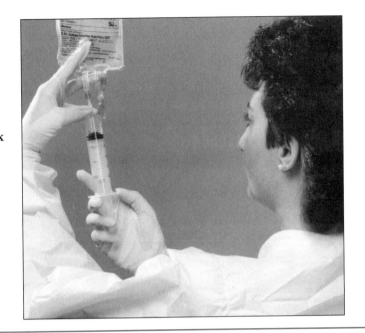

Use the syringe to flush the system with the sodium chloride solution. To do so, remove the injection cap from the patient line stopcock and attach the syringe (as shown).

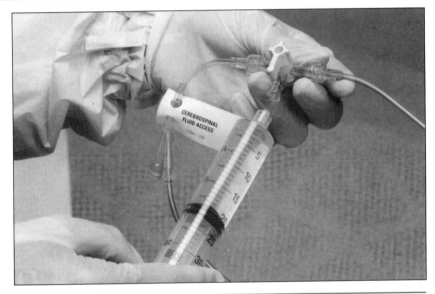

Turn the stopcock on the patient's line off to the short end of the line. Then flush the line through to the drip chamber. Allow a few drops to flow through the flow chamber (the manometer), the tubing, and the one-way valve into the drainage bag.

▶ *Clinical tip:* Fill the tubing and the manometer slowly to minimize air bubbles. If any air bubbles surface, be sure to force them from the system.

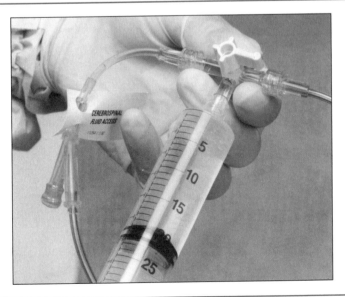

Loosen the red end plug on the patient's line. Turn the stopcock off to the long portion of the patient's line and flush the short portion, which connects to the intraventricular catheter. Then tighten the red end plug, and turn the stopcock on the patient's line off to the patient.

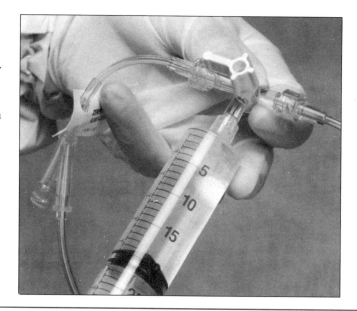

Attach the disposable transducer to the monitoring system. With the system shown here, the transducer may be attached to the stopcock on the patient's line. (It may also be attached to the main system stopcock, if preferred.) Follow your hospital's policy on the correct procedure. Attach the 20G needle to the syringe and fill the transducer with about 1 ml of the 0.9% sodium chloride solution. Then make sure that the free arm of the transducer is covered with a sterile luer-lock cap.

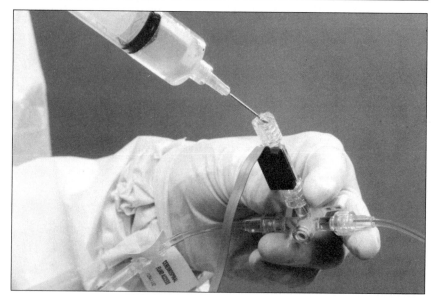

Check the setup for air bubbles or leaks. If you see any air bubbles, clear them from the system. If you notice any leaks, change the tubing or connectors.

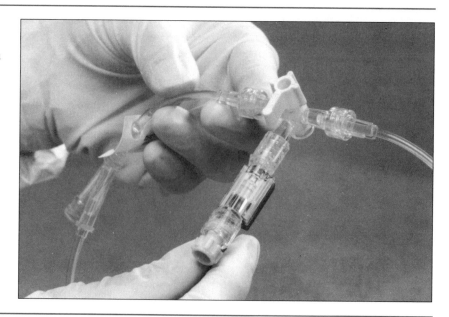

Hang the external drainage monitoring system on the I.V. pole. Be sure to close the slide clamp below the flow chamber and turn the stopcock on the patient's line off to the patient.

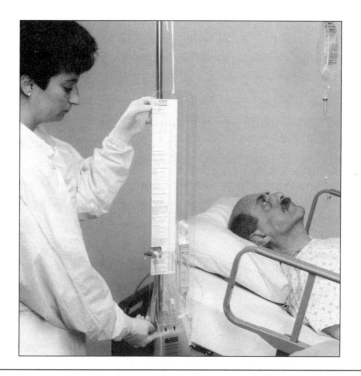

Lower the flow chamber and its inlet tube until the arrows point to zero. Then align the zero of the flow chamber with the center line of the patient's head (as shown). Locate this point, which is about 1″ (2.5 cm) above the external auditory meatus, using a level. This point corresponds to the level of the foramen of Monro.

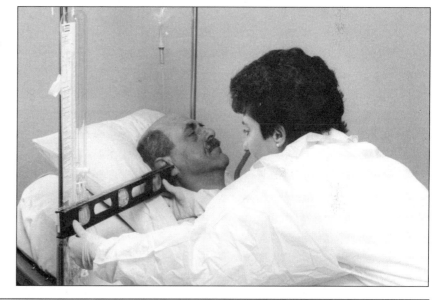

Following the manufacturer's instructions, zero the monitor. Make sure that the stopcock on the patient's line is turned off to the external catheter. Also be sure to remove the red end plug from the patient's line.

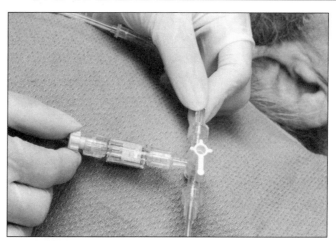

Assisting with catheter insertion

Place linen-saver pads under the patient's head. The surgeon will shave or clip the patient's hair at the insertion site. Afterward, carefully remove the linen-saver pads.

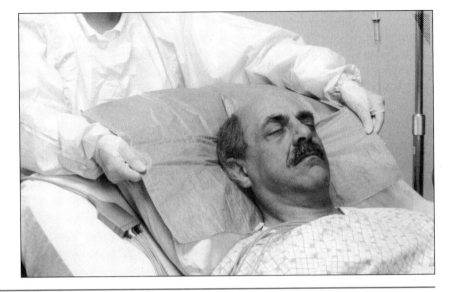

Next, you and the surgeon will put on sterile gowns, masks, and gloves. Any other person present for the procedure should wear a mask also.

The surgeon will cover the insertion area with a fenestrated drape to create a sterile field. Then as the surgeon inserts the catheter or bolt, steady the patient's head in your hands (as shown) and reassure him. Once the system is prepared, you may remove your mask. Assess the patient's level of consciousness, and watch for cardiac arrhythmias and abnormal breathing patterns.

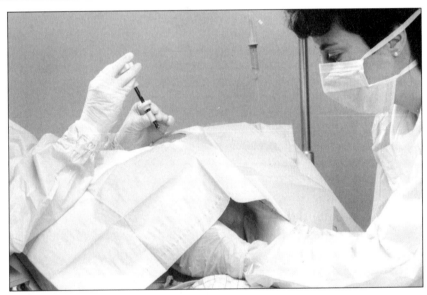

After the surgeon attaches the system, apply povidone-iodine ointment and precut sterile 4″ × 4″ gauze pads around the insertion site and the catheter.

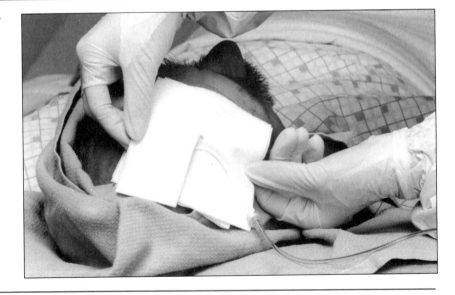

Wrap the site and the patient's head with sterile elastic gauze. As shown, use tape to secure the transducer stopcock (which is either on the patient's line or the main system, depending on the preferred connection site) at the level of the foramen of Monro.

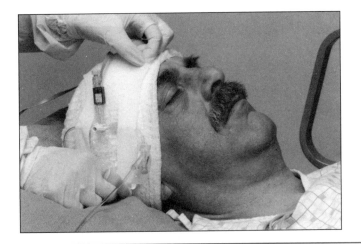

Align the ordered height of the flow chamber with the transducer stopcock. Tighten the locking bracket. Then turn the stopcock to the ordered position for monitoring or drainage, or for both monitoring and drainage. Document the procedure, noting the date and time, the insertion site, the initial ICP reading, and the patient's tolerance of the procedure. Also document the amount of drainage or the treatment required to obtain normal ICP.

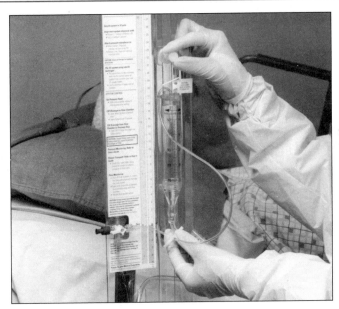

Setting up a direct pressure monitoring system

Commonly used for monitoring ICP in the ventricles, brain parenchyma, or subdura, the direct pressure monitoring system manufactured by Camino Laboratories has a fiber-optic transducer-tipped catheter. Other equipment you'll need includes a V420 direct pressure monitor, an external bedside monitor cable, a preamp cable, an ICP monitoring kit (which includes a fiber-optic catheter with pressure transducer and transducer connector), a zero adjustment tool, and all the equipment the doctor needs to insert an ICP monitoring device. The sterile drape may also be included in the kit.

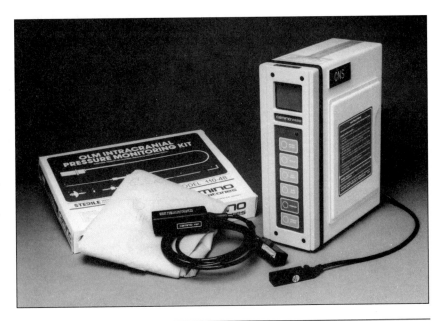

Turn on the monitor by pressing the START/STOP button on the front panel. Watch the monitor screen for a message indicating that the monitor is working. If no message appears, check to make sure that the circuit breaker switch on the back panel is in the up position.

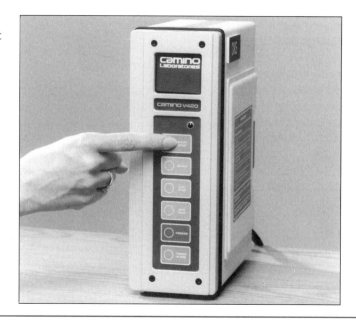

Connect the preamp cable to the V420 monitor by joining the two preamp cable couplers.

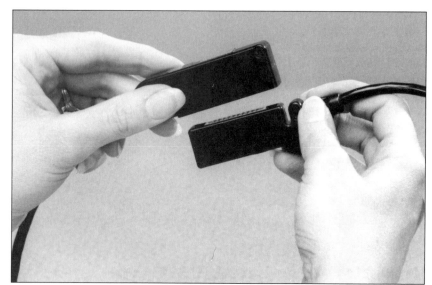

Using sterile technique, remove the fiber-optic catheter from the package. Place the catheter on a sterile drape on the overbed table. Now connect the nonsterile end of the fiber-optic catheter to the end of the preamp cable.

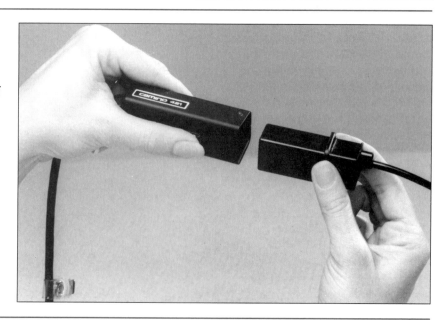

At this time, the monitor should display a short system test followed by the mean pressure display. When this appears, make sure that the mean pressure value reads "0." If it doesn't, use the zero adjustment tool to turn the screw on the bottom of the transducer connector until the mean pressure value reads "0." Be sure to do this before the surgeon inserts the catheter.

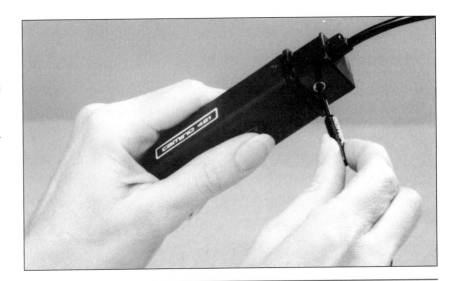

After the surgeon inserts the catheter, he will order the appropriate pressure scale. Press the SCALE button until the ordered scale appears. The choices are 10, 20, 50, 100, or 200 mm Hg.

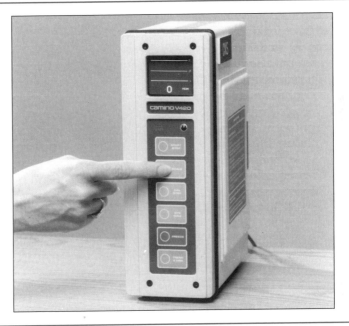

If the monitor is connected to an external bedside monitor, you'll need to calibrate the system so that the V420 monitor and the external bedside monitor are zeroed together. To do this, press CAL STEP (for "calibration step") on the V420 monitor until it reads "0." At the same time, press the ZERO button on the bedside monitor.

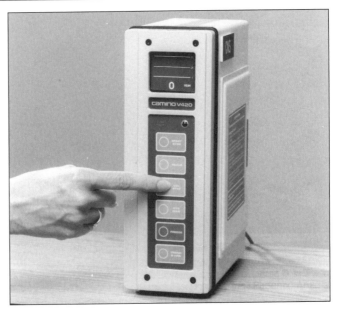

Correcting monitor problems

Many hospitals use a direct pressure monitoring system for evaluating intracranial pressure. If your hospital has this equipment and difficulties occur, check the chart below to help you identify and correct the problem. As needed, consult the manufacturer's instruction manual.

PROBLEM	CAUSE	INTERVENTIONS
Monitor display fails to appear.	• Circuit breaker switch in down position • Battery power too low	• Move the circuit breaker switch to the up position. • Verify that the battery is charged.
Low-battery (LOW BATT) indicator lights up.	• Failing battery charge	• Fully recharge the battery by connecting the monitor to an AC power source for about 12 hours. • Confirm that the circuit breaker switch is in the up position.
Monitor screen displays the warning message "CHECK CATHETER CONNECTION, +350 or more, −99."	• Loose connection in system	• Check the connection between the catheter and the preamp cable. • Check the connection between the preamp cable and the preamp extension cable. • Check the connection between the preamp extension cable and the V420 preamp extension cable receptacle. • As necessary, replace equipment components, such as the preamp cable, preamp extension cable, V420 monitor, or catheter.
Waveform appears too large or too small.	• Incorrect scale selection	• Press the SCALE key to change the scale selection.

PERFORMING I.C.P. MONITORING

To help maintain your patient's intracranial pressure (ICP) at an acceptable level, you'll need to measure his ICP regularly, care for the intracranial catheter site, and drain cerebrospinal fluid (CSF) to reduce pressure or provide a specimen for analysis. Bear in mind that ICP monitoring increases the risk of infection and neurologic complications from CSF loss. For these reasons, be sure to drain only the ordered amount of CSF, use strict aseptic technique, and maintain the integrity of the monitoring system.

Depending on the patient's condition, you may administer such medications as diuretics, corticosteroids, paralytic agents, and sedatives to reduce ICP. You may also use a hypothermia blanket to reduce the patient's temperature and to slow brain metabolism. If the patient is intubated, you may supply oxygen from a hand-held resuscitation bag or a ventilator to keep carbon dioxide levels down. This procedure constricts cerebral vessels, which helps reduce cerebral blood volume and ICP. (See *Providing routine care during ICP monitoring,* page 394.)

RECOGNIZING FACTORS THAT AFFECT I.C.P.

Stay alert for the following factors that can increase ICP, and take steps to correct them.
• *Body position.* Any position that obstructs venous return from the brain increases cerebral blood volume, as does any position that increases intra-abdominal, intrathoracic, or neck pressure.
• *Coughing.* Heightened intra-abdominal and intrathoracic pressures from coughing impede venous drainage from the brain.
• *Drug therapy.* Anesthetics, some antihypertensives, and other vasodilators, such as neuromuscular blockers that promote histamine release, may increase cerebral blood flow and ICP.
• *Emotional upset and pain.* Stimulation of the sympathetic nervous system increases blood pressure and cerebral blood flow.
• *Excessive activity.* Performing multiple procedures on a patient with elevated ICP increases blood pressure and cerebral blood flow. Activity—such as bathing, turning, venipuncture, and suctioning—can increase ICP enough to cause cerebral ischemia.
• *Hypercapnia.* Elevated carbon dioxide levels increase cerebral blood flow. Hypercapnia may

result from sleep, pulmonary disorders, sedation, shallow respirations, pressure on brain-stem respiratory centers, or an improperly calibrated ventilator.
• *Hypoxemia.* When oxygen levels decline to 50 mm Hg or less, cerebral vasodilation increases. Hypoxemia may result from insufficient oxygen concentration during oxygen therapy, insufficient ventilation during intubation or during and after suctioning, or partial or complete airway obstruction.
• *Increased cerebral metabolism.* Arousal from sleep, the rapid-eye-movement phase of sleep, seizure activity, and hyperthermia lead to increased ICP.
• *Isometric muscle contractions.* Isometric activities, such as pushing against the bed's footboard and shivering, raise systemic blood pressure.
• *Respiratory procedures.* Suctioning reduces oxygen levels, elevates carbon dioxide levels, and partially obstructs the airway with a catheter. Positive end-expiratory pressure raises intrathoracic pressure, which leads to increased ICP.
• *Valsalva's maneuver.* Increased intra-abdominal and intrathoracic pressures impede venous return from the brain. Straining during a bowel movement, moving in bed, and sneezing initiate this maneuver.

UNDERSTANDING C.P.P.

The maintenance of cerebral blood flow is essential to prevent cerebral ischemia and neuronal death. In a healthy person, autoregulation maintains cerebral blood flow by allowing the cerebral vessels to dilate and constrict in response to systemic blood pressure. In a neurologically impaired patient, autoregulation may break down. By calculating cerebral perfusion pressure (CPP), you can assess your patient's cerebral circulation.

To calculate CPP, subtract ICP from mean arterial pressure (MAP). To determine MAP, use this formula:

$$\text{MAP} = \frac{\text{diastolic}}{\text{pressure}} + \frac{\text{systolic} - \text{diastolic pressure}}{3}$$

Normal CPP ranges between 80 and 90 mm Hg. A sustained CPP under 40 mm Hg causes cerebral ischemia, and a sustained CPP under 30 mm Hg causes irreversible hypoxic changes, which lead to neuronal death.

Contributors to this section include *Ellie Z. Franges, RN, MSN, CCRN, CNRN,* and *Marie E. Wilson, RN, BSN, CCRN.* Ms. Franges is the director of Patient Care Services, CNS Unit, at Lehigh Valley Hospital, Allentown, Pa. Ms. Wilson is a clinical nurse III in the Intermediate Neuro ICU at Thomas Jefferson University Hospital, Philadelphia. The publisher thanks the following organizations for their help: *Pudenz-Schulte Medical Research Corp.,* Goleta, Calif.; *Delcrest Medical Products,* Blue Bell, Pa.; *Hewlett-Packard Co.,* Waltham, Mass.; *Hill-Rom,* Batesville, Ind.; *Lehigh Valley Hospital,* Allentown, Pa.; and *Doylestown (Pa.) Hospital.*

Providing routine care during ICP monitoring

Your nursing care can be a crucial factor in maintaining or reducing your patient's intracranial pressure (ICP). You can best manage elevated ICP (and possibly reduce it) with careful assessment and supportive care.

Create a calm environment
Because external stimuli may increase brain activity and thereby ICP, try to ensure serene surroundings for the patient. Greet him quietly. Speak softly and try to put him at ease. Dim the lights in the room or lower the window shades. Play soft background music if the patient finds it soothing. Instruct family members to use the same approach when visiting the patient.

Ensure safe surroundings
To protect the patient's limbs, head, and feet from potential injury, cover the side rails, headboard, and footboard with pads or bath blankets. If you use blankets, secure them with adhesive tape. Keep the side rails raised. Place an airway at the patient's bedside, or tape it to the wall above the bed, according to your hospital's policy. Keep suction equipment nearby in case you need to clear the patient's airway.

Monitor vital functions
• Use the Glasgow Coma Scale to assess the patient's level of consciousness. Check your assessment data against previous findings noted on his chart. Report significant changes to the doctor.
• Assess and document the patient's pupil size and reactivity every hour. Note any abnormal eye movements or deviations.
• Record the patient's blood pressure and pulse and respiratory rates at least every hour and more often if necessary. (If your patient has an arterial catheter in place to continuously monitor blood pressure, take pressure readings and provide site care as ordered.)
• Monitor the patient's temperature every 2 hours. Maintain a normal temperature range or mild hypothermia (90° to 98° F [32.2° to 36.7° C]) by giving tepid sponge baths, keeping bedclothes to a minimum, and lowering the room temperature. Administer antipyretics or use a hypothermia blanket, as ordered, if the patient has a fever. Take care, however, to keep the patient from shivering (which can raise

ICP). If indicated, remove the hypothermia blanket when his temperature rises 1° to 2° F (0.5° to 1° C) above normal.

Monitor fluid status
Because fluid intake can increase ICP, carefully assess intake and output, and report large differences between the two. If necessary, the doctor may order diuretics to combat fluid overload.

Position the patient carefully
• Keeping the patient's movement minimal, position him in the center of the bed. Elevate the head of the bed 30 to 45 degrees. Remove any pillows from behind his head to avoid jugular vein compression.
• Instruct the patient to keep his head midline and as still as possible. If he's unconscious, keep his head in a neutral position with sandbags or pillows.
• Instruct the patient to exhale when he turns or moves in the bed. This prevents initiation of Valsalva's maneuver, which increases ICP. When you turn the patient, use a small pillow or folded bath blanket to support his head in the midline position. Avoid having the patient assist in changing his position in bed (by pushing with his heels or arms, for example); such exertion will also initiate Valsalva's maneuver.
• Perform passive range-of-motion exercises to maintain muscle tone. Avoid isometric exercises, which may initiate Valsalva's maneuver.

Watch the monitor
Observe the monitor during all activities, and make sure that alarms are activated (not silenced) at all times. Check the monitoring system continually for leaks or blockages, and always handle the equipment aseptically. Plan nursing care by considering its effect on ICP. Don't perform several activities at a time if their cumulative effect would increase ICP. Watch the monitor for ICP spikes when caring for the patient, and suspend activity if necessary.

Caring for the intracranial catheter site

To change the dressing and clean the insertion site, you'll need a face mask, two pairs of sterile gloves, two sterile drapes, sterile 4″ × 4″ drain sponges, iodophor swabs, and adhesive tape.

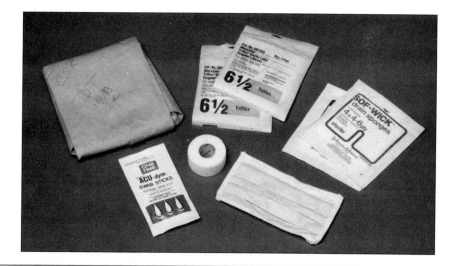

Explain the procedure to the patient. Wash your hands. Use one drape to set up a sterile field on a clean, flat surface, such as the patient's overbed table. Open the packages containing the gloves and the drain sponges, and drop these items on the sterile field. Put on the face mask and a pair of sterile gloves.

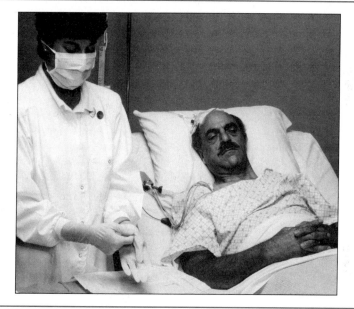

Next, remove the dressing over the insertion site. Enclose the dressing in your gloves as you remove them, and discard the gloves and dressing in a biohazard container.

▶ *Clinical tip:* To reduce the risk of infection, change only soiled, wet, or nonocclusive dressings. Don't change the dressing if it appears secure, dry, and clean.

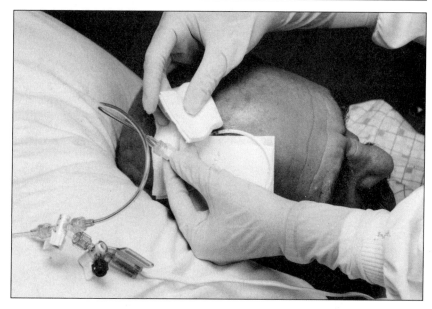

Remove your gloves and put on new sterile ones. Then place a sterile drape over the patient's head. Clean the intracranial catheter and the area around the insertion site with iodophor swabs. Use a circular motion, and work from the insertion site outward. Use each swab only once.

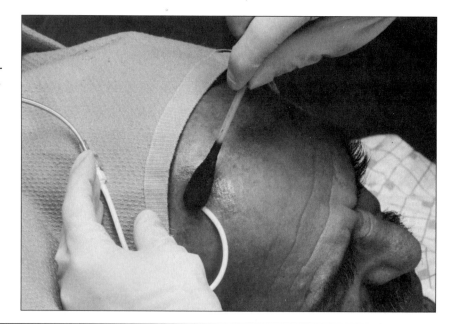

Remove the sterile drape and place sterile 4″ × 4″ drain sponges around the catheter. Secure the sponges with tape to create an occlusive dressing. Write the time, the date, and your initials on the tape. Document the procedure and include a description of the site and any apparent drainage.

▶ *Clinical tip:* Report any significant amount of clear or pale yellow drainage. Such drainage suggests leaking CSF.

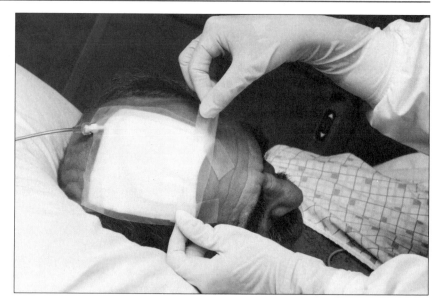

Measuring ICP

Although your patient's intracranial catheter is already connected to the monitoring equipment, you'll need additional items to measure his ICP: a level, a calculator, and gloves.

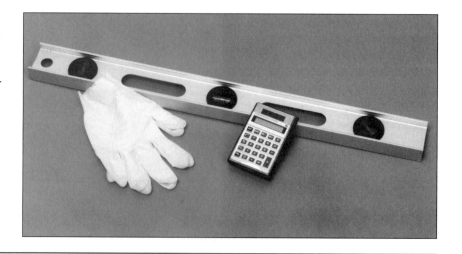

To ensure an accurate ICP measurement, position the patient in the center of the bed, and elevate the head of the bed 30 to 45 degrees. Remove any pillows from behind his head to prevent jugular vein compression. Instruct the patient to keep his head as still as possible and in a midline position (so that he looks straight ahead).

▶ *Clinical tip:* To keep an unconscious patient's head in a neutral position, place sandbags or pillows on each side of his head, if necessary.

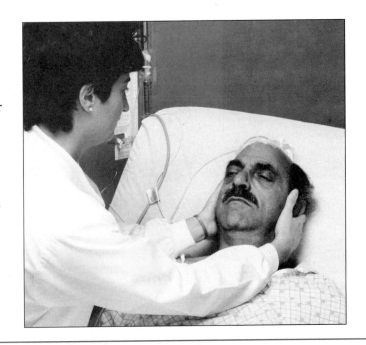

Wash your hands and align the zero of the monitoring system's flow chamber with the center line of the patient's head. Use a level to locate this point, which is about 1″ (2.5 cm) above the external auditory meatus and corresponds to the foramen of Monro.

▶ *Clinical tip:* To obtain an accurate ICP measurement, realign the equipment before you record each reading.

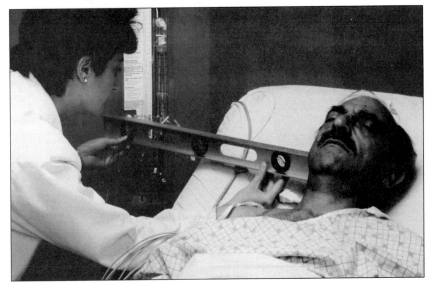

Following the manufacturer's guidelines, balance and calibrate the transducer. Maintain aseptic technique at all times. You'll need to balance and calibrate the transducer at least every 4 hours.

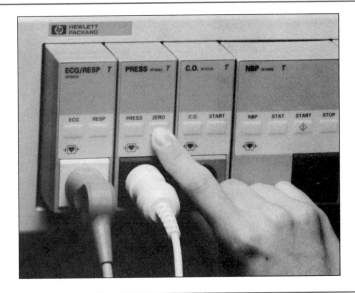

Put on your gloves and turn the main stopcock off to drainage.

▷ **Clinical tip:** Set the ICP monitoring system according to the doctor's order. The system may be closed to drainage, open to drainage, or opened periodically for drainage. For an accurate ICP measurement, the system must be closed to drainage.

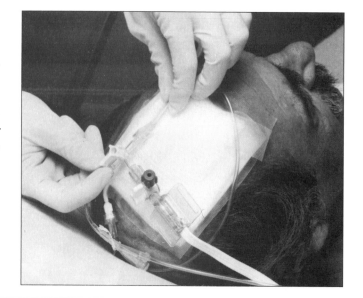

Observe the ICP waveform on the monitor. Note the waveform pattern and document the reading. Obtain printed recordings every shift to reflect general trends in ICP.

If you notice an abnormal waveform, make sure that the equipment is functioning correctly before reporting the abnormality. Then open the main stopcock to drainage.

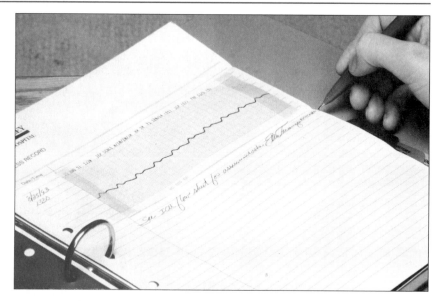

Take the patient's blood pressure or, if he has an arterial line in place to monitor blood pressure continuously, note the reading. Using a calculator, determine his CPP. Report insufficient CPP to the doctor immediately. Document your results and note CPP trends.

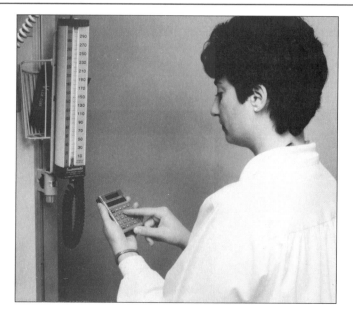

Draining CSF

First, ensure that the flow chamber of the ICP monitoring setup remains positioned according to the doctor's orders and that the patient's body is properly aligned. The doctor usually orders the flow chamber set between 5 and 10 cm H₂O, which slows drainage.

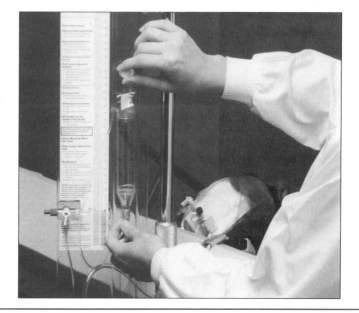

Note any specific orders regarding CSF drainage. For instance, the doctor may order 5 ml of CSF to be drained if the patient's ICP reaches 20 mm Hg.

To begin, put on gloves; then turn the main stopcock on to drainage. This allows CSF to collect in the graduated flow chamber. Document the time and the amount of CSF obtained.

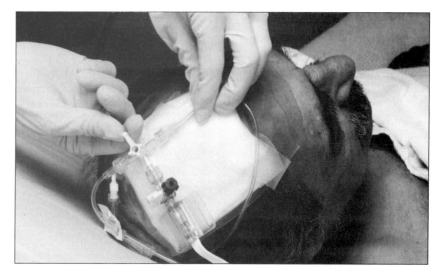

To stop CSF from draining into the flow chamber, turn the stopcock off to drainage.

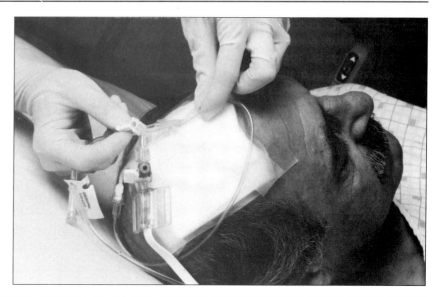

Release the clamp below the flow chamber to drain the CSF from this chamber into the drainage bag. Never empty the bag. Instead, replace it when full, using sterile technique.

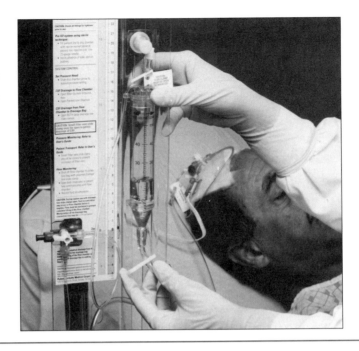

Collecting a CSF specimen

To obtain a CSF specimen, you'll need two 3-ml syringes with 22G needles, an iodophor swab, an alcohol sponge, sterile gloves, and sterile specimen tubes.

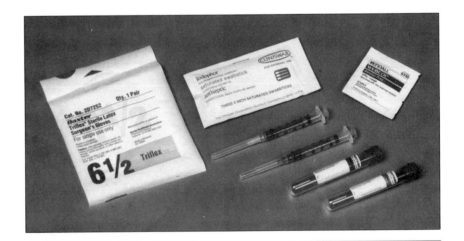

Wash your hands and put on the sterile gloves. Turn the stopcock of the patient's line on to drainage (off to the transducer).

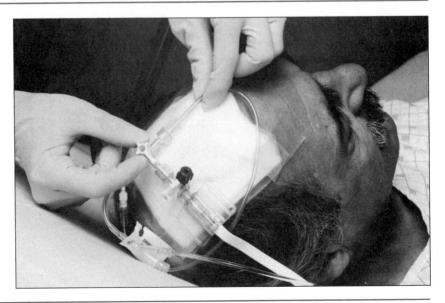

Clean the stopcock injection port on the patient's line with an iodophor swab (near right) and then with an alcohol sponge (far right).

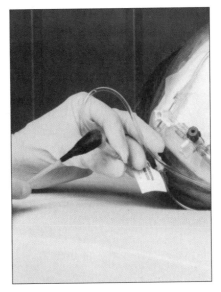
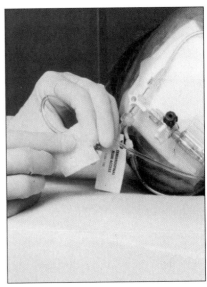

Using a 3-ml syringe, slowly withdraw 0.5 ml of CSF from the injection port. In case excess CSF components settle in the port, discard this specimen in a biohazard container and dispose of the syringe. Using the second syringe, withdraw 2 to 3 ml of CSF.

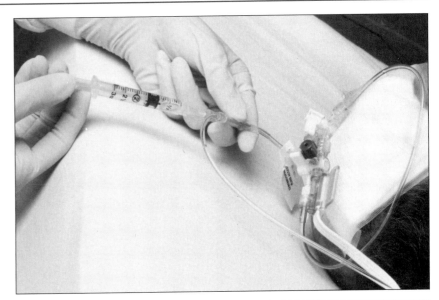

Empty this specimen into the tube. Turn the patient line stopcock off to drainage (on to the transducer). Note the return of the waveform to the monitor.

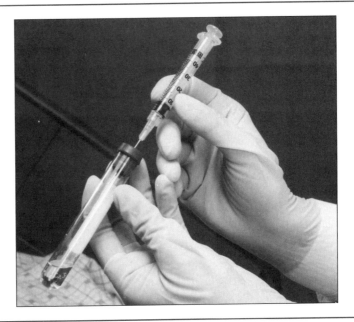

Reading ICP waveforms

When monitoring intracranial pressure (ICP), be alert for A, B, and C waves, which may help you recognize significant changes in your patient's condition. *A waves* are an ominous sign of intracranial decompensation and poor compliance. *B waves* correlate with changes in respiration; *C waves,* with changes in arterial pressure.

Normal waveform

A normal ICP waveform typically shows a steep upward slope (corresponding to systole) followed by a downward slope with a dicrotic notch (corresponding to diastole). In most cases, this waveform occurs continuously and indicates an ICP between 0 and 15 mm Hg — normal pressure.

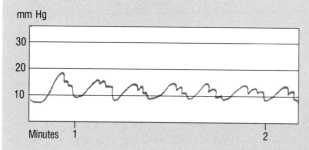

A waves

The most clinically significant ICP waveforms are A waves, which may reach elevations of 50 to 100 mm Hg, persist for 5 to 20 minutes, then drop sharply — signaling exhaustion of the brain's compliance mechanisms. A waves may come and go, spiking from temporary elevations in thoracic pressure or from any condition that increases ICP beyond the brain's compliance limits. Activities such as sustained coughing or straining with bowel movements can cause temporary elevations in thoracic pressure.

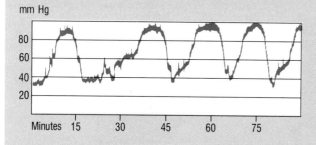

B waves

Rhythmic and sharp with a sawtooth pattern, B waves occur every 1½ to 2 minutes and may reach elevations of 50 mm Hg. Their clinical significance isn't clear, but they correlate with respiratory changes and may occur more frequently with decreasing compensation. B waves sometimes precede A waves; notify the doctor if B waves occur frequently.

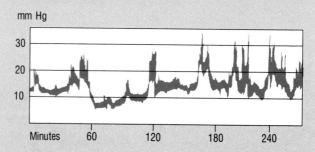

C waves

Like B waves, C waves are rapid and rhythmic, but not as sharp. Clinically insignificant, they may fluctuate with respirations or systemic blood pressure changes.

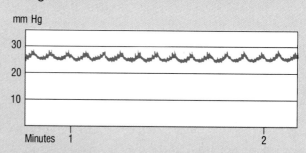

Waveform indicating system malfunction

A waveform that looks like the one shown below signals a problem with the transducer or monitor. Check for an obstruction in the catheter line, and determine whether the transducer needs rebalancing.

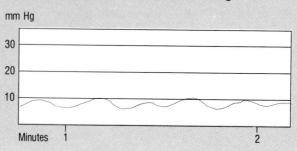

ASSISTING WITH LUMBAR PUNCTURE

In a lumbar puncture, the doctor inserts a sterile needle into the spinal subarachnoid space—usually between the third and fourth lumbar vertebrae. Besides assisting with the procedure, you'll maintain sterile technique and carefully position the patient.

The procedure may be performed to measure cerebrospinal fluid (CSF) pressure, detect blood in the CSF, obtain CSF specimens for laboratory analysis, or to inject dye or gas for contrast in radiologic studies of the brain and spinal cord. Lumbar puncture also allows administration of drugs or anesthetics and, rarely, reduction of intracranial pressure (ICP) by removing CSF.

The procedure is usually not performed on extremely agitated patients or on those with a lumbar deformity or an infection at the puncture site. Nor should it be performed in patients with increased ICP caused by space-occupying lesions; the rapid pressure reduction that follows CSF withdrawal may compress and herniate the brain stem.

The most common complication of lumbar puncture is a headache. Other potential complications include an adverse reaction to the anesthetic, fever, meningitis, epidural or subdural abscess, bleeding into the spinal canal, CSF leakage through the dura, local pain caused by nerve root irritation, edema or hematoma at the puncture site, and transient voiding difficulty. Brain stem herniation is the most serious complication. If the patient has a central nervous system (CNS) disorder, the doctor may withhold all sedatives and analgesics before the procedure to prevent masking CNS symptoms.

Gather the necessary equipment and take it to the patient's bedside. Most hospitals have disposable lumbar puncture trays containing most of the needed sterile equipment, including sterile gauze pads or sponges, a small adhesive bandage, a sterile fenestrated drape, a 3-ml syringe and a 25G sterile needle for injecting the anesthetic, a local anesthetic (usually 1% lidocaine), an 18G or a 20G 3½″ spinal needle with stylet, a manometer, a three-way stopcock, and three or four sterile, graduated collection tubes with stoppers. Other necessary equipment includes povidone-iodine solution, sterile gloves, clean gloves, a gown, a mask, and a mask with a face shield (for the doctor).

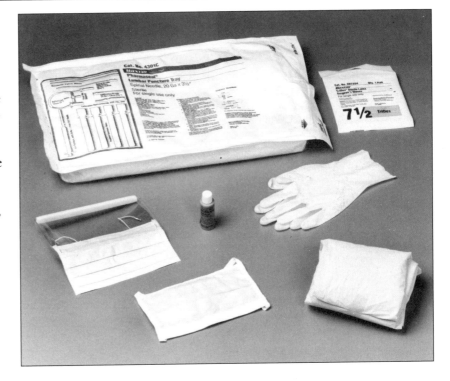

Ellie Z. Franges, RN, MSN, CCRN, CNRN, who contributed to this section, is the Director of Patient Care Services in the Neurologic Intensive Care Unit at Lehigh Valley Hospital, Allentown, Pa. The publisher thanks *Doylestown (Pa.) Hospital* and *Hill-Rom,* Batesville, Ind., for their help.

Reinforce the doctor's explanation of the procedure. Try to ease the patient's anxiety and ensure his cooperation. Inform him that he may experience a headache after lumbar puncture, but reassure him that you'll provide analgesics and other palliative measures.

Immediately before the procedure, provide privacy and instruct the patient to void. Wash your hands and put on a mask. Then open the lumbar puncture tray on an overbed table, taking care not to contaminate the sterile field when you open the wrapper.

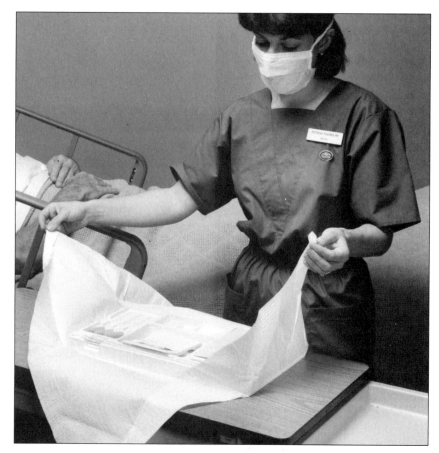

Help the patient lie on his side at the edge of the bed, with his chin tucked to his chest and his knees drawn up to his abdomen. This position widens the space between the vertebrae, easing needle insertion.

The procedure may also be performed with the patient in a sitting position with his chest lowered toward his knees.

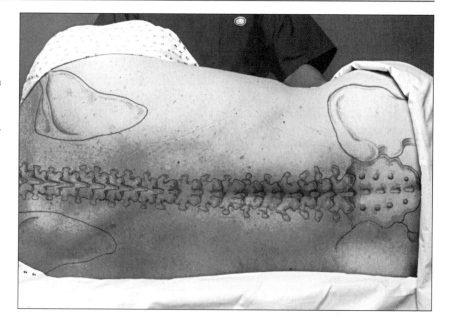

Stress the importance of remaining still during the procedure. To help the patient stay in position, place one of your hands behind his neck and the other behind his knees (as shown). Press gently and firmly. Maintaining this position will help to prevent accidental needle displacement.

During the procedure, watch closely for signs of an adverse reaction, including increased pulse or respiratory rate, pallor, clammy skin, and pain, numbness, or tingling in the legs. Alert the doctor if these or other unusual signs or symptoms occur.

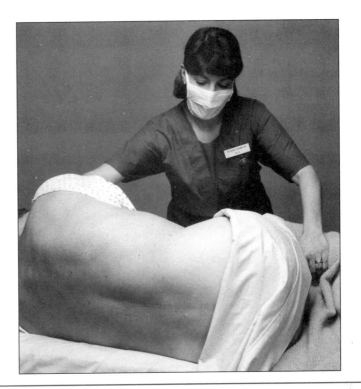

Once the doctor has the needle in place, she'll attach a manometer with a three-way stopcock to the needle hub to read the CSF pressure. If requested, help the patient extend his legs to provide a more accurate pressure reading. Avoid moving the patient's shoulders, however, because this could cause unwanted spinal rotation.

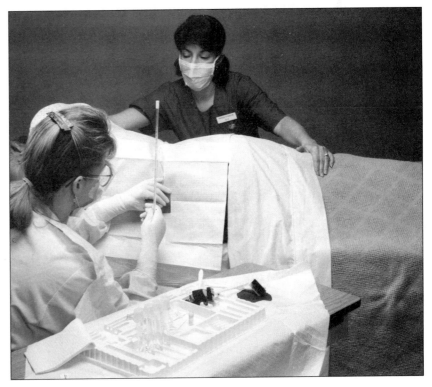

After reading the pressure, the doctor will detach the manometer and allow CSF to drain from the needle hub into the graduated collection tubes until each tube contains between 2 and 3 ml of CSF. Then she'll cap the tubes and place them in the lumbar puncture tray in the sequence collected.

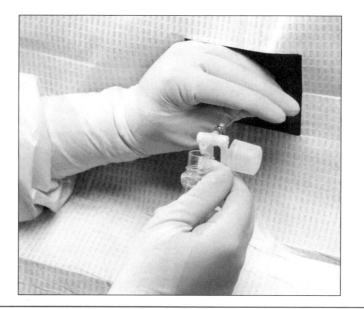

If the doctor suspects an obstruction in the spinal subarachnoid space, she may test for Queckenstedt's sign: First, she'll determine baseline CSF pressure to compare with later readings. Then she'll direct you to compress the patient's jugular vein for 10 seconds (as shown). This compression temporarily blocks blood flow from the cranium and increases ICP. If the subarachnoid space isn't obstructed, CSF pressure will rise.

The doctor then will take pressure readings at 10- to 30-second intervals until the pressure returns to baseline and stabilizes.

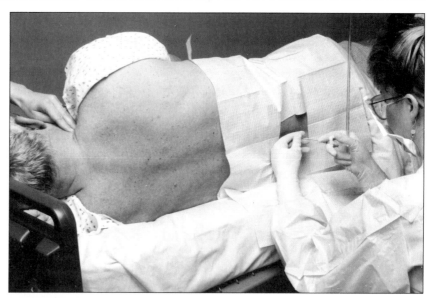

After the doctor collects the specimens and removes the needle, put on gloves, clean the puncture site with povidone-iodine solution, and apply a small adhesive bandage. Send labeled specimens to the laboratory immediately.

Remove your gloves, and help the patient into a supine position. He must remain in this position for 8 to 12 hours. Document the procedure, the patient's response, any drug administration, the number of specimen tubes collected, when you sent the specimen to the laboratory, and the color, consistency, and characteristics of the CSF specimen.

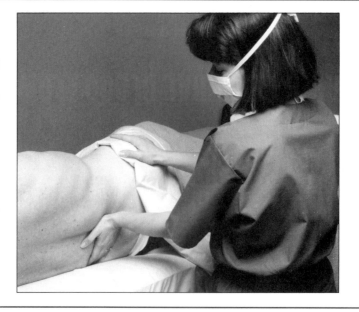

Monitoring Cerebral Blood Flow

Until recently, nurses estimated cerebral blood flow in neurologically compromised patients by calculating cerebral perfusion pressure. Today nurses may continuously monitor regional blood flow with a sensor implanted surgically on the cerebral cortex.

This sensor measures blood flow in the capillary bed by means of thermistors housed in the sensor. The thermistors consist of two metallic plates—one heated and one neutral. The sensor detects the temperature difference between the metallic plates. This difference is inversely proportional to cerebral blood flow: As cerebral blood flow increases, the temperature difference decreases—and vice versa.

BENEFITS OF MONITORING

Monitoring may be implemented whenever cerebral blood flow alterations are anticipated. It's most commonly used in patients with vascular tumors, subarachnoid hemorrhage from a cerebral aneurysm (in which vasospasm commonly restricts blood flow), or trauma associated with intracranial hypertension. It's also used with arteriovenous malformations.

COMPLICATIONS

Like intracranial pressure monitoring, cerebral blood flow monitoring has drawbacks, such as the possibility of infection. To help prevent infection, administer prophylactic antibiotics as prescribed, and maintain a sterile dressing around the sensor insertion site. Another potential complication, cerebrospinal fluid (CSF) leakage, may occur at the insertion site. To prevent this, the surgeon usually places an additional suture at the site.

PATIENT PREPARATION

Before the patient undergoes surgery, make sure that he (or a responsible party) understands the procedure and signs an informed consent form.

To allay the patient's fears, explain how the cerebral blood flow sensor is inserted. In brief, the surgeon performs a craniotomy (or creates a burr hole) through which he tunnels the sensor to the cerebral cortex. Next, he inserts the metallic plates of the sensor so that they're in continuous contact with the surface of the cerebral cortex. Then, working backward, he closes the insertion site, replacing the bone flap and suturing the scalp.

Tell the patient how long the sensor will remain in place and that it can be removed at the bedside. Mention that the insertion site will be covered with a dry, sterile dressing while the sensor is in place.

Setting up the sensor monitor

In most cases, the surgeon sets up the monitoring system after inserting the cerebral blood flow sensor. If he doesn't, you may be asked to do so. If you are, first assemble the following equipment at the bedside: a monitor (such as the Micro Saber Plus monitor from Flowtronics, Inc. shown here) and a sensor cable with an attached sensor.

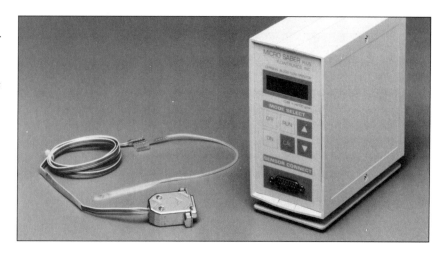

Ellie Z. Franges, RN, MSN, CCRN, CNRN, and *Marie E. Wilson, RN, BSN, CCRN,* contributed to this section. Ms. Franges is a clinical nurse specialist in neurosciences at Lehigh Valley Hospital, Allentown, Pa. Ms. Wilson is a clinical nurse III in the Intermediate Neuro ICU at Thomas Jefferson University Hospital, Philadelphia. The publisher thanks *Flowtronics, Inc.,* Phoenix, Ariz., and *Hill-Rom,* Batesville, Ind., for their help.

Attach the distal end of the sensor cable (from the patient's head) to the monitor port labeled SENSOR CONNECT.

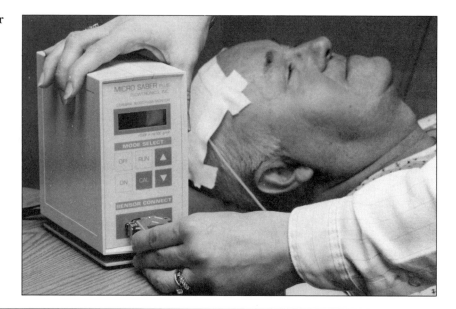

When the sensor cable is securely in place, press the ON key to activate the monitor.

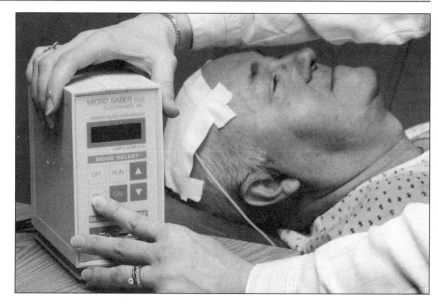

Next, calibrate the system by pressing the CAL key. You should see the red light appear on the CAL button.

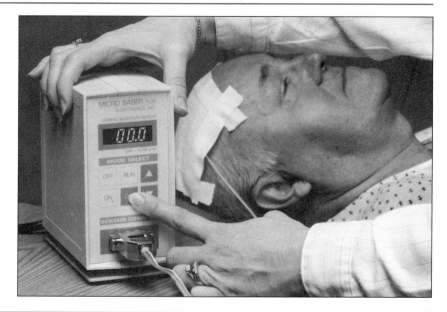

Ideally, you'll begin by calibrating the sensor to 00.0 by pressing the directional arrows (▲ and ▼). Readouts of ±0.1 are also acceptable.

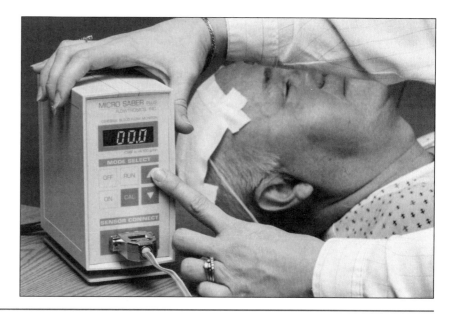

Press the RUN key to display the cerebral blood flow reading.

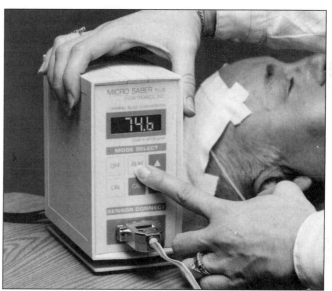

Observe the monitor's digital display and document the baseline value. Record the cerebral blood flow rate hourly. Be sure to watch for trends and correlate values with the patient's clinical status.

▶ **Clinical tip:** Be aware that stimulation or activity may cause a 10% increase or decrease in cerebral blood flow. If you detect a 20% increase or decrease, suspect poor contact between the sensor and the cerebral cortex.

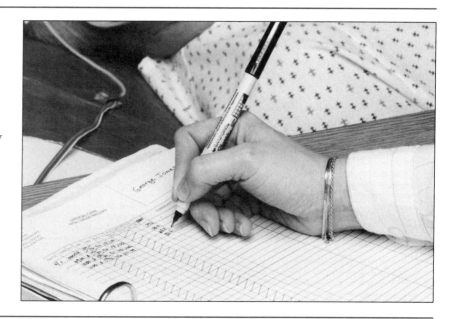

Caring for the insertion site

Assemble the following equipment at the patient's bedside: a linen-saver pad, sterile 4″ × 4″ gauze pads, clean gloves, sterile gloves, and povidone-iodine solution. You also may need povidone-iodine ointment, depending on your hospital's policy.

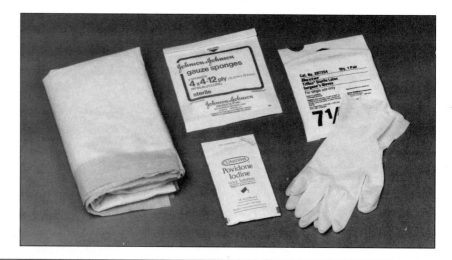

Explain the procedure to the patient; then wash your hands. Don clean gloves and remove the dressing from the sensor insertion site. Observe the site for CSF leakage, a potential complication. Then remove and discard your gloves according to hospital protocol.

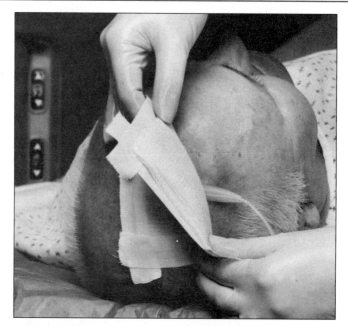

Now put on sterile gloves. Using aseptic technique, clean the insertion site with a gauze pad soaked with povidone-iodine solution. Clean the site, starting at the center and working outward in a circular pattern.

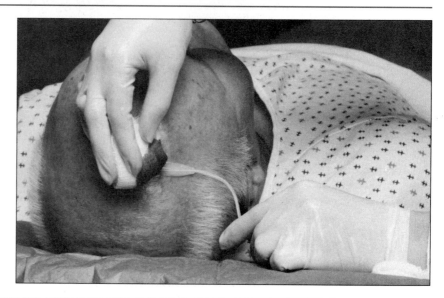

Using a new gauze pad soaked with povidone-iodine, clean the exposed part of the sensor from the insertion site to the end of the sensor. Apply povidone-iodine ointment to the insertion site, if hospital policy permits.

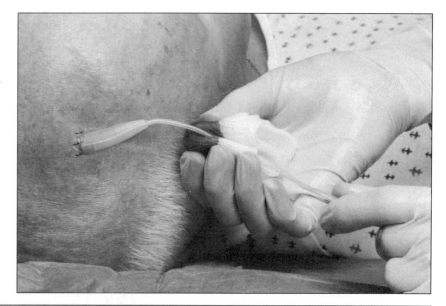

Next, place sterile 4″ × 4″ gauze pads over the insertion site to completely cover it. Tape all edges securely to create an occlusive dressing. Finally, document the dressing change, being sure to describe the site's appearance precisely.

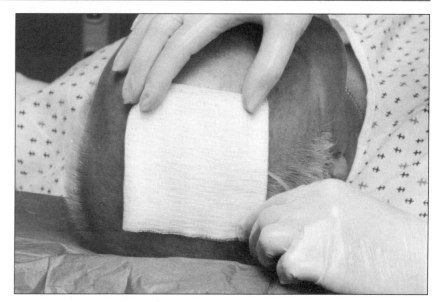

Removing the sensor

In most cases, the cerebral blood flow sensor remains in place for about 3 days when used for postoperative monitoring. To remove the sensor, assemble the following equipment at the patient's bedside: a sterile suture removal tray, 1″ adhesive tape, sterile 4″ × 4″ gauze pads, clean gloves, sterile gloves, and suture material.

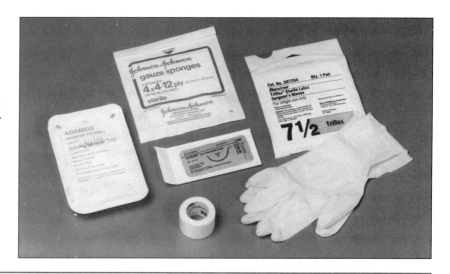

Explain the procedure to the patient; then wash your hands. Don clean gloves, remove the old dressing, and dispose of the gloves and the dressing properly.

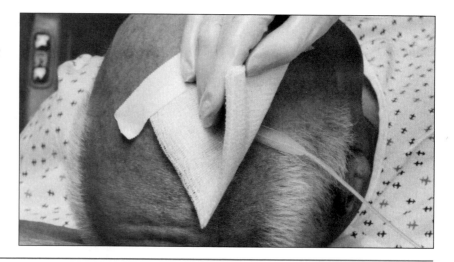

Open the suture removal tray and the package of suture material. The surgeon removes the anchoring sutures and then gently removes the sensor from the insertion site. After he closes the wound with stitches, don sterile gloves, apply a folded gauze pad to the site, and tape it in place. Carefully observe and document the condition of the site, including any leakage.

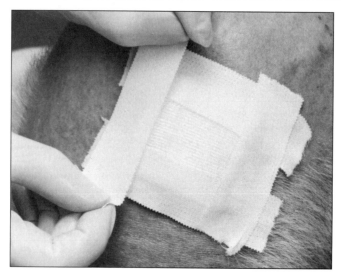

 INSIGHTS AND INTERPRETATIONS

Analyzing cerebral blood flow rates

A crucial part of cerebral blood flow monitoring involves watching for trends and correlating monitored values with the patient's clinical condition.

Normal cerebral blood flow
Normal values range from 60 to 90 ml of blood flow per 100 g of brain tissue per minute. However, you'll need to establish acceptable ranges for each patient based on his neurologic condition. Cerebral blood flow fluctuates according to metabolic demand, so a comatose patient may have half the normal cerebral blood flow value.

Abnormal cerebral blood flow
The following conditions may produce abnormal cerebral blood flow:
• An induced barbiturate coma in a patient whose

EEG waveform reflects burst suppression may result in cerebral blood flow as low as 10 to 20 ml/100 g/minute.
• A vasospasm in a patient with a subarachnoid hemorrhage may result in cerebral blood flow less than 40 ml/100 g/minute.
• Imminent hyperemia in a patient who's awake may be signaled by a high-normal cerebral blood flow range of 80 to 90 ml/100 g/minute (or more).
• The sensor's incomplete contact with the cerebral cortex (possibly as the result of a small hematoma) may result in readings that are 20% above or below baseline.

Diagnostic Tests

PERFORMING 12-LEAD ELECTROCARDIOGRAPHY

A valuable diagnostic tool, 12-lead electrocardiography (ECG) graphically records the heart's electrical activity. In this procedure, electrical impulses created by the heart's conduction system can be monitored by electrodes attached to the skin. These electrodes sense the electric currents and transmit them to an instrument that produces a record of cardiac activity. The printed record, or waveform, is the electrocardiogram.

UNDERSTANDING LEADS

To assess cardiac activity using a standard 12-lead ECG, you'll position a series of electrodes on the patient's extremities and chest wall. The 12 leads include three bipolar limb leads (I, II, and III), three unipolar augmented limb leads (aV_R, aV_L, and aV_F), and six unipolar precordial, or chest, leads (V_1, V_2, V_3, V_4, V_5, and V_6). By recording data from 12 different leads, or perspectives, this type of ECG provides a composite picture of the heart's electrical activity. Because each lead displays cardiac electrical activity from a different perspective, the waveform resulting from a particular lead will have its own characteristic pattern.

Limb leads

The six limb leads reflect electrical activity in the heart's frontal plane. In this plane—a vertical view through the middle of the heart from top to bottom—electrical activity is recorded from the anterior to the posterior axis.

Leads I, II, and III are called bipolar because they require two electrodes—one positive and one negative. These leads record the potential difference (the work required to transport an electric charge from one point to another) between the two electrodes. Lead I records the potential difference between the right arm and the left arm. Lead II records the potential difference between the right arm and the left leg. Lead III records the potential difference between the left arm and the left leg. (See *Einthoven's triangle*, page 416.)

Augmented limb leads aV_R, aV_L, and aV_F are called unipolar because they have only one electrode—the positive pole. The negative pole is computed by the ECG machine. Without augmentation,

the tracings from these leads would be quite small. The ECG machine automatically enlarges (or augments) the deflections to make them more readable. When the positive pole is the right arm, the lead is known as the aV_R (augmented vector right) lead; when the positive pole is the left arm, the lead is known as the aV_L (augmented vector left) lead; when the positive pole is the left leg, the lead is known as the aV_F (augmented vector foot) lead.

Chest leads

The six unipolar precordial leads provide information on electrical activity in the heart's horizontal plane—a transverse view through the middle of the heart, dividing it into upper and lower portions. In this plane, electrical activity can be seen from a superior or an inferior approach.

These leads are placed at six sites over the anterior surface of the chest and connected to the positive terminal of the ECG machine. The negative electrode, called the indifferent electrode, is connected to the arms and left leg at the same time.

Leads V_1 and V_2 monitor the right side of the heart, so they're often referred to as the right precordial leads. In contrast, leads V_3 through V_6 are called the left precordial leads because they monitor the heart's left side.

By reviewing the ECG tracings from all the leads, you'll obtain a fairly complete view of the electrical activity in the heart's inferior, anterior, and lateral portions. The leads are grouped together and called inferior leads, anterior leads, or lateral leads based on the area they scan. The inferior leads are leads II, III, and aV_F; the anterior leads, leads V_1, V_2, V_3 and V_4; and the lateral leads, leads I, aV_L, V_5, and V_6. Lead aV_R doesn't provide a specific view of the heart but does reflect changes in electrical activity.

OPERATING THE RECORDER

The ECG machine can be a multichannel or a single-channel recorder. For a multichannel recording, you'll attach all electrodes to the patient at once, and the machine will print a simultaneous view of all leads. For a single-channel recording, you'll systematically attach and remove selected electrodes, stopping and starting the tracing each time.

Contributors to this section include *Marilyn Sawyer Sommers, RN, PhD, CCRN,* an assistant professor at the University of Cincinnati College of Nursing and Health Sciences, and *Paulette Dorney, RN, MSN, CCRN,* an instructor in the Department of Critical Care Staff Development at North Penn Hospital, Lansdale, Pa. The publisher thanks *Doylestown (Pa.) Hospital* and *Hewlett-Packard Co.,* Waltham, Mass., for their help.

Einthoven's triangle

The axes of the three bipolar limb leads (I, II, and III) form a triangle, known as Einthoven's triangle, that is the model for the standard limb leads in electrocardiography. Because the electrodes for these leads are placed about equidistant from the heart, the triangle is equilateral.

The axis of lead I extends from shoulder to shoulder, with the right arm lead being the negative electrode and the left arm lead being the positive electrode. The axis of lead II runs from the negative right arm lead electrode to the positive left leg lead electrode. The axis of lead III extends from the negative left arm lead electrode to the positive left leg lead electrode.

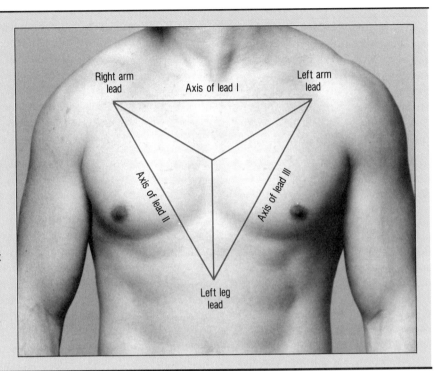

Using a multichannel ECG machine

Begin by gathering the necessary equipment. You'll need a multichannel ECG machine, such as the one shown at right. You'll also need recording paper, pregelled disposable electrodes (or reusable electrodes with suction bulbs and rubber straps and electrode paste or gel), and 4″ × 4″ gauze pads or a moist cloth towel. Optional equipment includes a drape, shaving supplies, and a marking pen.

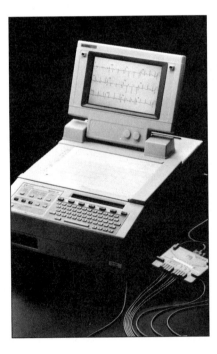

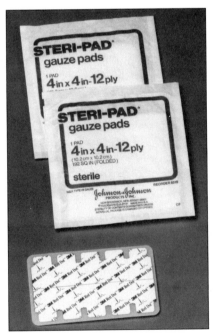

Inform the patient that his doctor has ordered an ECG and explain the procedure. Tell the patient that the procedure will take about 10 minutes and that it's a safe and painless way to evaluate cardiac function. Set up the equipment at the patient's bedside.

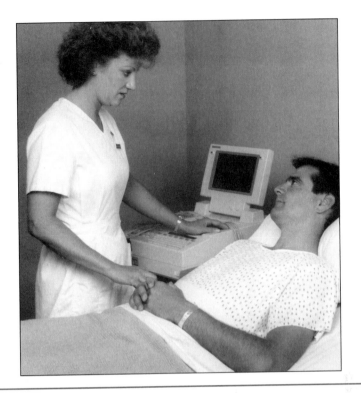

Plug the cord into a grounded outlet, and place the patient in a supine position. If he can't tolerate lying flat, help him to semi-Fowler's position. Uncover his chest, and expose his arms and legs. Always maintain his privacy.

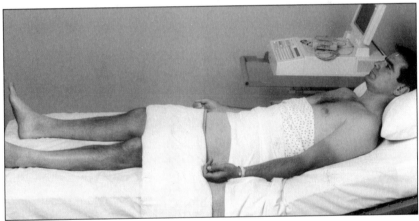

Attach the limb leads to hair-free sites on the arms and legs. A flat, fleshy site is best; try to avoid bony or muscular areas. The inner aspect of the wrist and the inner aspect of the ankle are usually good contact sites. Clean each site to remove skin oil and to increase contact with the electrodes, following the electrode manufacturer's guidelines for skin preparation.

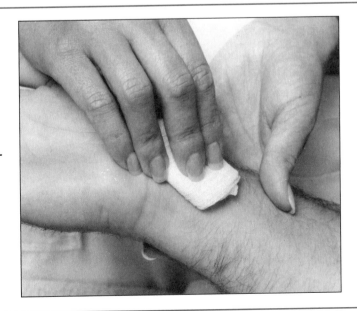

Apply electrode paste or gel, or the disposable electrodes (as shown), to the inner aspects of the wrists and the medial aspects of the ankles. If you're using paste or gel, rub it into the skin. If you're using disposable electrodes, peel off the contact paper and apply them to the site. Position leg electrodes with the lead connections pointing up.

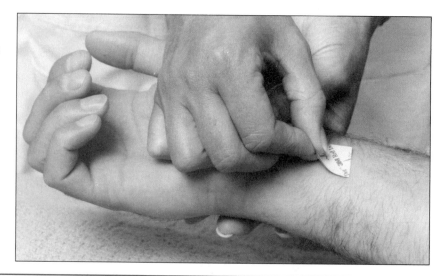

Connect the limb leadwires to the electrodes. Make sure that metal parts are clean to ensure a good electrical connection.

▶ *Clinical tip:* The tip of each leadwire is lettered and color coded for easy identification. The white (or RA) leadwire goes to the right arm; the green (or RL) leadwire, to the right leg; the red (or LL) leadwire, to the left leg; the black (or LA) leadwire, to the left arm; and the brown (or V_1 to V_6) leadwires, to the chest.

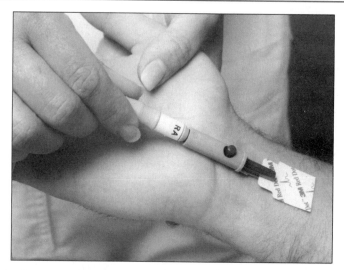

Prepare the anterior chest sites as you did the extremities. Attach the chest leads to the six anterior chest sites (as shown). If the patient is a woman, place the chest electrodes below the breast tissue.

Make sure that all leads are securely attached; then turn on the machine. Tell the patient to relax, lie still, and breathe normally. Advise him not to talk when you record his ECG because muscle movement may distort the ECG tracing.

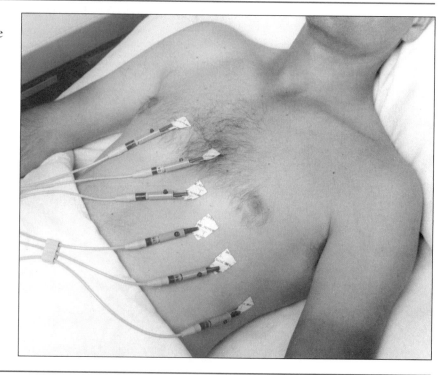

Make sure that the ECG paper speed selector is set to the standard 25 mm/second. Then, if necessary, enter the appropriate patient identification data. Calibrate or standardize the machine according to the manufacturer's recommendation. The machine will record a normal standardization mark—a square that's the height of 2 large squares or 10 small squares on the recording paper.

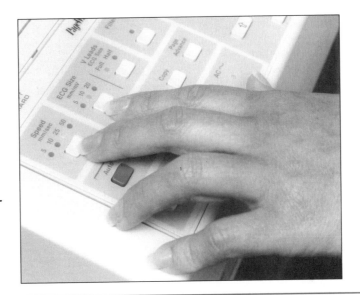

Press the AUTO button and record the ECG. Observe the tracing quality. The machine will record all 12 leads automatically, recording three consecutive leads simultaneously. When the machine finishes recording the 12-lead ECG, turn it off. Remove the electrodes and clean the patient's skin. Use a moist cloth towel or a 4" × 4" gauze pad to remove any residual paste or gel from the patient's skin.

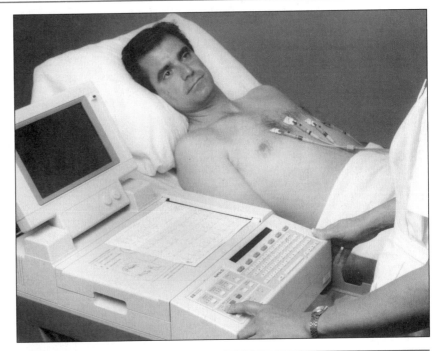

Help the patient into his gown and cover him. Raise the head of the bed, and assist him to a comfortable position. Then document the procedure. Note any changes in his condition, such as chest pain or shortness of breath. Also note any unusual electrode placements—necessitated by a dressing in place or an I.V. line, for example. Write his name and room number, the date and time, and his doctor's name on the ECG strip, and place the strip in his chart.

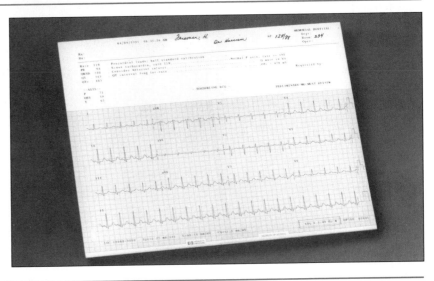

Using a single-channel ECG machine

Before you begin, obtain the single-channel ECG machine, recording paper, pregelled disposable electrodes (or reusable electrodes with rubber straps [with or without suction bulbs] and electrode paste or gel), and 4″ × 4″ gauze pads (or skin preparation pads). Optional equipment includes a drape, shaving supplies, a marking pen, and a moist cloth towel.

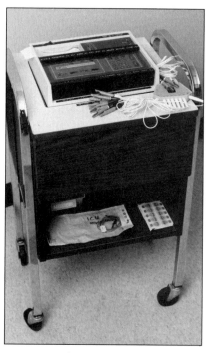

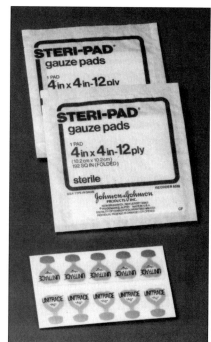

Explain the procedure to the patient, and assemble the equipment at his bedside. Place him in a supine position. If necessary for comfort, elevate the head of the bed slightly. Then uncover his arms and legs, and drape him appropriately. Always maintain his privacy.

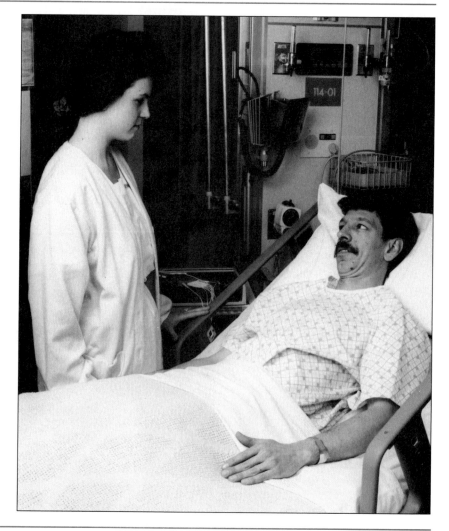

Select sites for limb lead attachment that are flat, fleshy, and hair-free; avoid bony and muscular areas. The inner aspects of the wrists and the medial aspects of the ankles are good choices. Following the manufacturer's guidelines for skin preparation, clean the sites to remove skin oil and improve electrode contact.

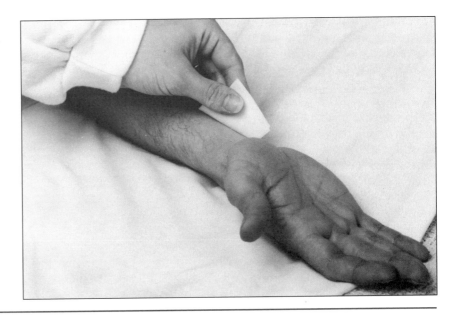

Apply the disposable electrodes to each of the four limbs. (If you're using reusable electrodes, apply the electrode paste or gel to each electrode before applying it to the skin.)

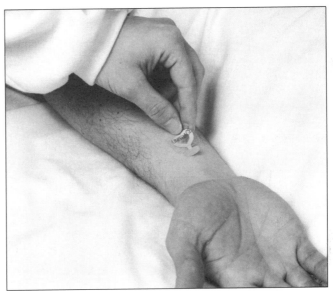

Clip each limb leadwire to the limb electrodes, matching each limb leadwire to the corresponding electrode. Each leadwire is color coded (and possibly letter coded) as follows: white (RA) for right arm, green (RL) for right leg, red (LL) for left leg, and black (LA) for left arm.

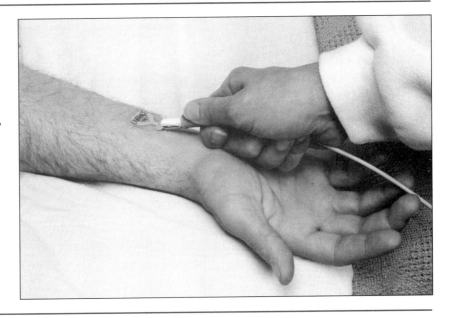

Alternatively, if you have reusable electrodes, place the metal electrodes on top of the paste or gel.

▶ *Clinical tip:* If you're using paste or gel, secure the electrode promptly after applying the conductive medium to prevent it from drying before use. Never substitute alcohol or acetone pads for the electrode paste or gel because these pads impair electrode contact with the skin and thus transmission of electrical impulses. Secure the electrode with a rubber strap. Avoid pulling the rubber strap too tightly; this could cause muscle spasms that would distort the ECG tracings. Then connect the limb leadwires to the electrodes (as shown).

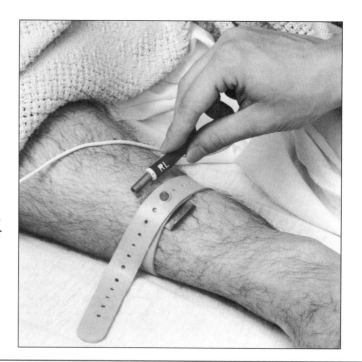

After connecting the machine to its power source, turn it on by pressing the ON-OFF switch. Then standardize or calibrate the machine according to the manufacturer's instructions. Watch for the standardization marks to appear on the ECG tracing (as shown).

▶ *Clinical tip:* To provide a consistent frame of reference throughout the procedure, standardize the machine after you run each lead. Some machines do this automatically.

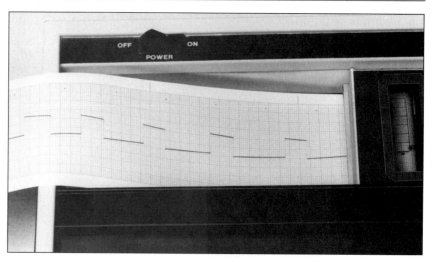

Now you're ready to run the first six leads: I, II, III, aV_R, aV_L, and aV_F. To begin, press the lead I button and run a 6-second strip. Label the strip with the appropriate lead according to your hospital's policy. (*Note:* Some machines, such as the one shown here, automatically mark the strip.)

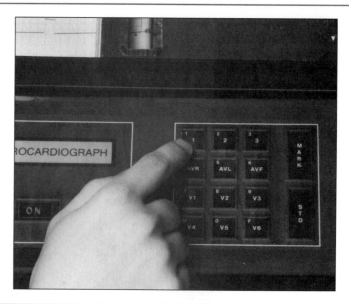

Press each remaining standard limb lead button (leads II and III) and the augmented limb lead buttons (leads aV$_R$, aV$_L$, and aV$_F$), and run a 6-second strip for each lead. Label the strip with the appropriate lead.

▷ **Clinical tip:** If you observe ectopic beats or rhythm changes, run longer strips so that the doctor can observe these irregularities at greater length.

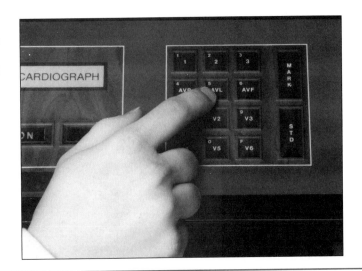

Now expose the patient's chest, being sure to preserve his privacy. Apply the chest leads as indicated at right. If you're using a suction bulb electrode, place the electrode gel or paste at the proper position for lead V$_1$. Then squeeze the rubber bulb of the electrode between your fingers, and place the bulb over the gel. Release your fingers.

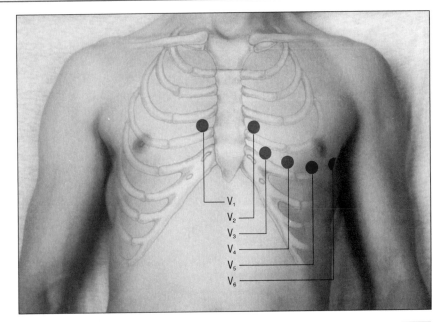

Clip the chest leadwires, which are color coded brown, to the chest electrodes (as shown). Before recording the ECG, make sure that all the leadwires are attached properly and that the electrodes adhere to the chest.

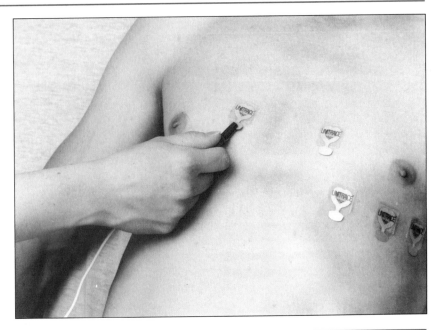

To record cardiac electrical activity from the chest leads, press the V₁ button and run a 6-second strip. Then press the V₂ button and run another 6-second strip. Continue this procedure until you record all six chest leads. (*Note:* If your machine uses a suction bulb electrode, you'll have to reposition this electrode each time you record a lead.)

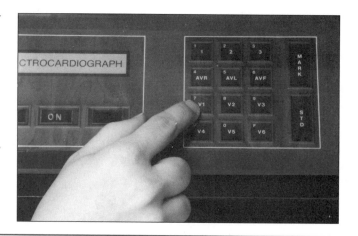

When the ECG is complete, remove the electrodes from the patient's skin. Clean his skin with the moist cloth towel or a 4″ × 4″ gauze pad. Then disconnect the leadwires from the electrodes.

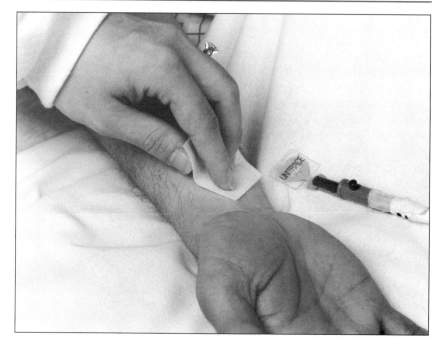

Document the procedure. On the ECG strip, write the patient's name and room number, the date and time, and his doctor's name.

▶ *Clinical tip:* Include any other special information about your patient. For instance, note whether he has an artificial pacemaker or feels any chest pain during the ECG. Also document any unusual electrode placements.

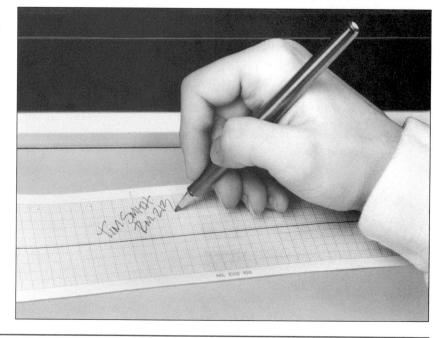

Twelve-lead ECG: A closer look

The 12-lead electrocardiogram (ECG) shows cardiac electrical activity from 12 different directions in relation to the wave of depolarization (shown in color). The waveform from the standard limb leads (I, II, and III) and the three augmented limb leads (aV$_R$, aV$_L$, and aV$_F$) represents the direction of electrical potential throughout the heart (indicated below by arrows). Abnormal waveforms from a particular lead reflect possible damage or dysfunction in that area.

The six precordial leads (V$_1$, V$_2$, V$_3$, V$_4$, V$_5$, V$_6$) represent the direction that electrical potential takes in the ventricles (also shown by directional arrows below at right). Again, waveform abnormalities suggest areas for further investigation.

The chart below lists each lead and the corresponding direction of electrical potential and view of the heart. A normal ECG waveform from that lead also appears.

Keep in mind that a normal ECG waveform has the following characteristics:
• P wave deflection is usually positive but may be diphasic or inverted in leads III, aV$_L$, and V$_1$, and may be inverted in aV$_R$.
• PR intervals are constant in all leads.
• QRS complex deflection changes with the lead, but duration remains constant.
• ST-segment deflection is isoelectric or with minimal deviation.
• T wave deflection should be upright in most leads. This wave is inverted in lead aV$_R$. Occasionally, deflection is biphasic or inverted in leads III, aV$_L$, and V$_1$.

Limb lead vectors

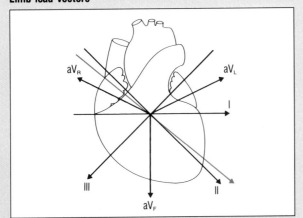

Precordial lead vectors

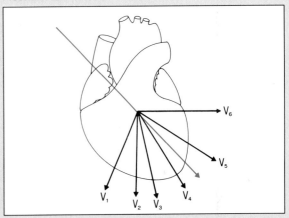

LEAD	DIRECTION OF POTENTIAL	VIEW	NORMAL WAVEFORM
I	Between left arm (positive) and right arm (negative)	Lateral wall	
II	Between left leg (positive) and right arm (negative)	Inferior wall	
III	Between left leg (positive) and left arm (negative)	Inferior wall	

(continued)

Twelve-lead ECG: A closer look (continued)

LEAD	DIRECTION OF POTENTIAL	VIEW	NORMAL WAVEFORM
aV$_R$	Right arm to heart	No specific view	
aV$_L$	Left arm to heart	Lateral wall	
aV$_F$	Left leg to heart	Inferior wall	
V$_1$	Fourth intercostal space, right sternal border, to heart	Anteroseptal wall	
V$_2$	Fourth intercostal space, left sternal border, to heart	Anteroseptal wall	
V$_3$	Midway between V$_2$ and V$_4$ to heart	Anterior wall	
V$_4$	Fifth intercostal space, midclavicular line, to heart	Anterior wall	
V$_5$	Fifth intercostal space, anterior axillary line, to heart	Lateral wall	
V$_6$	Fifth intercostal space, midaxillary line, to heart	Lateral wall	

PERFORMING A RIGHT CHEST-LEAD E.C.G.

Unlike a standard 12-lead electrocardiogram (ECG), used primarily to evaluate left ventricular function, a right chest-lead ECG reflects right ventricular function and provides clues to damage or dysfunction in this chamber. You may need to perform a right chest-lead ECG for a patient with an inferior wall myocardial infarction (MI) and suspected right ventricular involvement. Between 25% and 50% of patients with this type of MI have right ventricular involvement. And many of these patients have high creatine kinase levels.

Early identification of a right ventricular MI is essential because its treatment differs from that for other MIs. For instance, in left ventricular MI, treatment involves withholding I.V. fluids or administering them judiciously to prevent congestive heart failure. Conversely, in right ventricular MI, treatment usually requires administration of I.V. fluids to maintain adequate filling pressures on the right side of the heart. This helps the right ventricle eject an adequate volume of blood at an adequate pressure.

To perform a multichannel ECG for right chest leads, you'll need the following equipment: a multichannel ECG machine and paper, pregelled disposable electrodes, and several 4″ × 4″ gauze pads. You may also need a moist cloth or towel, shaving supplies, a drape, and a marking pen.

Take the assembled equipment to the patient's room. Then wash your hands.

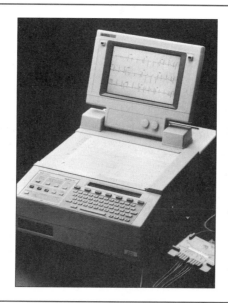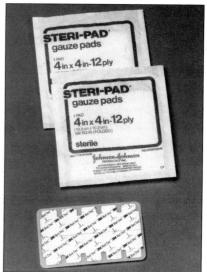

Inform the patient that the doctor has ordered a right chest-lead ECG, and describe the procedure. Explain that it involves placing electrodes on his wrists, ankles, and chest. Reassure him that the test is painless and takes only a few minutes, during which he'll need to lie quietly on the bed.

After plugging the ECG machine's cord into a grounded outlet, check the settings. The standard setting for paper speed is 25 mm/second; for amplitude, 1 mV/10 mm.

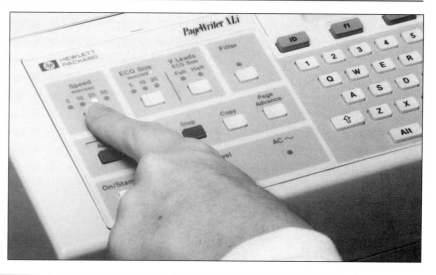

Contributors to this section include *Linda S. Baas, RN, PhD, CCRN, Carol Ann Knauff, RN, MSN, CCRN*, and *Karen E. Michael, RN, MSN*. Ms. Baas is an assistant professor at the University of Cincinnati College of Nursing and Health. Ms. Knauff is a critical care educator at Grand View Hospital, Sellersville, Pa. Ms. Michael is a case manager with Greater Atlantic Health Service, Philadelphia. The publisher thanks *Hill-Rom*, Batesville, Ind., and *Hewlett-Packard Co.*, Waltham, Mass., for their help.

Place the patient in a supine position or, if he has difficulty lying flat, in semi-Fowler's position. Provide privacy and expose his arms, legs, and chest. Use a drape or folded sheet to cover his pelvic area. (Cover a female patient's chest with a drape until you apply the chest leads.)

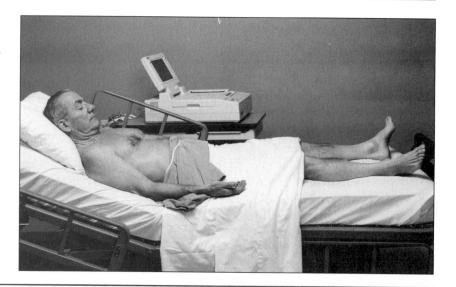

Examine the patient's wrists and ankles to select the best areas for the electrodes (near right). Choose flat and fleshy (not bony or muscular), hairless areas, such as the inner aspects of the wrist and ankle. Clean the sites with a gauze pad to promote good skin contact.

Follow the manufacturer's recommendations for electrode placement, if provided. If you're using disposable electrodes, peel off the contact paper and apply the electrodes to the chosen sites (far right).

▶ *Clinical tip:* For best results, place the electrodes symmetrically on the limbs. If the patient's wrist or ankle is covered by a dressing, or if the patient is an amputee, choose an area that's available on both sides.

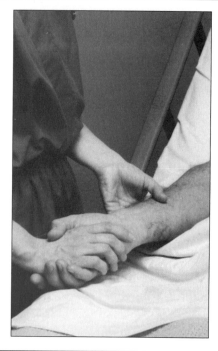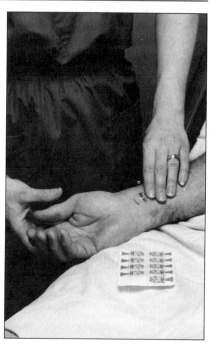

Connect the leadwires to the electrodes. The leadwires are color coded and lettered. Place the white or right arm (RA) wire on the right arm; the black or left arm (LA) wire on the left arm; the green or right leg (RL) wire on the right leg; and the red or left leg (LL) wire on the left leg.

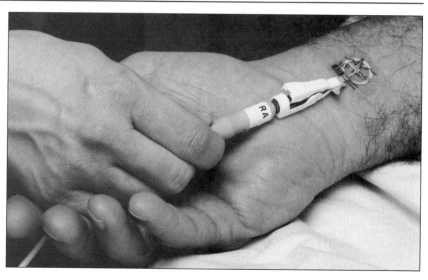

Examine the patient's chest to locate the correct sites for chest-lead placement. If the patient is a woman, you'll place the electrodes under the breast tissue.

▷ *Clinical tip:* If the patient's chest is very hairy, you may need to shave a small area for each electrode to ensure adequate skin contact.

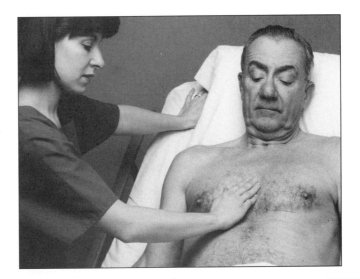

Use your fingers to feel the spaces between the patient's ribs (the intercostal spaces). Start at the second intercostal space on the left (the notch felt at the top of the sternum, where the manubrium joins the body of the sternum). Count down two spaces to the fourth intercostal space.

Apply a disposable electrode to that site, and attach leadwire V_{1R} to the electrode.

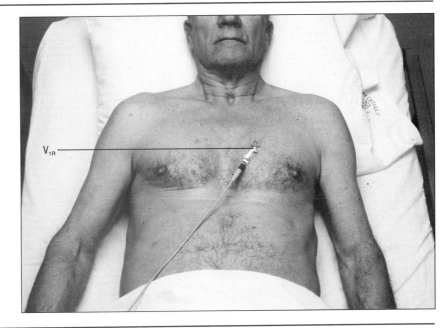

Move your fingers across the sternum to the fourth intercostal space on the right side of the sternum. Apply a disposable electrode to that site and attach lead V_{2R}.

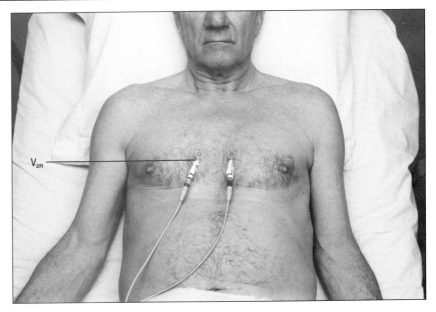

Move your finger down to the fifth intercostal space and over to the midclavicular line. Place a disposable electrode here and attach lead V_{4R}.

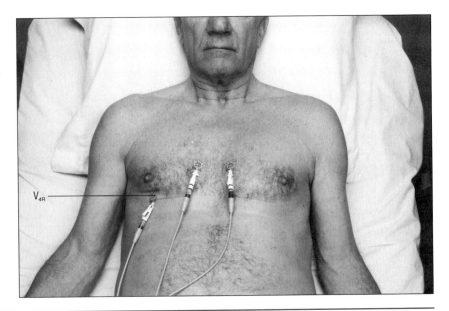

Visually draw a line between V_{2R} and V_{4R}. Apply a disposable electrode midway on this line and attach lead V_{3R}.

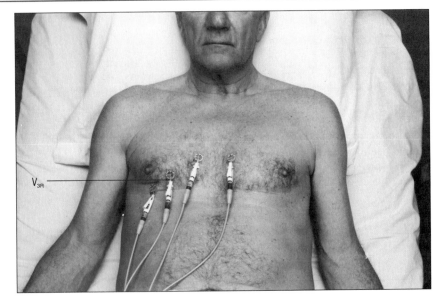

Move your finger horizontally from V_{4R} to the right midaxillary line. Apply a disposable electrode to this site and attach lead V_{6R}.

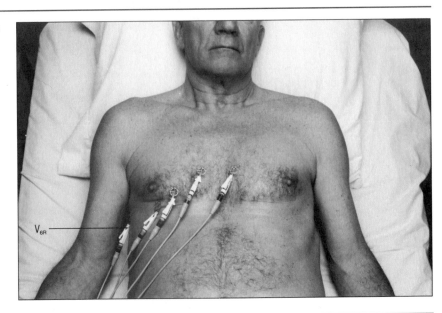

Move your fingers along the same horizontal line to the midpoint between V_{4R} and V_{6R}. This is the right anterior midaxillary line. Apply a disposable electrode to this site and attach lead V_{5R}.

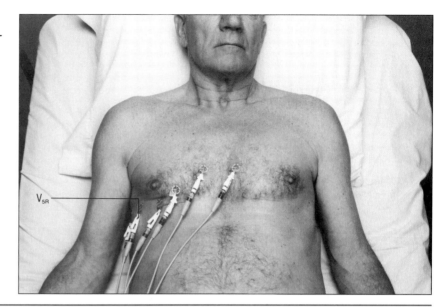

Turn on the ECG machine. Ask the patient to breathe normally but not to talk during the recording so that muscle movement won't distort the tracing. Enter any appropriate patient information required by the machine you're using.

If necessary, standardize the machine. This will cause a square tracing of 10 mm (two large squares) to appear on the ECG paper when the machine is set for 1 mV (1 mV = 10 mm).

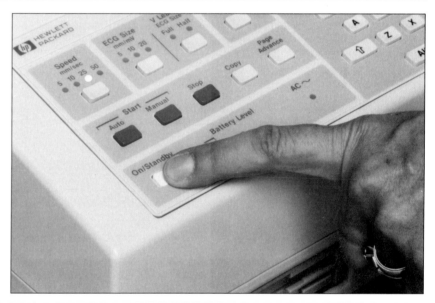

Press the AUTO key. The ECG machine will record all 12 leads automatically. Check your hospital's policy for the number of readings to obtain. (Some hospitals require at least two ECGs so that one copy can be sent out for interpretation while the other remains at the bedside.)

When you're finished recording the ECG, turn off the machine. Clearly label the ECG with the patient's name, the date, and the time. Also label it "RIGHT CHEST ECG" to distinguish it from a standard 12-lead ECG. Remove the electrodes and help the patient get comfortable before you document the procedure.

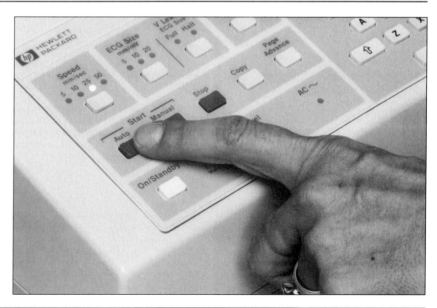

PERFORMING A POSTERIOR-LEAD E.C.G.

Because of the location of the heart's posterior surface, changes associated with myocardial damage aren't apparent on a standard 12-lead electrocardiogram (ECG). To help identify posterior involvement, some practitioners recommend adding posterior leads to the 12-lead ECG. Despite lung and muscle barriers, posterior leads may provide clues to a posterior wall infarction so that appropriate treatment can begin.

Usually, the posterior-lead ECG is performed with a standard ECG and only involves recording the additional posterior leads—V_7, V_8, and V_9. Rarely, the doctor may request right-sided posterior leads V_{7R}, V_{8R}, and V_{9R}.

To perform a posterior-lead ECG, you'll need a multichannel or single-channel ECG machine with recording paper, disposable pre-gelled electrodes, and a few $4'' \times 4''$ gauze pads. You may also need a moist cloth, a drape, shaving supplies, and a marking pen.

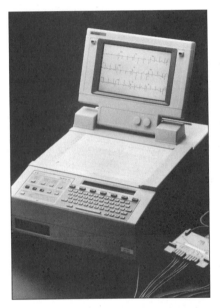
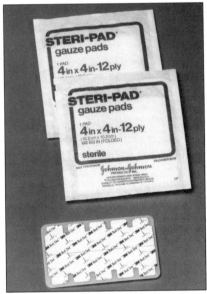

Explain the procedure to the patient, and wash your hands. Help him onto his right side and expose his back (as shown). Use the drape as needed for privacy.

Locate the three sites—V_7, V_8, and V_9—for electrode placement on the patient's back. You'll find these sites along the same horizontal line opposite anterior leads V_4, V_5, and V_6: V_7 is on the posterior axillary line, V_8 is on the left midscapular line, and V_9 is left of the spinal column.

▶ *Clinical tip:* The number of leads may vary according to the cardiologist's preference. (If right posterior leads are requested, position the patient on his left side. These leads, known as V_{7R}, V_{8R}, and V_{9R}, are located at the same landmarks on the right side of the patient's back.)

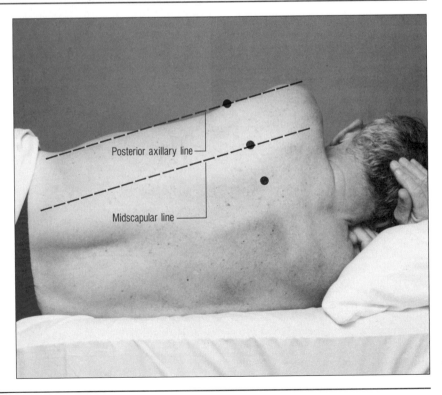

Posterior axillary line —
Midscapular line —

Prepare the electrode sites according to the manufacturer's instructions. To ensure good skin contact, shave the site if the patient has considerable back hair.

If you're using a multichannel ECG machine, begin by attaching a disposable electrode to the V_1 position on the left posterior axillary line, fifth intercostal space. Then attach the V_4 leadwire to the V_7 electrode (as shown).

▶ *Clinical tip:* Some ECG machines won't operate unless you connect all leadwires. In that case, you may need to connect the limb leadwires and the leadwires for V_1, V_2, and V_3.

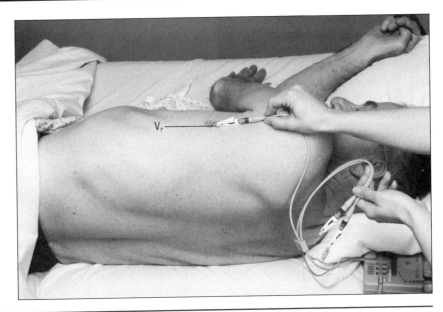

Next, attach a disposable electrode to the patient's back at the V_8 position on the left midscapular line, fifth intercostal space, and attach the V_5 leadwire to this electrode.

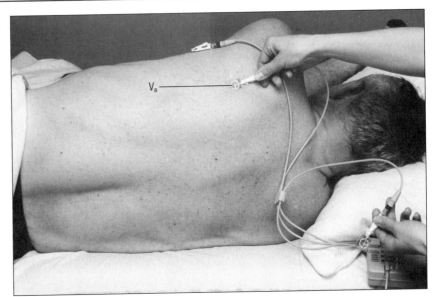

Finally, attach a disposable electrode to the patient's back at the V_9 position, just left of the spinal column at the fifth intercostal space. Then attach the V_6 leadwire to the V_9 electrode.

If you're using a single-channel ECG machine, put electrode gel at locations for electrodes V_7, V_8, and V_9. Then connect the brown V leadwire to the V_7 electrode and record this lead. Move the brown leadwire to the V_8 position and record the V_8 lead. Finally, move the leadwire to the V_9 position and record the V_9 lead.

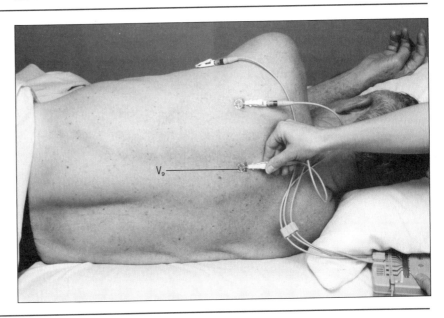

Turn on the machine. Make sure that the paper speed is set for 25 mm/second. If necessary, standardize the machine. Press AUTO and the machine will record.

▶ **Clinical tip:** For a multi-channel ECG machine, all leads will print out a straight line except for V_4, V_5, and V_6. Relabel these V_7, V_8, and V_9, respectively.

For a single-channel ECG machine, turn the selector knob to "V" and record the V_7 lead. Reposition the electrode to the V_8 position and record the lead. Repeat for the V_9 position.

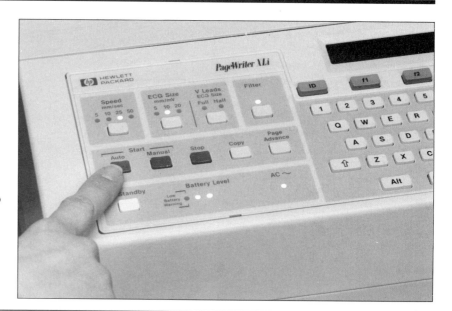

When the ECG is complete, remove the electrodes and clean the patient's skin with a gauze pad or a moist cloth. If you think the patient may need more than one posterior-lead ECG, use the marking pen to mark the electrode sites on his skin to permit an accurate comparison for future tracings.

Document the procedure in your nurse's notes. Make sure that the patient's name, age, room number, date, time, and doctor's name are clearly written on the ECG, along with the relabeled lead tracings.

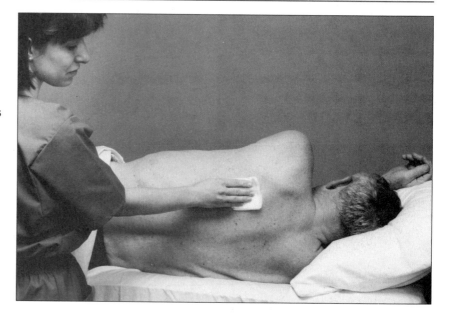

PERFORMING SIGNAL-AVERAGED E.C.G.

A simple, noninvasive test, signal-averaged electrocardiography (ECG) uses a computer to identify late electrical potentials (tiny impulses that follow normal ventricular depolarization). It may help identify patients who have a high risk of sudden death from sustained ventricular tachycardia (VT). Identifying such patients allows the doctor to take preventive measures, such as drug therapy. Test results may also help determine whether the patient is a candidate for invasive procedures, such as electrophysiologic testing or angiography.

Patients who are prone to VT—after myocardial infarction, for example—or those who have unexplained syncope or nonischemic congestive cardiomyopathy typically have late electrical potentials. Although researchers have known about this conduction abnormality for years, they hadn't been able to detect it until the recent development of signal-averaged ECG.

Of course, screening for late potentials isn't foolproof. Some patients with VT may not have late potentials because reentry abnormalities don't always cause this arrhythmia. Or some patients may have late potentials of such low amplitude that the abnormality will be obscured despite signal averaging.

What's more, the test isn't indicated for patients with prolonged QRS complexes (which may conceal late potentials) that result from such conduction abnormalities as bundle-branch blocks, Wolff-Parkinson-White syndrome, or paced ventricular rhythms.

HOW SIGNAL AVERAGING WORKS

The signal-averaged ECG is a noise-free surface ECG recording from three specialized leads for several hundred beats. The computer-assisted tracing results from three processes—amplification, signal averaging, and filtering.

Amplification enlarges late electrical potentials so that they can be recognized. However, it also enlarges other electrical activity or "noises," such as external interference and respiratory and skeletal muscle movement.

At the same time, the computer processes the signals from a series of heartbeats to produce one representative QRS complex without artifacts. Its averaging process cancels out noise that doesn't occur as a repetitive pattern or with the same consistent timing as the QRS complex.

To complete the process, high-pass and low-pass filters reduce additional noise that occurs, for instance, during the ST segment and the T wave. Without this filtering, late electrical potentials would remain hidden. Filtering, however, can't eliminate the noise caused by muscle movement, so you'll need to keep the patient still during the test. (See the patient-teaching aid *Learning about a signal-averaged electrocardiogram,* page 442.) You'll also need to prepare his skin adequately and keep in mind that a slow heart rate and frequent ventricular ectopic beats or aberrant beats may increase the time needed to produce a signal-averaged ECG.

Gather the necessary equipment and take it to the patient's bedside. You'll need a specialized ECG machine (such as the model from Arrhythmia Research Technology at right), electrodes, alcohol sponges, and possibly a razor. You'll also need an IBM-compatible computer to store and print the results.

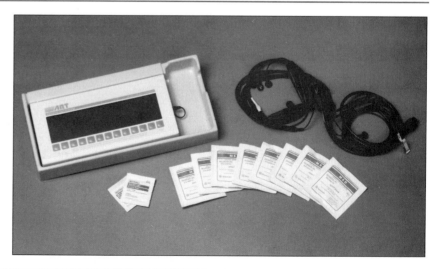

Contributors to this section include *Lynn Lansdowne, RN,C, MSN, CCRN,* Director of Critical Care and Education at Pocono Medical Center, East Stroudsburg, Pa., and *Marylin Schactman, RN, MSN, CCRN,* Assistant Vice-President of Nursing at St. Francis Hospital, Roslyn, N.Y. The publisher thanks *Arrhythmia Research Technology, Inc.,* Austin, Tex., and *Hill-Rom,* Batesville, Ind., for their help.

Explain the procedure to the patient. Tell him that this test records the heart's electrical activity and can identify abnormal rhythms early, when they can be treated. Emphasize that he shouldn't talk or move his head, arms, or body during the procedure. Reassure him that the test takes only about 10 minutes and that no electrical current will enter his body.

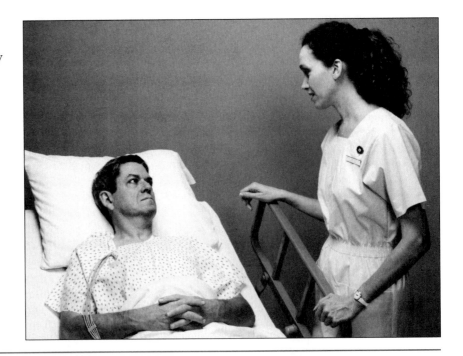

Place the machine close to the patient's bed. If he's connected to a cardiac monitor, remove the monitoring electrodes to accommodate the new electrodes and leadwires and to minimize electrical interference on the signal-averaged tracing. Unplug all unnecessary equipment to decrease extraneous electrical noise.

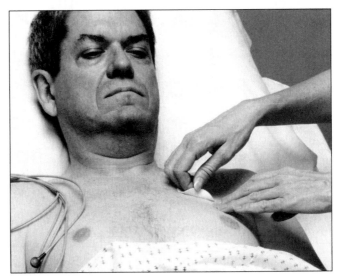

Place the patient in a supine position with his arms at his sides. Drape him appropriately (as shown). Ask him to relax his arms and legs, and keep him warm to minimize shivering or trembling, which can cause electrical interference. Make sure his feet aren't touching the bed's footboard, which can also cause interference.

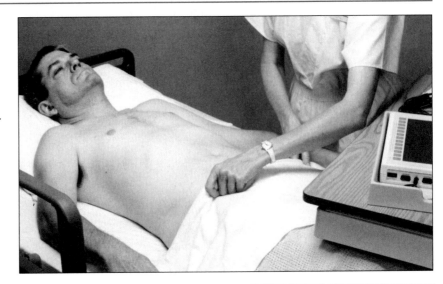

Using an alcohol sponge, prepare the patient's skin for electrode placement (as shown). After the skin dries, lightly scrape it with the edge of the electrode so that the slightly rough surface promotes contact with the electrode.

Avoid applying an electrode to hairy skin. If necessary, shave the area first.

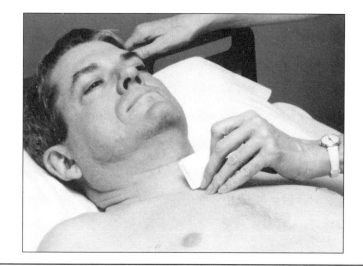

To place electrodes on the patient's chest, select flat, fleshy areas and avoid large muscles or bony prominences. Place the positive X electrode at the left fourth intercostal space, midaxillary line; the negative X electrode at the right fourth intercostal space, midaxillary line; the positive Y electrode at the left iliac crest; the negative Y electrode at the superior aspect of the manubrium of the sternum; the positive Z electrode at the fourth intercostal space, left sternal border (standard V_2 position); and the ground (G) electrode on the lower right at the eighth rib.

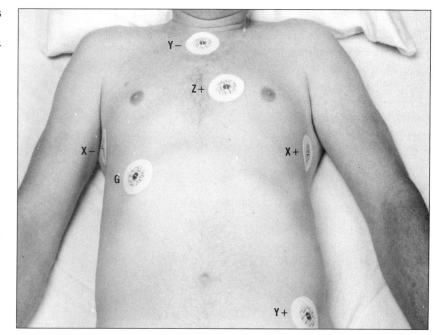

Then have the patient turn over or sit up. Place the negative Z electrode on his back, directly posterior to the positive Z electrode.

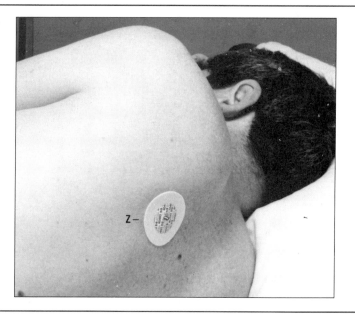

Alternatively, your hospital may use the following electrode placements: the positive X electrode at the left fourth intercostal space, midaxillary line; the negative X electrode at the right fourth intercostal space, midaxillary line; the positive Y electrode at the standard V_3 position; the negative Y electrode at the second intercostal space along the left side of the sternum; the positive Z electrode at the standard V_2 position; and the ground electrode on the lower right side at the eighth rib.

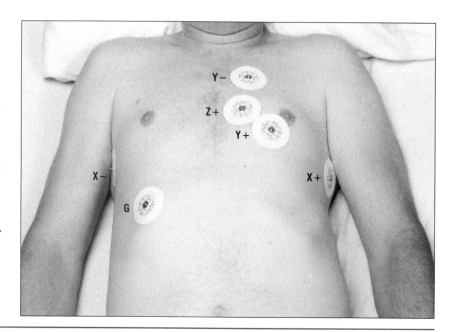

To position the negative Z electrode, have the patient turn over or sit up. Place this electrode on his back, directly posterior to the positive Z electrode. Then help him into a supine position.

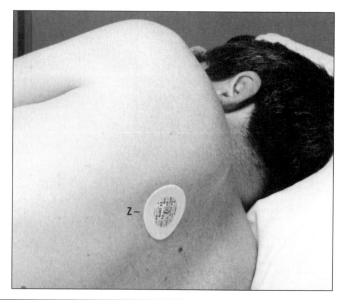

Connect the leadwires to the electrodes. Instruct the patient to lie still with his arms at his sides. Tell him to relax and breathe normally. Also tell him to avoid talking except to inform you if he needs to move, cough, or sneeze. That way, you can stop the recording temporarily.

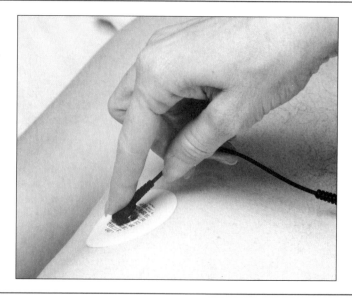

Turn on the machine by pressing the ON/OFF key. Now press the HIR key (as shown) to record a signal-averaged ECG tracing. Check to see that the baseline tracing doesn't show any noise interference. Examine the pattern of the tracing.

Note: To obtain a reliable signal-averaged ECG, check that the patient isn't having ectopic beats.

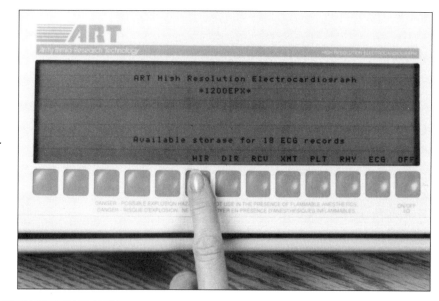

Press the START key. The patient's heart rate will be displayed at the top of the screen. The ECG machine will also store the number of beats recorded and display this number next to the patient's heart rate.

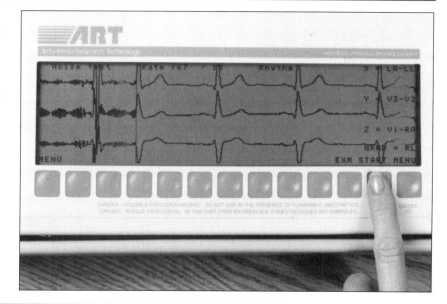

Once you've recorded 50 beats (the monitor will display 50 cycles), press the EXM key to view the current averaged data. Note that once you press the EXM key, the screen will display new codes (as shown).

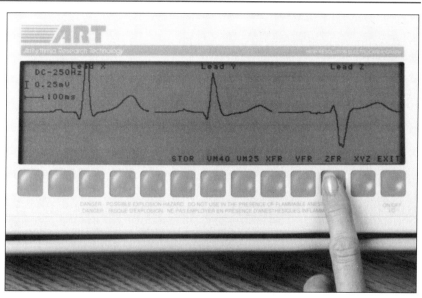

Then press the UM40 key to filter the tracing. Verify that the noise level is 0.3 microvolts (μV) or less and continue recording. Record at least 200 beats.

▶ **Clinical tip:** If the noise level exceeds 0.3 μV, check the electrode connections and make sure that the patient isn't holding onto the bed rails or pressing against the footboard. If you can't decrease the noise level, stop the recording, remove the electrodes, and begin the procedure again.

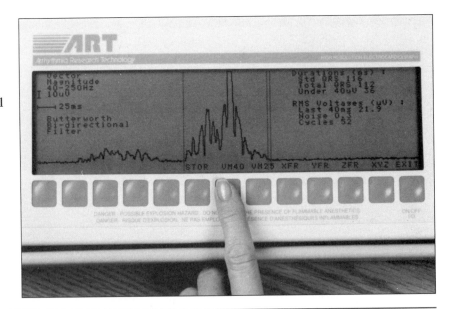

After you've recorded 200 beats with a noise level of 0.3 μV or less, press the STOR key to store the information. Then enter the patient's identifying data into the machine, and turn it off. Remove the electrodes from the patient (as shown) and cover him. Process the information from the signal-averaging apparatus as directed by the operator's manual, and print a tracing for interpretation and documentation.

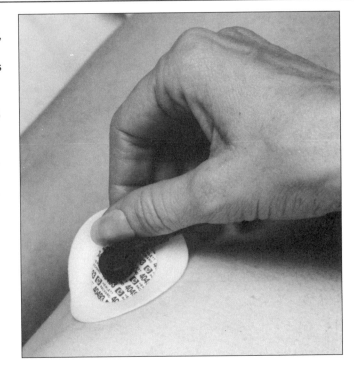

Detecting late potentials

Because late electrical potentials have a low amplitude, you'll need to look closely at a patient's signal-averaged electrocardiogram (ECG) to detect them. Occurring at the end of or just after the QRS complex and lasting from 20 to 60 milliseconds (msec) into the ST segment, late potentials range in amplitude from 1 to 20 microvolts (μV).

Compare the signal-averaged ECGs shown here.

In both examples, the upper tracings reflect cardiac activity from leads Z, X, and Y at high gain; the lower tracings illustrate the filtered QRS complex.

The tracing at left illustrates the absence of late potentials; the tracing at right shows late potentials (see arrow) lasting about 60 msec with a maximum amplitude under 10 μV. The right lower tracing also indicates that the patient has ventricular tachycardia.

Signal-averaged ECG without late potentials

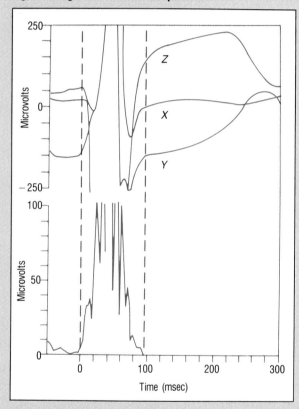

Signal-averaged ECG with late potentials

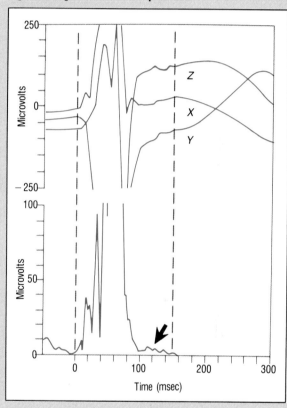

Waveforms provided by Arrhythmia Research Technology, Inc., Austin, Tex.

Learning about a signal-averaged electrocardiogram

Dear Patient:

Your doctor has ordered a test called a *signal-averaged electrocardiogram*. This test records the electrical activity of your heart. It uses special computerized equipment to study many of your heartbeats and to create an image of one typical heartbeat. The doctor will then review this typical heartbeat to detect very small electrical signals called *late potentials*. This test can help detect certain heart problems early, when they can be treated most effectively. Here are important steps you can take to make sure that test results are accurate.

What happens before the test
Listen to the nurse's directions about remaining perfectly still when she tells you to. The test takes only a few minutes.

What happens during the test
First, the nurse will clean and rub areas on your chest and back briskly with an alcohol pad. This may redden your skin. If necessary, she may shave the area.

Next, she'll place several small disks called *electrodes* on your skin. She'll

attach several electrodes to your chest and one to your back. Then she'll attach thin wires to the electrodes. Don't be concerned: The electrodes will not produce an electric shock.

During the test, keep these directions in mind:
• Remember to lie as still as possible during the test.
• Rest your arms at your sides.
• Don't talk.
• Try to breathe normally.
• Stay relaxed.
• Close your eyes if you want to.
• If you think you have to move, cough, sneeze, or scratch your nose, signal the nurse so that she can stop the test before losing the information that has already been collected. When you feel settled, she'll resume the test.

What happens after the test
Because this test is simple and painless, you won't need any special follow-up care. However, you may feel a minor tugging sensation on your skin when the nurse removes the electrodes.

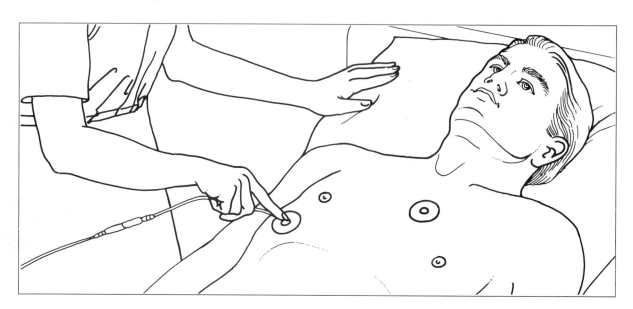

OBTAINING AN ATRIAL ELECTROGRAM

When a patient has suspected atrial fibrillation or atrial flutter—arrhythmias that commonly occur after cardiac surgery—the doctor may request an atrial electrogram for confirmation. This test records the heart's electrical activity from electrode wires positioned on atrial tissue during open-heart surgery. The recording amplifies the signal for atrial activity and reduces the signal for ventricular activity. Atrial electrograms are useful when a standard 12-lead electrocardiogram (ECG) fails to clearly identify and record atrial rhythm.

Junctional rhythms and ventricular tachycardia can also be detected on an atrial electrogram, which may be obtained from either unipolar or bipolar electrode wires.

Recording a unipolar atrial electrogram

Obtain the necessary equipment and take it to the patient's bedside. You'll need clean gloves, double-ended alligator clips, sterile 3″ × 3″ gauze pads, and tape (near right), as well as a 5-lead bedside monitor (far right) or a 12-lead ECG machine.

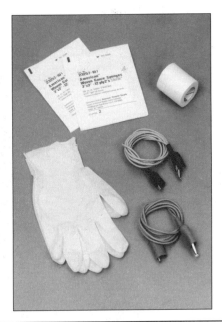
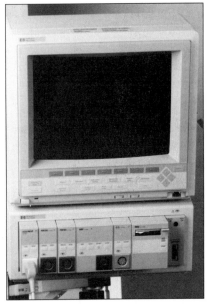

Locate the atrial pacing wires, which lie to the right of the patient's sternal incision. Put on gloves and remove the dressing from these wires (as shown). By wearing gloves, you observe universal precautions and protect yourself from microshock when handling pacemaker wires.

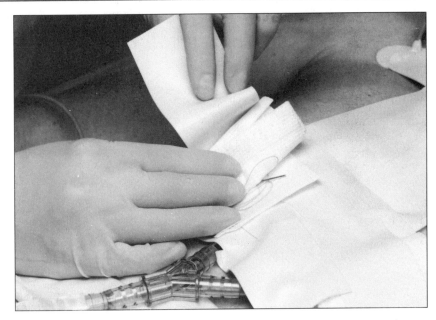

Connect one atrial wire to one end of a double-ended alligator clip. Then attach the opposite end of the alligator clip to the V lead of the bedside monitor (as shown). Leave the remaining four ECG leads attached to the patient.

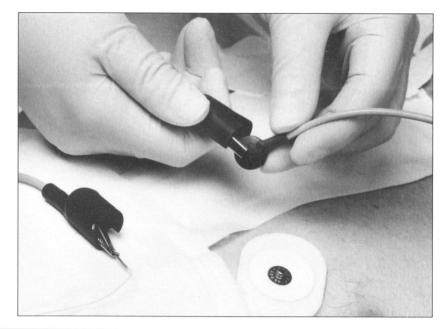

Display lead II and a V lead on the bedside monitor. Lead II is the standard lead for an ECG tracing. The V lead tracing produces the atrial electrogram (as shown). Record a dual-channel ECG strip from lead II and the V lead.

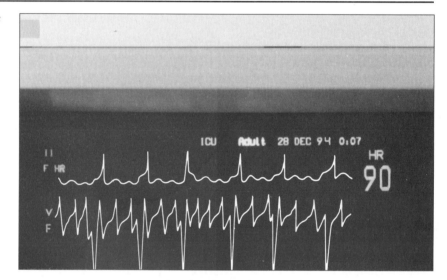

Remove the alligator clips from the atrial wire (as shown), and re-wrap the atrial wires in a sterile 3″ × 3″ gauze pad before taping the bundle in place on the patient's chest. Label the dressing "ATRIAL WIRES" or "A."

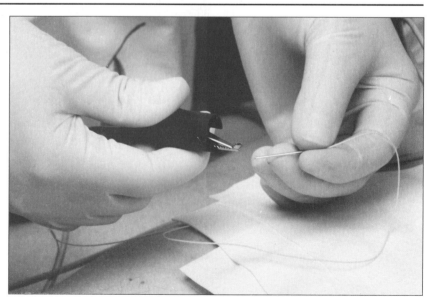

Return the V lead electrode to its original location on the chest. Then remove and dispose of your gloves and wash your hands.

Interpret the rhythm strip and notify the doctor of any abnormalities.

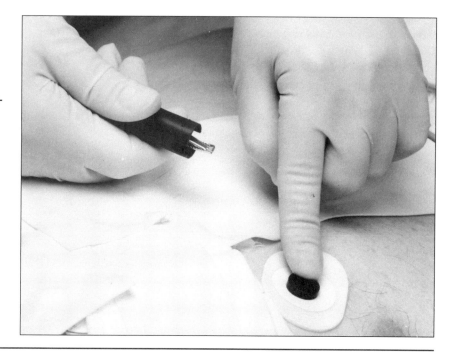

Recording a bipolar atrial electrogram

Wash your hands and put on gloves. Locate the atrial wires to the right of the patient's incision. Remove the dressing from the atrial wires.

You'll need two alligator clips. Connect one end of the first alligator clip to the left arm (LA) ECG leadwire and the other end to the atrial wire. Connect one end of the second alligator clip to the right arm (RA) leadwire and the other end to the remaining atrial wire (as shown).

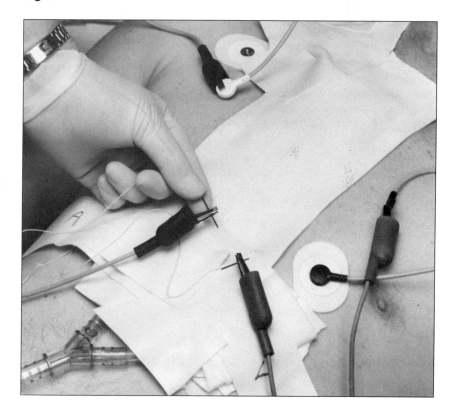

Display lead I and a V lead on the bedside monitor. Lead I produces the atrial electrogram, and the V lead produces the standard ECG. Record a dual-channel rhythm strip displaying both leads.

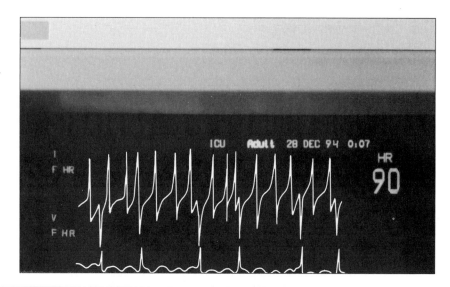

Remove the alligator clips. Then redress the atrial wires by wrapping them in a 3″ × 3″ gauze pad and taping the bundle in place. Label the dressing "ATRIAL WIRES" or "A."

Return the RA and LA electrodes to their original locations on the patient's chest (as shown). Interpret the rhythm strip and notify the doctor if the tracings are abnormal. Keep in mind that the bipolar simultaneous recording provides the best tracing of atrial activity.

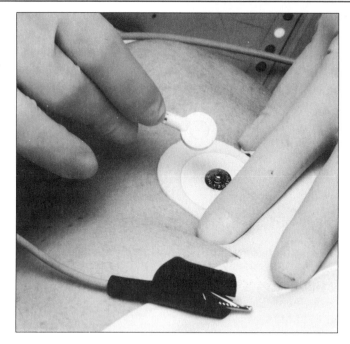

LEARNING ABOUT A.B.G. ANALYSIS

When a patient has respiratory difficulty, one of the first tests his doctor may order is arterial blood gas (ABG) analysis. ABG analysis measures the pressure exerted by both oxygen (O_2) and carbon dioxide (CO_2) in a mixture of gases in circulating blood. This value, called a partial pressure, is denoted by the letter "P" before the name of the measured gas—for example, PO_2 and PCO_2.

By measuring pH and the levels of O_2, CO_2, and bicarbonate (HCO_3^-) in blood, you can evaluate how effectively the patient's lungs exchange gases. These levels also help you gauge the effectiveness of respiratory therapy.

Some patients, particularly those who are critically ill, require monitoring of arterial O_2 and CO_2 levels as well as arterial oxygen saturation (SaO_2). This monitoring may be done intermittently, as discussed in this section, or continuously.

Either way, you'll need to know how to perform specific procedures—monitoring O_2 or CO_2 levels in arterial or venous blood, for example—to ensure optimal respiratory status for every patient.

NORMAL VALUES

PaO_2 denotes oxygen tension, or the partial pressure of oxygen in arterial blood. It reflects the amount of oxygen delivered to the bloodstream from the lungs. PaO_2 normally ranges from 80 to 100 mm Hg.

$PaCO_2$ signifies carbon dioxide tension, or the partial pressure exerted by carbon dioxide in arterial blood. Primarily influenced by lung changes and respiratory pattern, this value indicates how efficiently the lungs eliminate carbon dioxide. $PaCO_2$ typically ranges from 34 to 46 mm Hg.

A measure of blood acidity, pH reflects hydrogen ion concentration. Arterial blood's pH should be between 7.34 and 7.45.

Primarily affected by metabolic changes, HCO_3^- indicates the amount of bicarbonate ion or alkaline substance dissolved in the blood. The normal range is from 22 to 26 mEq/liter.

A measure of oxygen-saturated hemoglobin (oxyhemoglobin), SaO_2 represents the percentage of oxygen carried by hemoglobin. SaO_2 should range from 95% to 100%.

SAMPLING SITES

Typically, you'll tap the radial artery to obtain an arterial blood sample, although you may use the brachial or femoral arteries. In most cases, a doctor performs a femoral artery puncture; however, a specially trained nurse may also do this.

If the patient requires frequent ABG analyses, an indwelling intra-arterial line may be inserted to eliminate the pain and risk of multiple vessel punctures. Or a venous-arterial management protection (VAMP) device may be used. This device permits repeated blood sampling while reducing the staff's exposure to blood and minimizing the patient's blood loss.

NURSING CONSIDERATIONS

Although ABG findings help you evaluate overall respiratory and metabolic status, they usually must be interpreted along with the findings of other tests, such as pulmonary function studies or cardiac output measurements.

Keep in mind that the accuracy of ABG results hinges on proper technique for specimen collection. For instance, inaccurate results can stem from failure to properly heparinize a syringe before drawing the sample, exposing the sample to air, or inadvertently drawing venous as well as arterial blood.

Also keep in mind that some medications may alter ABG results. For example, sodium bicarbonate, ethacrynic acid, hydrocortisone, metolazone, prednisone, and thiazide may elevate $PaCO_2$ levels. Acetazolamide, methicillin, nitrofurantoin, and tetracycline may lower $PaCO_2$ levels.

Another measure to ensure an accurate ABG analysis involves timing the blood sample. If the patient has had an intermittent positive-pressure breathing treatment, a change in the concentration of delivered oxygen, or suctioning, for example, wait about 20 minutes before drawing blood. This allows time for the blood gases to stabilize.

Joanne Patzek DaCunha, RN, MSN, who contributed to this section, is the associate clinical director at Springhouse Corporation. The publisher also thanks the following organizations for their help: *Baxter Healthcare Corp., Edwards Critical Care Division*, Irvine, Calif.; *Doylestown (Pa.) Hospital; Hill Rom*, Batesville, Ind.; and *Hopkins Medical Products*, Baltimore.

OBTAINING AN ARTERIAL SAMPLE

To obtain an arterial blood sample, you'll need to prepare the equipment. And, if you'll be drawing blood from the radial artery, you'll need to perform Allen's test. The following pages show you how to accomplish these necessary tasks and obtain an arterial blood sample.

Setting up the equipment

Begin by obtaining a prepackaged ABG kit or assembling the following: a 10-ml plastic syringe specially made for drawing ABG samples, a 1-ml ampule of aqueous heparin (1:1,000) if the syringe is not heparinized, a 20G 1½" needle, a 22G 1" needle, an alcohol sponge, a povidone-iodine sponge, two 2" × 2" gauze pads, a rubber cap for the syringe hub and a rubber stopper for the needle, a plastic bag for ice, a label, a rolled washcloth, and an adhesive bandage. If the patient has an indwelling arterial line, obtain an unheparinized 5-ml syringe.

You'll also need clean gloves, ice, and a laboratory request form if your hospital uses them. Write on the form (or enter into the computer) the amount of oxygen the patient is receiving (if any), the type of oxygen delivery device, the patient's rectal temperature, and his respiratory rate.

If the patient is on a ventilator, note the fraction of inspired oxygen (FIO_2), tidal volume, and rate. Then wash your hands and open the ABG kit. Remove the sample label and complete it appropriately. Fill the plastic bag with ice.

If the patient will have a VAMP device (shown at right), you'll need to obtain it.

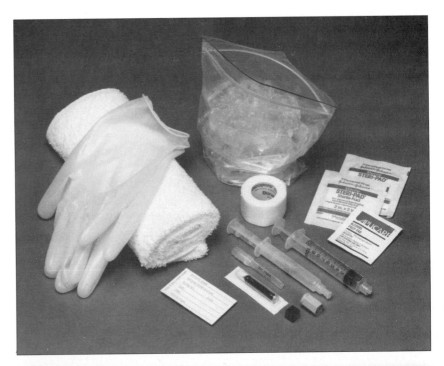

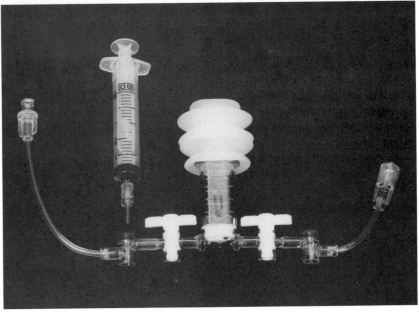

First, put on gloves. Then heparinize the 10-ml syringe to prevent the drawn blood from clotting. Attach the 20G needle to the syringe and open the heparin ampule. Draw all of the heparin into the syringe. Next, hold the syringe upright, rotate the barrel, and slowly pull back the plunger to about two-thirds of the barrel length or to the 7-ml mark if the syringe is marked (as shown near right).

Slowly depress the plunger, expelling all but about 0.1 ml of heparin. Replace the 20G needle with the 22G needle. Uncap the 22G needle, and eject the remaining heparin (as shown far right). Recap the needle, take the equipment to the patient's bedside, and explain the procedure to him.

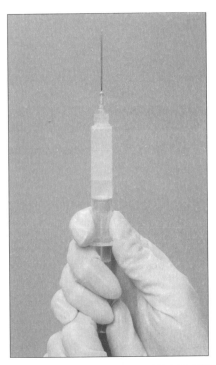 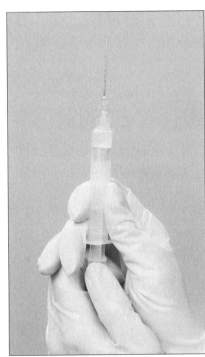

Performing Allen's test

To make sure that the ulnar artery can supply the patient's hand with blood if the radial artery occludes, perform Allen's test: Place the patient's arm palm side up on the bedside table. Put a rolled washcloth under his wrist, and ask him to clench his fist. With the index and middle fingers of both hands, press on the patient's radial and ulnar arteries. Apply enough pressure to occlude arterial flow. Maintain this pressure briefly.

Keeping your fingers in place, ask the patient to unclench his fist and relax his hand (as shown). Because you'll be impeding blood flow, the palm will be blanched.

Next, remove your fingers from the ulnar artery only. Oxygenated blood should flood the hand, causing the hand to flush with color. If this happens, you can safely perform the radial artery puncture. If the hand doesn't flush, don't perform the puncture. Instead, repeat the test on the other hand. If that hand also fails to color, collect the sample from the brachial artery.

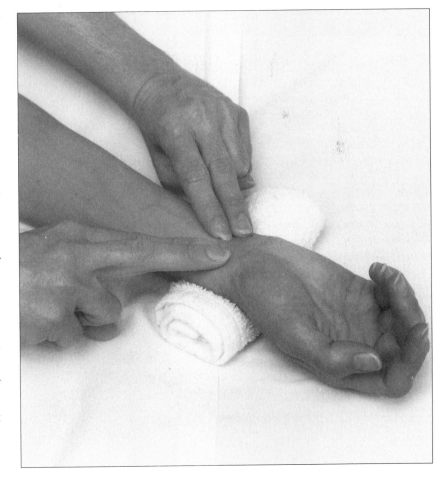

Drawing blood from the radial artery

Wash your hands and put on gloves. Palpate the patient's wrist to locate the radial artery. Then, using a povidone-iodine sponge, clean the puncture site. Wipe in a circular motion, starting at the center and swirling outward. Allow the area to dry.

Using the same circular motion, wipe the site with the alcohol sponge. Allow the skin to dry.

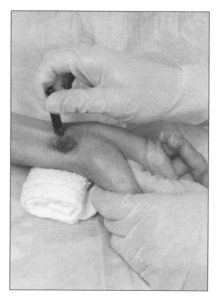 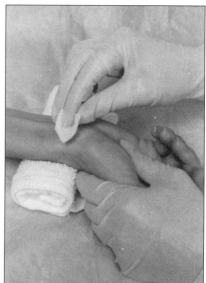

Using your index or middle finger, again palpate the artery. Then pick up the 22G needle, making sure that the bevel of the needle points upward. Hold the syringe over the site, with the needle at a 45-degree angle over the radial artery.

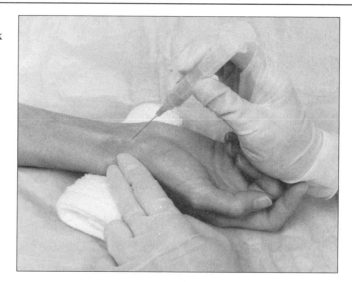

If you're drawing blood from the brachial artery, hold the needle at a 60-degree angle over the artery.

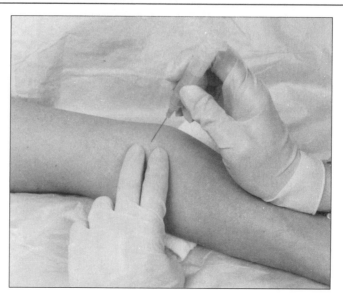

Without changing the angle of the needle, puncture the skin and arterial wall in one motion. Follow the path of the artery. Be careful not to exert too much pressure, which could cause you to puncture the opposite wall of the artery (resulting in a hematoma) or to nick the periosteum (causing severe pain).

Unless the patient has severe hypotension, the blood should fill the syringe without your having to pull back on the plunger. Collect about 5 ml of blood in the syringe.

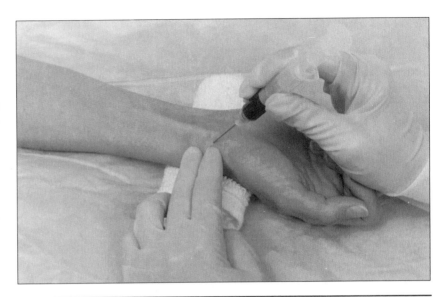

Remove the syringe from the artery. Immediately press a gauze pad against the puncture site, and apply firm pressure for at least 5 minutes—10 minutes if the patient is receiving anticoagulant therapy. If necessary, have a co-worker apply pressure to the site while you prepare the sample for the laboratory. Place an adhesive bandage on the site when the bleeding stops.

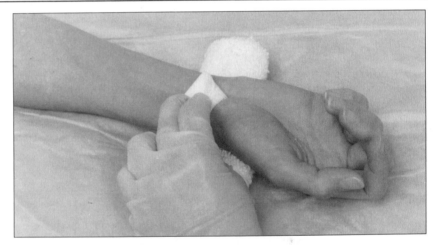

Check the syringe for air bubbles, which can alter PaO₂ values. To remove any bubbles, place a 2″ × 2″ gauze pad over the needle, hold the syringe upright, and slowly eject some of the blood.

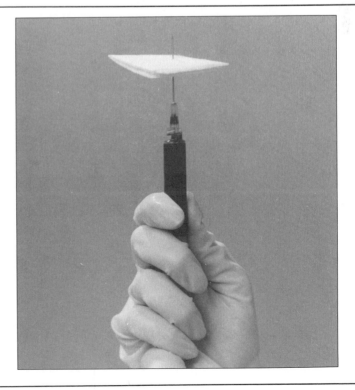

Insert the needle into a rubber stopper. Or remove the needle and place a rubber cap directly on the syringe hub (as shown). This prevents leaks and protects the sample from contact with air, both of which may alter test results.

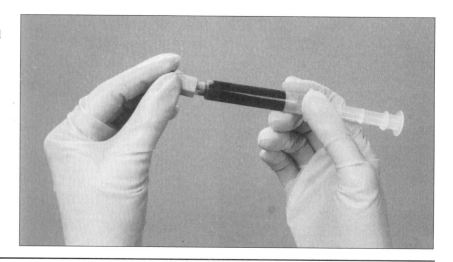

Drawing blood from an arterial line

Before you can draw blood from an arterial line, you'll first need to flush the line. To do so, turn the stopcock handle toward the syringe port and activate the continuous fast-flush device.

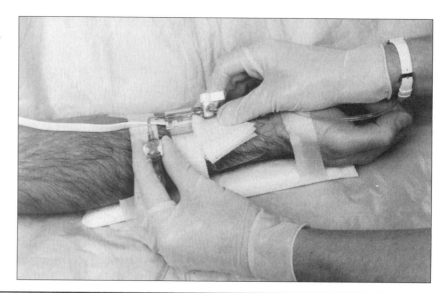

Next, unscrew the stopcock cap and attach the unheparinized 5-ml syringe. Turn the stopcock handle toward the continuous fast-flush device, and allow blood to flow into the syringe. Pull back on the plunger as necessary to withdraw 5 ml of blood.

Return the stopcock to the upright position. Remove and properly discard the syringe.

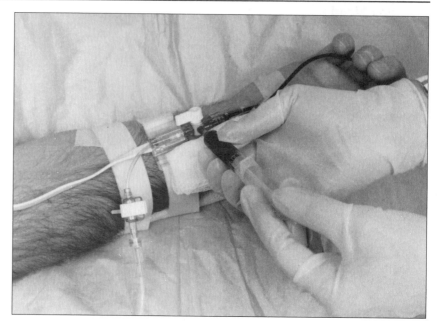

Attach the 10-ml syringe to the stopcock port, making sure that the port holds no air bubbles. Then turn the stopcock handle back toward the continuous fast-flush device and allow blood to flow into the syringe. Pull back on the plunger of the syringe as necessary to withdraw 3 to 5 ml of blood.

Return the stopcock handle to the upright position and remove the syringe. Put the rubber cap on the syringe hub (as shown), and slip the syringe into the ice-filled bag. Label the bag and send it to the laboratory.

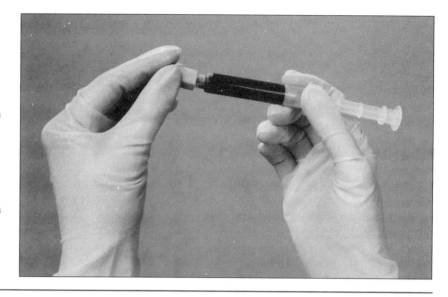

Next, place a 2″ × 2″ gauze pad over the syringe port. Turn the stopcock handle toward the patient, and activate the fast-flush device to clear blood from the syringe port (as shown). Replace the cap on the syringe port, and position the stopcock handle in the upright position. Again activate the fast-flush device to completely clear the arterial line.

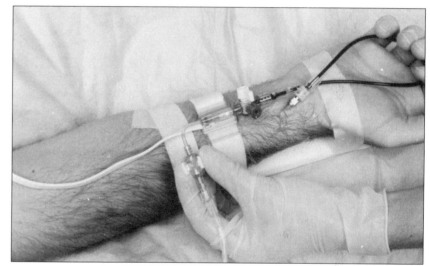

Drawing blood from a VAMP device

To draw blood from a VAMP device that *isn't* included in the patient's pressure tubing setup, you'll first need to connect the VAMP to the tubing between the insertion site and the pressure transducer (as shown).

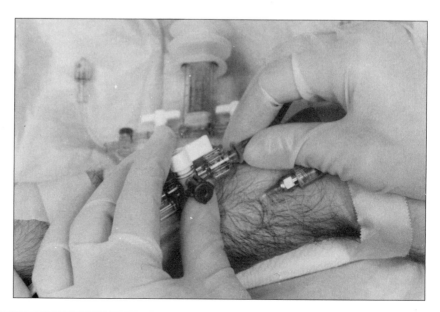

Next, turn the stopcock handle toward the flush solution. If you're using a VAMP device that you attached to an existing line, grasp the top of the plunger and pull up until the blood fills the reservoir (as shown).

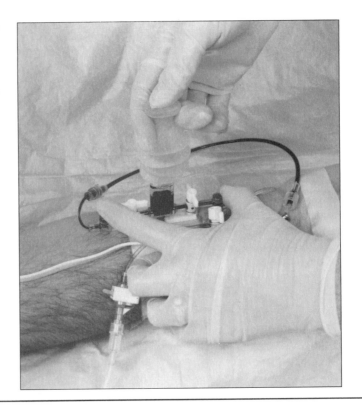

If you're using a VAMP device that's part of the tubing, squeeze the sides of the flexure at the top while pulling the flexure upward. The reservoir should fill with solution that clears the arterial line.

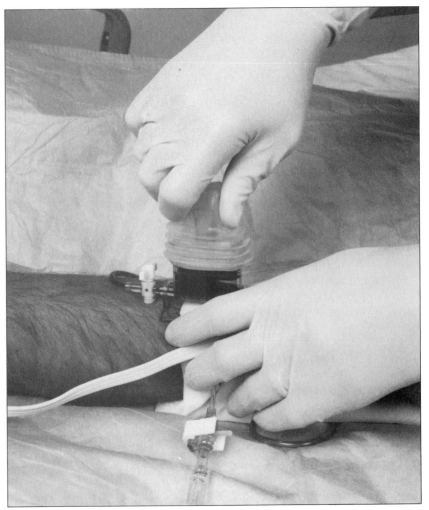

Push a preheparinized syringe with a blunt cannula straight down over the sample site (as shown). Pull back on the plunger and collect 3 to 5 ml of blood. Remove the syringe and place it in an ice-filled bag. Label the bag and send it to the laboratory.

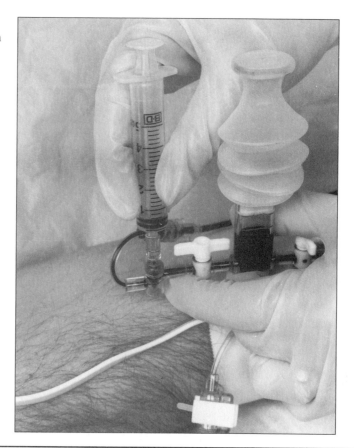

Depress the reservoir pump to reinfuse the blood (as shown). Return the stopcock handle to the upright position, and activate the continuous fast-flush device to clear the line.

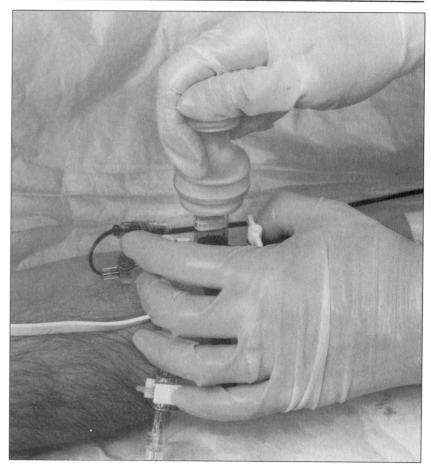

USING A VASCULAR INTERMITTENT ACCESS SYSTEM

A vascular intermittent access (VIA) system enables you to monitor blood chemistry results in a critically ill patient by automatically withdrawing a small amount of blood from an arterial or venous line and then reinfusing the sample into the patient. In 1 minute, the VIA system can measure and display a patient's hematocrit, pH, and oxygen, carbon dioxide, potassium, calcium, sodium, and glucose levels.

The VIA system has clear-cut advantages: It measures changes in blood gas and electrolyte levels almost as they occur, thereby allowing a quick response to abnormalities. What's more, it allows you to take measurements as often as every 8 minutes without drawing blood manually or risking many of the problems that accompany an indwelling sensor.

The VIA system travels easily with the patient, making it suitable for use in the operating room, intensive care unit, emergency department, and other special care units.

Setting up the VIA system

Begin by gathering the necessary equipment. If you're using VIA Medical Corporation's 1-01 system (shown at right), assemble a VIA monitor with a sensor cable, a calibration kit (specifically, the VIA Cal Kit), and a VIA sensor kit.

The calibration kit contains an isotonic I.V. solution (usually lactated Ringer's solution) and prefilled syringes containing the additives needed for calibrating the VIA system and maintaining the I.V. line. The sensor kit contains a VIA sensor, an I.V. infusion set, and surgical tape.

You'll also need to gather gloves, alcohol swabs, a sharps container for used needles, an I.V. pole, and a pole clamp (model 117).

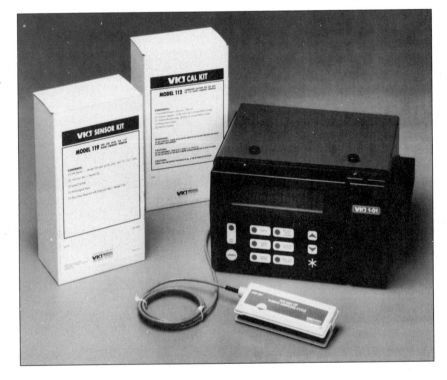

Carol Ann Knauff, RN, MSN, CCRN, and *Karen E. Michael, RN, MSN,* contributed to this section. Ms. Knauff is a critical care educator at Grand View Hospital, Sellersville, Pa. Ms. Michael is a case manager for Greater Atlantic Health Service, Philadelphia. The publisher thanks *VIA Medical Corp.,* San Diego, for its help.

Wash your hands. Then open the calibration kit and prepare the isotonic I.V. solution. Double-check that the contents match those on the package label.

Using an alcohol swab, clean the medication port of the I.V. bag containing lactated Ringer's solution. Then inject the contents of the pre-filled syringes into the bag. Clean the medication port with a new alcohol swab before each injection. Use the 5-ml syringe to withdraw the dextrose solution from the ampule and inject it into the bag. Discard the used syringe and needle unit in the sharps container.

Now complete the medication label and attach it to the I.V. bag (as shown). Shake the bag for at least 10 seconds to ensure thorough mixing.

▶ *Clinical tip:* Be sure to prepare the calibration solution immediately before use.

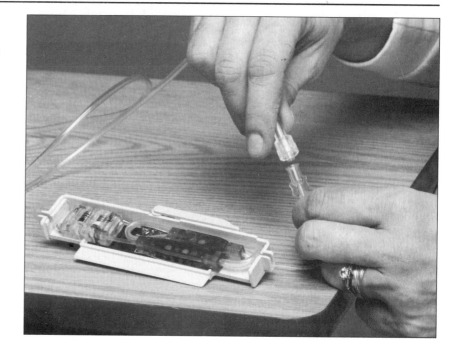

Take the equipment to the patient's bedside and explain the procedure. Attach the VIA sensor set to the distal end of the infusion set by twisting the luer-lock connection.

Close the regulating clamp on the infusion set. Then insert the spike into the I.V. bag (as shown). Hang the bag from the I.V. pole, and squeeze the drip chamber until it fills about halfway.

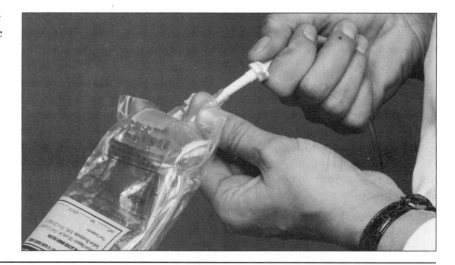

Hold the sensor disk between your thumb and index finger to keep the membrane flat. Prime the infusion set and the sensor set by slowly opening the regulating clamp and allowing about 10 ml of fluid to flow freely through the sensor tubing into a sink or a refuse container. Tap the tubing gently, as needed, to expel unwanted air. When no air bubbles remain, close the regulating clamp.

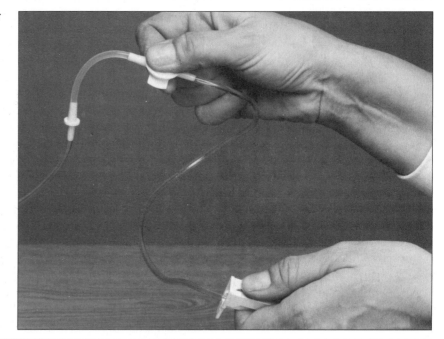

Operating the VIA system

Turn on the monitor by pressing the ON/OFF key. (The screen will display the current software version number, confirming that the monitor is on.)

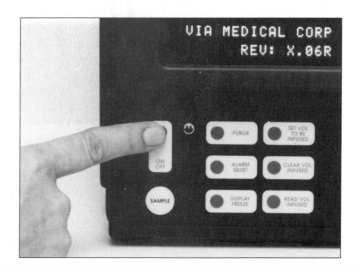

Watch the display screen for the words "SELECT MODE." Choose one of the four modes by pressing the up or down arrow. In most cases, you'll select mode 1 (as shown).

▶ *Clinical tip:* On the VIA 1-01 system, mode 1— STANDARD MODE—is used for normal monitoring of blood chemistry values. This is the default mode. You can select other modes as needed.

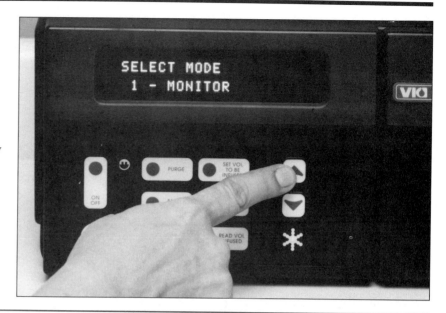

After selecting the mode, press the * (asterisk) key to advance the instructions. The monitor screen will display cues (or prompts) for continuing.

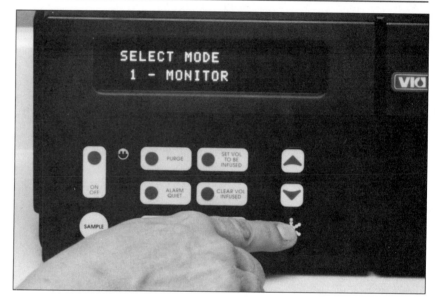

Open the door on the right of the monitor by sliding the latch to the right. Then pull the anti-free-flow lever down to open the pump mechanism.

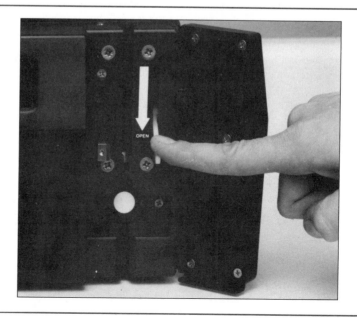

Setting up the pump

Holding the silicone portion of the tubing, place the tubing adapter into the top of the tubing retainer in the pump compartment.

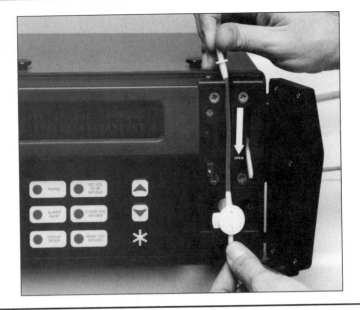

Hold the sensor disk so that the flat side faces the monitor. Pull down slightly and hook the disk under its retainer in the monitor.

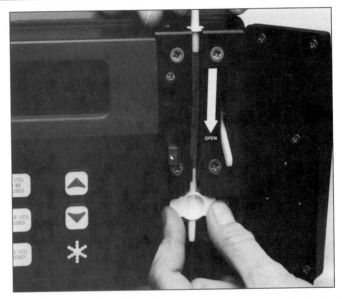

Holding the sensor disk in place, push the anti-free-flow lever up to close the pump.

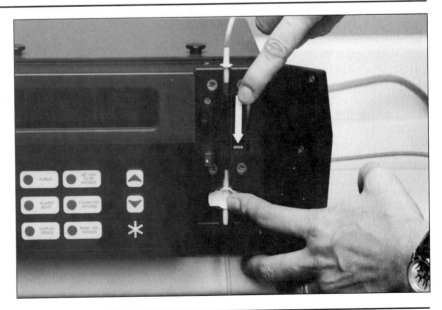

Now shut the monitor door.

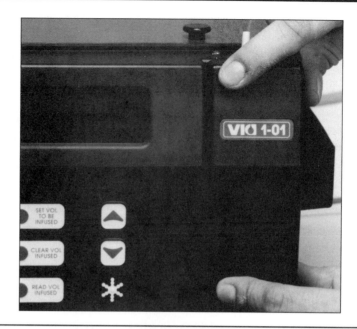

Programming the sensor system

Open the regulating clamp on the I.V. tubing all the way. (If the infusion set is properly positioned, the solution won't flow on its own.) Check the drip chamber (as shown) to make sure that the solution isn't flowing.

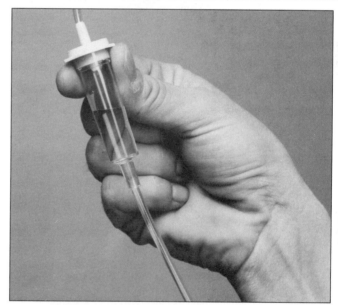

Continue to advance the programming instructions by pressing the * key. When the previously infused volume appears on the screen, you may clear it by pressing the CLEAR VOL INFUSED key for 1 second (as shown).

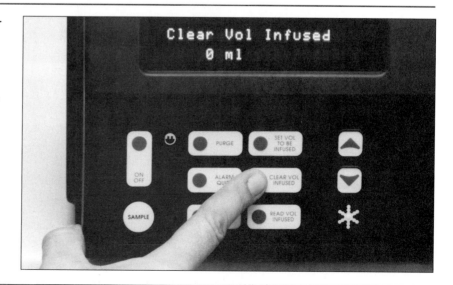

Select the intended infusion volume (in 50-ml increments from 50 to 1,000 ml) by pressing the up and down arrows until the desired total appears. Simultaneously press the SET VOL TO BE INFUSED key.

▶ *Clinical tip:* To prevent the system from running dry and to give yourself adequate time to prepare a new I.V. solution, enter a volume that's 50 ml less than the volume in the I.V. bag. This accounts for fluid in the tubing and fluid lost in priming. Once the selected volume infuses, an alarm will sound. The solution will continue to infuse at a rate of 10 ml/ hour—the keep-vein-open rate.

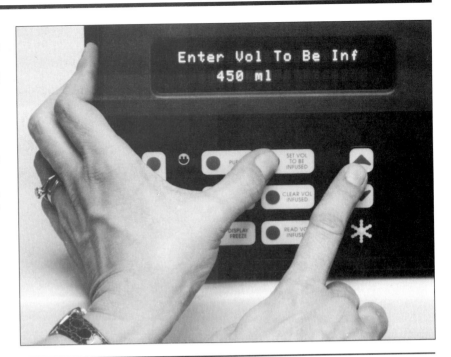

Connecting the system to the patient

Before connecting the system to the patient, perform an initial two-point calibration check of the sensor. Remember to perform this check each time you use a new sensor. (Refer to the operator's manual for complete instructions.)

Use a four-way stopcock to connect the end of the I.V. tubing from the sensor set to the patient's arterial line. Secure all luer-lock connections and be careful not to introduce air into the line.

▶ *Clinical tip:* If you're using an arterial pressure monitoring line with the VIA system, attach it to the stopcock on the extension set. The flush solutions used in the arterial pressure monitoring system (the existing arterial line) and in the VIA system must be the same.

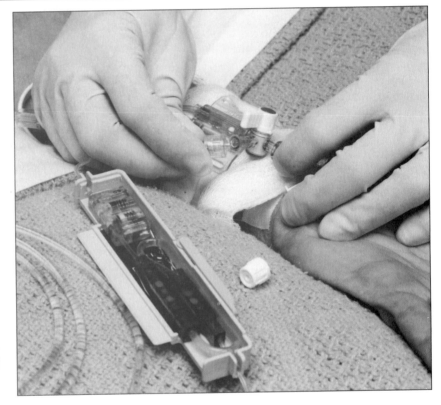

Again, press the ✳ key. This starts the infusion and maintains the flow rate at 10 ml/hour. The display screen will alternately present two messages—one identifying the flow rate ("Flow 10 ml/hr"), and the other, the measurable values ("pH = pCO_2 = pO_2 = Hct = Glu = K = Ca = Na = "). The actual values will follow the equal signs when the blood is tested.

Also appearing on the screen will be a pinwheel-like character that spins clockwise to indicate forward-flowing I.V. solution.

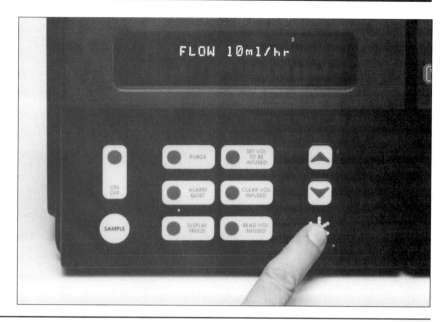

Connect the monitor's sensor cable to the sensor set of the infusion tubing by lining up the cable with the sensor set and sliding it in place.

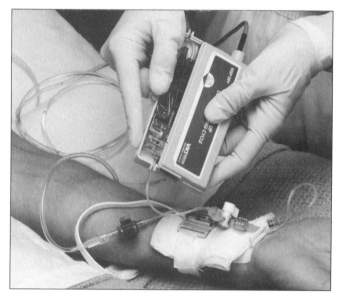

Position the sensor upright and horizontal on the patient's arm, as indicated by the label on the sensor cable, and secure it with surgical tape (as shown).

▶ *Clinical tip:* Leave slack in the line with a loop of tubing between the sensor set and the insertion site. This prevents tugging at the insertion site if you accidentally pull on the I.V. tubing or sensor cable.

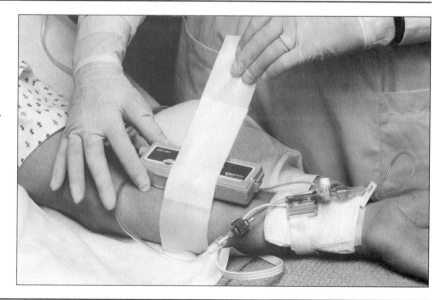

Secure all of the tubing and the cable lines to the patient's wrist so that they won't accidentally dislodge or pull out. As needed, use an armboard to stabilize the patient's wrist. Also, remind the patient to keep his wrist on top of his bed linens at all times.

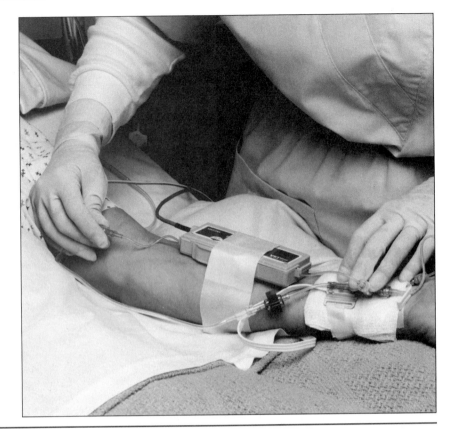

Testing blood

To start a sampling cycle and measure an electrolyte level, press the SAMPLE key. During the sampling cycle, the following steps occur automatically: The VIA system calibrates its sensors, and the word "CALIBRATING" and a countdown time appear on the screen (until the system segregates and analyzes a blood sample). After 8 seconds, the pumping system reverses its action and withdraws about 1.2 ml of blood, and the word "SAMPLING" appears as shown. (The pinwheel spins counterclockwise to indicate the reverse flow.)

As the patient's blood comes in contact with the sensors, the word "ANALYZING" appears on the screen. The word "PURGING" will appear on the screen when the system returns the blood and I.V. solution to the patient.

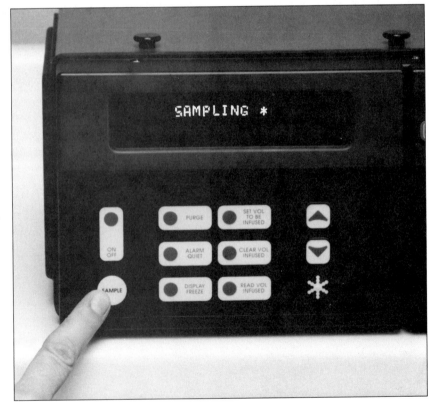

Finally, blood chemistry values appear on alternating screens. To hold the display for 30 seconds, press the DISPLAY FREEZE key (as shown). To resume the alternating display, press the same key again. Record the results promptly because they appear for only 5 minutes, after which they automatically clear from the system. If your monitor has an attached printer, however, you can print the results along with the date and time.

Be sure to document the whole procedure and the patient's response.

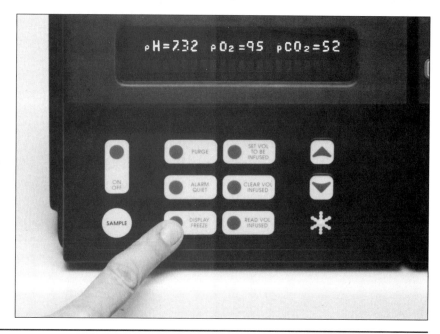

Using additional features

If necessary, you can temporarily suspend the infusion by pressing the ∗ key. The infusion will stop for 1 minute, after which an alarm will sound and the word "TIMEOUT" will appear on the display screen. To restart the infusion, press the ∗ key again.

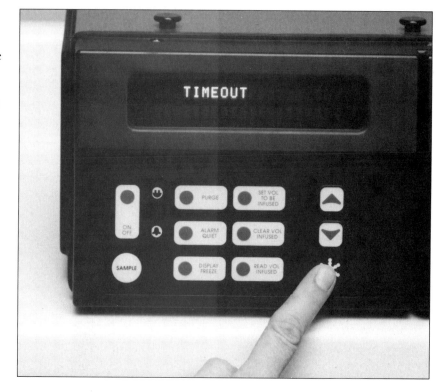

You can purge the I.V. line manually during the infusion by pressing the PURGE key. The system will then purge at the rate of 900 ml/hour for as long as the key remains depressed. The accumulated volume purged will be displayed on the screen.

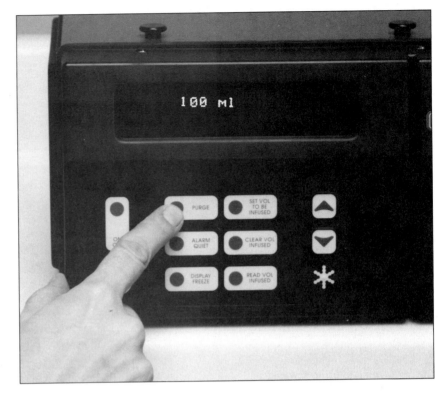

TROUBLESHOOTING

Responding to VIA system alarms

The vascular intermittent access (VIA) system is equipped with several alarms that are activated when a problem occurs, thus alerting you to the need to readjust the equipment. The exact alarm messages displayed on the VIA monitor appear in the left-hand column. The malfunctions they indicate are listed in the center column, and suggested interventions for correcting them are given in the right-hand column.

ALARM MESSAGE	MALFUNCTION	NURSING INTERVENTIONS
SAMPLE ERR – CHECK LINE	• The sensor does not detect blood. • Fluid and blood may have mixed to dilute the blood sample. • An occlusion distal to the sensor set may have occurred. • The needle of the vascular access device may be too small (if it's in a peripheral vein), or the access device may be lodged against the vein wall.	• Check the fluid volume in the line from the catheter to the sensor; it shouldn't exceed 1.2 ml. • Ensure that neither fluid nor medication from another source mixes with the VIA system's blood sample. • Inspect the tubing for kinks and patency. Make sure that all stopcocks are properly positioned. • Use at least an 18G needle or catheter, and check it for proper positioning.
TUBING OCCLUDED	• In-line flow is restricted, and in-line pressure has reached the maximum set limit.	• Inspect the line from the monitor to the patient. Look for closed roller clamps, closed stopcocks, or kinks. Eliminate any obstruction.
DOOR OPEN	• The pump door may be ajar.	• Observe the anti-free-flow lever to make sure that it's in the up (closed) position. Then close the pump door securely.
INFUSION SET OUT	• The I.V. infusion set was incorrectly inserted or removed.	• Check placement of the silicone tubing in the tubing retainer and placement of the sensor disk in the disk retainer.
AIR IN LINE	• The air sensor detects air in the tubing.	• Check the tubing for evidence of air in the line (bubbles). Eliminate the air according to hospital protocol.
I.V. SET MISLOADED	• The I.V. set was improperly inserted in the pump.	• Close the roller clamp. Open the monitor door and remove the I.V. tubing from the pump. Then reload the I.V. infusion set in the pump.
TIMEOUT	• The system isn't infusing solution and no key has been pressed in over 1 minute (or a key has been pressed for more than 1 minute).	• Press the * key to cancel the timeout. • Press the * key again if the monitor was on hold. This will restart the infusion.
BATTERY DEPLETED	• The charge is low.	• Plug the monitor into an AC power outlet.
FIX ME	• An internal malfunction occurred. (See the operator's manual for the number or letter code corresponding to the specific malfunction.)	• Switch the power off and on. If the "FIX ME" message recurs, remove the monitor and have it serviced.

TESTING GASTRIC CONTENTS

You can test gastric contents at the patient's bedside with pH test strips and a Gastroccult slide. Common studies include a determination of gastric pH (or acidity) and detection of occult blood, signifying a bleeding or related disorder. Obtain gastric aspirate from the patient's nasogastric (NG) tube or from regurgitated matter.

 Clinical tip: If you've just administered medication through the NG tube, wait 30 min-utes before obtaining a gastric contents specimen.

You must measure gastric pH immediately; in contrast, the test for occult blood can be performed up to 4 days after specimen collection.

Keep in mind that the test findings may be inconclusive. Many foods, including incompletely cooked meat, raw fruits, and certain vegetables, can cause a false-positive test result.

For gastric pH and occult blood testing, take the following equipment to the patient's bedside: gloves, a linen-saver pad, a piston syringe, an emesis basin, a Gastroccult slide, developer, and an eyedropper.

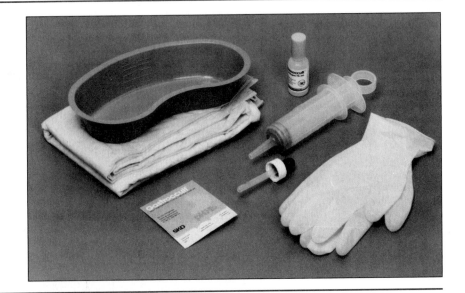

Wash your hands and explain the procedure to the patient. Place the emesis basin on the overbed table and open the piston syringe package. Put on the gloves. If necessary, disconnect the NG tube from the suction unit.

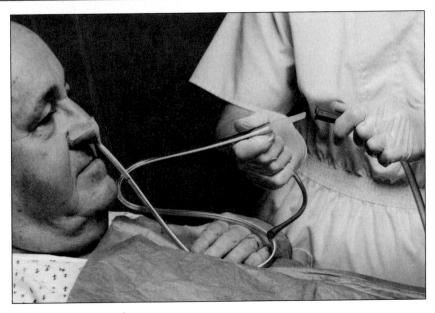

Insert the piston syringe into the tube and aspirate 10 ml of gastric contents. This specimen is likely to contain the tube residue, so discard it according to hospital protocol. Then obtain another 10-ml specimen and place it in the emesis basin.

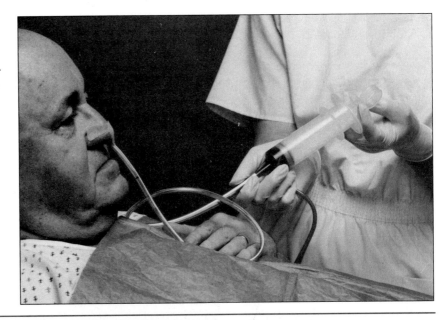

To test gastric acidity with a Gastroccult slide, use an eyedropper to place a drop of aspirate on the slide in the pH test circle. In 30 seconds, the aspirate will change color. Compare the color on the slide with the color key provided (as shown).

You can also test gastric acidity by dipping a pH strip into the gastric aspirate and comparing the color on the strip with the color key.

Once you've finished the test, discard the gastric contents according to hospital protocol. Document the test and the results.

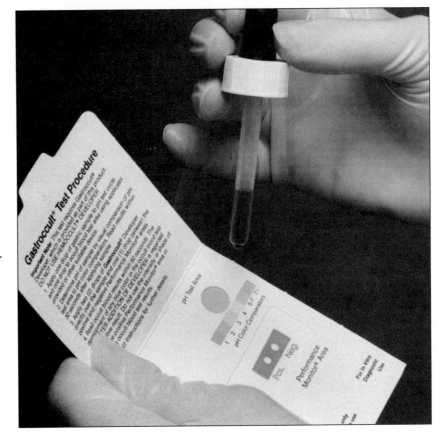

To test for occult blood, place a drop of gastric aspirate on a Gastroccult slide (near right). Apply two drops of developer directly over the sample and one drop between the positive and negative circles in the performance monitor area (far right). Use only the developer recommended by the Gastroccult slide manufacturer.

Wait 60 seconds before observing the slide. A blue tint over the sample and between the positive and negative circles denotes a positive result. No color change in either area indicates a negative result. Document the test and the results.

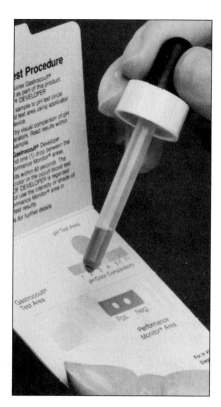

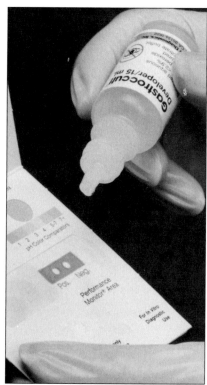

INDEX

i refers to an illustration; t refers to a table.

i refers to an illustration; t refers to a table.

i refers to an illustration; t refers to a table.